Glioblastoma, Part II: Molecular Targets and Clinical Trials

Editor

LINDA M. LIAU

NEUROSURGERY CLINICS OF NORTH AMERICA

www.neurosurgery.theclinics.com

Consulting Editors
RUSSELL R. LONSER
DANIEL K. RESNICK

April 2021 • Volume 32 • Number 2

ELSEVIER

1600 John F. Kennedy Boulevard • Suite 1800 • Philadelphia, Pennsylvania, 19103-2899

http://www.theclinics.com

NEUROSURGERY CLINICS OF NORTH AMERICA Volume 32, Number 2
April 2021 ISSN 1042-3680, ISBN-13: 978-0-323-81305-1

Editor: Stacy Eastman
Developmental Editor: Ann Gielou Posedio

Neurosurgery Clinics of North America (ISSN 1042-3680) is published quarterly by Elsevier Inc., 360 Park Avenue South, New York, NY 10010-1710. Months of issue are January, April, July, and October. Business and Editorial Offices: 1600 John F. Kennedy Blvd., Suite 1800, Philadelphia, PA 19103-2899. Customer Service Office: 11830 Westline Industrial Drive, St. Louis, MO 63146. Periodicals postage paid at New York, NY, and additional mailing offices. Subscription prices are $438.00 per year (US individuals), $1,013.00 per year (US institutions), $470.00 per year (Canadian individuals), $1,059.00 per year (Canadian institutions), $545.00 per year (international individuals), $1,059.00 per year (international institutions), $100.00 per year (US students), $255.00 per year (international students), and $100.00 per year (Canadian students). International air speed delivery is included in all *Clinics* subscription prices. All prices are subject to change without notice. **POSTMASTER:** Send address changes to *Neurosurgery Clinics of North America*, Elsevier Periodicals Customer Service, 11830 Westline Industrial Drive, St. Louis, MO 63146. **Customer Service: 1-800-654-2452 (US and Canada). From outside the US and Canada, call: 1-314-453-7041. Fax: 1-314-453-5170. E-mail: JournalsCustomerService-usa@elsevier.com (for print support) and journalsonlinesupport-usa@elsevier.com (for online support).**

Reprints. For copies of 100 or more, of articles in this publication, please contact the Commercial Reprints Department, Elsevier Inc., 360 Park Avenue South, New York, NY 10010-1710. Tel. 212-633-3874; Fax: 212-633-3820; E-mail: reprints@elsevier.com.

Neurosurgery Clinics of North America is covered in *MEDLINE/PubMed (Index Medicus), EMBASE/Excerpta Medica, and Current Contents/Clinical Medicine (CC/CM).*

Contributors

CONSULTING EDITORS

DANIEL K. RESNICK, MD, MS
Professor and Vice Chairman, Program
Director, Department of Neurosurgery,
University of Wisconsin-Madison School of
Medicine and Public Health, Madison,
Wisconsin

RUSSELL R. LONSER, MD
Professor and Chair, Department of
Neurological Surgery, The Ohio State
University Wexner Medical Center, Columbus,
Ohio

EDITOR

LINDA M. LIAU, MD, PhD, MBA, FAANS
W. Eugene Stern Professor & Chair of
Neurosurgery, UCLA Department of
Neurosurgery, David Geffen School of
Medicine at UCLA, University of California, Los
Angeles, Los Angeles, California

AUTHORS

OSORIO LOPES ABATH NETO, MD, PhD
Laboratory of Pathology, National
Cancer Institute, National Institutes of
Health, Bethesda, Maryland; Division of
Neuropathology, Department of
Pathology, University of Pittsburgh
Medical Center, Pittsburgh, Pennsylvania

OLUWATOSIN O. AKINTOLA, MBBS, MS
Clinical Fellow, Center for Neuro-Oncology,
Dana-Farber Cancer Institute, Massachusetts
General Hospital Cancer Center, Boston,
Massachusetts

KENNETH ALDAPE, MD
Laboratory of Pathology, National Cancer
Institute, National Institutes of Health,
Bethesda, Maryland

TRAVIS J. ATCHLEY, MD
Department of Neurosurgery, The University of
Alabama at Birmingham, Birmingham,
Alabama

ZEV A. BINDER, MD, PhD
Department of Neurosurgery, Glioblastoma
Translational Center of Excellence, Center for
Cellular Immunotherapies, The Abramson
Cancer Center, Perelman School of Medicine,
University of Pennsylvania, Philadelphia,
Pennsylvania USA

RANJIT S. BINDRA, MD, PhD
Department of Therapeutic Radiology, Yale
School of Medicine, New Haven, Connecticut

ORIETA CELIKU, PhD
Neuro-Oncology Branch, Staff Scientist,
National Cancer Institute, National Institutes of
Health, Bethesda, Maryland

GUSTAVO CHAGOYA, MD
Department of Neurosurgery, The University of
Alabama at Birmingham, Birmingham,
Alabama

DAVID J. DANIELS, MD, PhD
Department of Neurosurgery, Mayo Clinic,
Rochester, Minnesota

GALAL A. ELSAYED, MD
Department of Neurosurgery, The University of Alabama at Birmingham, Birmingham, Alabama

DAGOBERTO ESTEVEZ-ORDONEZ, MD
Department of Neurosurgery, The University of Alabama at Birmingham, Birmingham, Alabama

GREGORY K. FRIEDMAN, MD
Department of Neurosurgery, Department of Pediatrics, Division of Pediatric Hematology-Oncology, The University of Alabama at Birmingham, Birmingham, Alabama

MARK R. GILBERT, MD
Chief and Senior Investigator, Neuro-Oncology Branch, National Cancer Institute, National Institutes of Health, Bethesda, Maryland

CHRISTOPHER S. HONG, MD
Department of Neurosurgery, Yale School of Medicine, New Haven, Connecticut

RUPESH KOTECHA, MD
Department of Radiation Oncology, Miami Cancer Institute, Baptist Health South Florida; Herbert Wertheim College of Medicine, Florida International University, Miami, Florida

KATHERINE E. KUNIGELIS, MD
Fellow in Neurosurgical Oncology, Department of Neuro-Oncology, Neuro-Oncology Program, Moffitt Cancer Center, Tampa, Florida

NICHOLAS M. B. LASKAY, MD
Department of Neurosurgery, The University of Alabama at Birmingham, Birmingham, Alabama

JUSTIN LEE, BA
UCLA Department of Neurosurgery, David Geffen School of Medicine at UCLA, University of California, Los Angeles, Los Angeles, California

NALIN LEELATIAN, MD, PhD
Department of Pathology, Yale School of Medicine, New Haven, Connecticut

LINDA M. LIAU, MD, PhD, MBA, FAANS
W. Eugene Stern Professor & Chair of Neurosurgery, UCLA Department of Neurosurgery, David Geffen School of Medicine at UCLA, University of California, Los Angeles, Los Angeles, California

ANIL K. MAHAVADI, MD
Department of Neurosurgery, The University of Alabama at Birmingham, Birmingham, Alabama

JAMES M. MARKERT, MD, MPH
James Garber Galbraith Professor, Chair, Department of Neurosurgery, Neurosurgery, Pediatrics, and Cell, Developmental and Integrative Biology, The University of Alabama at Birmingham, Birmingham, Alabama

MINESH P. MEHTA, MD
Department of Radiation Oncology, Miami Cancer Institute, Baptist Health South Florida; Herbert Wertheim College of Medicine, Florida International University, Miami, Florida

JENNA MINAMI, BS
Graduate Student Researcher, Department of Molecular and Medical Pharmacology, University of California, Los Angeles, California

DANIELLE MORROW, BS
PhD Candidate, Graduate Student Researcher, Department of Molecular and Medical Pharmacology, University of California, Los Angeles, Los Angeles, California

YAGMUR MUFTUOGLU, MD, PhD
Department of Neurosurgery, David Geffen School of Medicine, University of California, Los Angeles, Los Angeles, California

BRIAN NA, MD
Department of Pediatrics, Division of Hematology/Oncology, University of California, Los Angeles, Los Angeles, California

DAVID A. NATHANSON, PhD
Associate Professor, Department of Molecular and Medical Pharmacology, David Geffen School of Medicine, University of California, Los Angeles, Los Angeles, California

DONALD M. O'ROURKE, MD
Department of Neurosurgery, John Templeton, Jr. M.D. Professor in Neurosurgery, Glioblastoma Translational Center of Excellence, Center for Cellular Immunotherapies, The Abramson Cancer

Center, Perelman School of Medicine, University of Pennsylvania, Philadelphia, Pennsylvania

FRANK PAJONK, MD, PhD
Department of Radiation Oncology, David Geffen School of Medicine, Jonsson Comprehensive Cancer Center, University of California, Los Angeles, Los Angeles, California

MATTHEW S. PARR, MD
Department of Neurosurgery, The University of Alabama at Birmingham, Birmingham, Alabama

SOPHIE M. PEETERS, MD
Department of Neurosurgery, University of California, Los Angeles, Los Angeles, California

SAGE P. RAHM, MD
Department of Neurosurgery, The University of Alabama at Birmingham, Birmingham, Alabama

DAVID A. REARDON, MD
Clinical Director, Center for Neuro-Oncology, Dana-Farber Cancer Institute, Professor of Medicine, Harvard Medical School, Boston, Massachusetts

ARSALAAN SALEHANI, MD
Department of Neurosurgery, The University of Alabama at Birmingham, Birmingham, Alabama

MATTHEW A. SMITH-COHN, DO
Neuro-Oncology Branch, Clinical and Research Neuro-Oncology Fellow, National

Cancer Institute, National Institutes of Health, Department of Neurology, The Johns Hopkins University School of Medicine, Baltimore, Maryland

MARTIN C. TOM, MD
Department of Radiation Oncology, Miami Cancer Institute, Baptist Health South Florida; Herbert Wertheim College of Medicine, Florida International University, Miami, Florida

THILAN TUDOR, BA
Department of Neurosurgery, Glioblastoma Translational Center of Excellence, Center for Cellular Immunotherapies, The Abramson Cancer Center, Perelman School of Medicine, University of Pennsylvania, Philadelphia, Pennsylvania

BENJAMIN R. UY, MD, PhD
UCLA Department of Neurosurgery, David Geffen School of Medicine at UCLA, University of California, Los Angeles, Los Angeles, California

MICHAEL A. VOGELBAUM, MD, PhD
Program Leader of Neuro-Oncology, Chief of Neurosurgery, Department of Neuro-Oncology, Neuro-Oncology Program, Moffitt Cancer Center, Tampa, Florida

ANTHONY C. WANG, MD
Department of Neurosurgery, University of California, Los Angeles, Los Angeles, California

Contents

Molecular Considerations

> The definition of glioblastomas has continually evolved from a reliance on strict morphologic features to a combination of histologic and molecular criteria, as the understanding of the genetic basis of these tumors expands. Modern pathologic workup of glioblastomas includes intraoperative evaluations with tissue-sparing techniques, histologic assessment with immunohistochemical markers, and comprehensive molecular characterization aiming at personalized targeting of genetic abnormalities. Machine learning analysis of DNA methylation profiles is a breakthrough technology that has bolstered central nervous system tumor classification and discovery and is particularly beneficial for the diagnosis and subtyping of glioblastomas.

> Glioblastomas (GBMs) exhibit altered metabolism to support a variety of bioenergetic and biosynthetic demands for tumor growth, invasion, and drug resistance. Changes in glycolytic flux, oxidative phosphorylation, the pentose phosphate pathway, fatty acid biosynthesis and oxidation, and nucleic acid biosynthesis are observed in GBMs to help drive tumorigenesis. Both the genetic landscape of GBMs and the unique brain tumor microenvironment shape metabolism; therefore, an understanding of how both intrinsic and extrinsic factors modulate metabolism is becoming increasingly important for finding effect targets and therapeutics for GBM.

> Mismatch repair (MMR) is a highly conserved DNA repair pathway that is critical for the maintenance of genomic integrity. This pathway targets base substitution and insertion-deletion mismatches, which primarily arise from replication errors that escape DNA polymerase proof-reading function. Here, the authors review key concepts in the molecular mechanisms of MMR in response to alkylation damage, approaches to detect MMR status in the clinic, and the clinical relevance of this pathway in glioblastoma multiforme treatment response and resistance.

> Next-generation sequencing of pediatric gliomas has revealed the importance of molecular genetic characterization in understanding the biology underlying these

tumors and a breadth of potential therapeutic targets. Promising targeted therapies include mTOR inhibitors for subependymal giant cell astrocytomas in tuberous sclerosis, BRAF and MEK inhibitors mainly for low-grade gliomas, and MEK inhibitors for NF1-deficient BRAF:KIAA fusion tumors. Challenges in developing targeted molecular therapies include significant intratumoral and intertumoral heterogeneity, highly varied mechanisms of treatment resistance and immune escape, adequacy of tumor penetrance, and sensitivity of brain to treatment-related toxicities.

Clinical Trials

Glioblastoma remains incurable despite advances in surgery, radiation, and chemotherapy, underscoring the need for new therapies. The genetic heterogenicity, presence of redundant molecular pathways, and the blood-brain barrier have limited the applicability of molecularly targeted agents. The therapeutic benefit seen with a small subset of patients suggests, however, that patient selection is critical. Recent investigations show that molecularly targeted synthetic lethality is a promising complementary approach. The article provides an overview of the challenges of molecularly targeted therapy in adults with glioblastoma, including current trials and future therapeutic directions.

The standard of care treatment for glioblastoma is surgical resection followed by radiotherapy to 60 Gy with concurrent and adjuvant temozolomide with or without tumor-treating fields. Advanced imaging techniques are under evaluation to better guide radiotherapy target volume delineation and allow for dose escalation. Particle therapy, in the form of protons, carbon ions, and boron neutron capture therapy, are being assessed as strategies to improve the radiotherapeutic ratio. Stereotactic, hypofractionated, pulsed-reduced dose-rate, and particle radiotherapy are re-irradiation techniques each uniquely suited for different clinical scenarios. Novel radiotherapy approaches, such as FLASH, represent promising advancements in radiotherapy for glioblastoma.

Peptide and dendritic cell vaccines activate the immune system against tumor antigens to combat brain tumors. Vaccines stimulate a systemic immune response by inducing both antitumor T cells as well as humoral immunity through antibody production to cross the blood–brain barrier and combat brain tumors. Recent trials investigating vaccines against peptides (ie, epithelial growth factor receptor variant III, survivin, heat shock proteins, or personalized tumor antigens) and dendritic cells pulsed with known peptides, messenger RNA or unknown tumor lysate targets demonstrate the potential for therapeutic cancer vaccines to become an important therapy for brain tumor treatment.

The glioblastoma tumor microenvironment is highly immunosuppressed. This immunosuppressive state is engineered by inhibitory molecules secreted by tumor cells that limit activation of immune effector cells, drive T-cell exhaustion, and enhance the immunosuppressive action of tumor-associated myeloid cells. Immunotherapeutic approaches have sought to combat glioblastoma microenvironment immunosuppression with agents such as immune checkpoint inhibitors. Although immune checkpoint blockade in glioblastoma has yielded disappointing results thus far, there is significant interest in the combination of immune checkpoint blockade with other approaches to enhance response.

CAR T Cells   249

Thilan Tudor, Zev A. Binder, and Donald M. O'Rourke

Chimeric antigen receptor T (CAR-T) cells, an immunotherapy that demonstrates marked success in treatment of hematologic malignancies, are an emergent therapeutic for patients with glioblastoma (GBM). GBM CAR-T trials have focused on targeting well-characterized antigens in the pathogenesis of GBM. Early stage trials demonstrate initial success in terms of safety and tolerability. There is preliminary evidence of antitumor activity and localization of the CAR-T product to tumoral sites. There are mixed results regarding patient outcomes. Ongoing GBM CAR-T trials will target novel antigens, explore CAR-T combination therapy, design multivalent CAR constructs, and assess the impact of lymphodepletion before CAR-T delivery.

Immunovirotherapy for the Treatment of Glioblastoma and Other Malignant Gliomas   265

Dagoberto Estevez-Ordonez, Gustavo Chagoya, Arsalaan Salehani, Travis J. Atchley, Nicholas M.B. Laskay, Matthew S. Parr, Galal A. Elsayed, Anil K. Mahavadi, Sage P. Rahm, Gregory K. Friedman, and James M. Markert

Glioblastoma multiforme (GBM) represents one of the most challenging malignancies due to many factors including invasiveness, heterogeneity, and an immunosuppressive microenvironment. Current treatment modalities have resulted in only modest effect on outcomes. The development of viral vectors for oncolytic immunovirotherapy and targeted drug delivery represents a promising therapeutic prospect for GBM and other brain tumors. A host of genetically engineered viruses, herpes simplex virus, poliovirus, measles, and others, have been described and are at various stages of clinical development. Herein we provide a review of the advances and current state of oncolytic virotherapy for the targeted treatment of GBM and malignant gliomas.

Targeting Glioma Stem Cells   283

Yagmur Muftuoglu and Frank Pajonk

Only a small fraction of the tumor cell population, glioma-initiating cells (GICs) help glioblastoma propagate, invade, evade immune recognition, repair DNA in response to radiation more efficiently, remodel the microenvironment for optimal growth, and actively pump out chemotherapies. Recent data hint that efforts toward GIC characterization and quantification can help predict patient outcomes, and yet the different subpopulations of GICs remain incompletely understood. A better understanding of GIC subtypes and functions proves critical for engineering targeted therapies. Challenges for doing so are discussed, and dopamine receptor antagonists are introduced as new means to enhance the efficacy of the current standard-of-care against GICs.

Therapies for glioblastoma face several physiologic hurdles. The blood-brain barrier (BBB) and blood-brain-tumor barrier (BTB) present impediments to therapeutic delivery of drugs to the central nervous system. Strategies to disrupt or bypass the native BBB are necessary to deliver therapeutic agents. Techniques to bypass the BBB/BTB include implantable controlled-release polymer systems, intracavitary drug delivery, direct injection of viral vectors, and infusion via convection-enhanced delivery. Ideal methods and agents to accomplish the goal providing survival benefit are yet to be determined. Further development of methods to break down or bypass the BBB and BTB is necessary for patients with glioblastoma.

NEUROSURGERY CLINICS OF NORTH AMERICA

SERIES OF RELATED INTEREST

Neurologic Clinics
https://www.neurologic.theclinics.com/
Neuroimaging Clinics
https://www.neuroimaging.theclinics.com/

THE CLINICS ARE AVAILABLE ONLINE!
Access your subscription at:
www.theclinics.com

Preface

Glioblastoma: Molecular Mechanisms and Clinical Trials

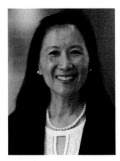

Linda M. Liau, MD, PhD, MBA, FAANS
Editor

Despite growing basic research on the molecular genetics and mechanisms of brain tumor biology and new clinical trials for brain tumors, glioblastoma has remained a formidable foe. In this issue of *Neurosurgery Clinics of North America*, an authoritative panel of researchers and clinicians critically reviews the current state-of-the-field to provide a comprehensive guide to modern molecular considerations and clinical trials for glioblastoma, with hopes of enhancing future research in this area. The contributors detail many of the key laboratory experiments and clinical protocols that are currently being investigated, integrate the available information from previous and ongoing research, and help define the current status of the field.

Topics range from an overview of glioblastoma pathology and molecular markers (Aldape) to new insights into the molecular mechanisms of tumor resistance, such as targeting metabolic vulnerabilities (Nathanson) and exploiting the role of DNA mismatch repair in treatment response in glioblastoma (Bindra and colleagues). In addition to adult glioblastoma, an updated synopsis of the molecular landscape and emerging targets in pediatric gliomas is also provided (Wang and colleagues). This issue also includes an exciting overview and update on many vanguard clinical trial strategies for treating brain tumors, including molecularly targeted trials (Smith-Cohn and colleagues), novel radiation protocols (Mehta and

colleagues), brain tumor vaccines (Liau), immune checkpoint blockade (Akintola and Reardon), CAR-T cell therapeutics (O'Rourke and colleagues), oncolytic virotherapy (Markert), and targeting cancer stem cells (Pajonk). Finally, we conclude with a discussion about the challenges and opportunities for the therapeutic delivery of agents to tumors in the central nervous system (Vogelbaum and Kunigelis).

Cutting-edge and comprehensive, this issue aims to bring together many of the important and emerging advances in our understanding of glioblastoma and illustrates in powerful detail some of the new applications for translating new scientific knowledge in the field to novel clinical trials. I am grateful to my many colleagues who have contributed their valuable time and effort to writing articles for this issue, and also, to Dr Russel Lonser and Dr Daniel Resnick for inviting me to be a Guest Editor for this collective work on a topic that I am particularly passionate about.

Linda M. Liau, MD, PhD, MBA, FAANS
UCLA Department of Neurosurgery
David Geffen School of Medicine at UCLA
300 Stein Plaza, Suite 564
Los Angeles, CA 90095-6901, USA

E-mail address:
LLIAU@mednet.ucla.edu

neurosurgery.theclinics.com

Neurosurg Clin N Am 32 (2021) xiii
https://doi.org/10.1016/j.nec.2021.03.001
1042-3680/21/© 2021 Published by Elsevier Inc.

Molecular Considerations

Morphologic and Molecular Aspects of Glioblastomas

Osorio Lopes Abath Neto, MD, PhD[a,b], Kenneth Aldape, MD[a,*]

KEYWORDS

- Glioblastoma • GBM • Pathology • Molecular testing • Methylation profiling

KEY POINTS

- The definition of glioblastomas has continually evolved from a reliance on strict morphologic features to a combination of histologic and molecular criteria, as the understanding of the genetic basis of these tumors expands.
- Modern pathologic workup of glioblastomas includes intraoperative evaluations with tissue-sparing techniques, histologic assessment with immunohistochemical markers, and comprehensive molecular characterization aiming at personalized targeting of genetic abnormalities.
- Machine learning analysis of DNA methylation profiles is a breakthrough technology that has bolstered central nervous system tumor classification and discovery and is particularly beneficial for the diagnosis and subtyping of glioblastomas.

INTRODUCTION

Glioblastomas have been frustratingly refractory to significant therapeutic progress over the last century and remain associated with a dismal prognosis.[1] However, the development of technologies that speed up molecular research has paved the way to significant advances in the understanding of the biology of this class of tumors and opened the horizon for the introduction of potential targeted therapies. As the knowledge expands, concepts and definitions need revisions.

It is now accepted that the original descriptions of glioblastoma *multiforme* represent an amalgam of various neoplasms with diverse, even sometimes mutually exclusive, genetic abnormalities and biologic behaviors. The very concept of glioblastoma has evolved through time, starting with the dropping of the "multiforme" qualifier. With the seminal discovery of *IDH1* gene mutations as drivers of prognosis of glioblastomas,[2] a major split in the classification of glioblastomas into 2

major types, IDH-mutant and IDH-wildtype, was introduced in the 2016 edition of the World Health Organization (WHO) classification of tumors of the central nervous system (CNS), for the first time incorporating molecular criteria into the very definition of glioblastomas.[3]

For the next edition of the WHO classification, slated for release in 2021, glioblastomas are poised to be even further defined on a molecular basis.[4] Lower-grade glial neoplasms that show molecular features of glioblastomas have been shown to behave in a similar fashion and will thus be sanctioned to be called as such.[5] The incorporation of artificial-intelligence techniques to classify CNS tumors based on methylome profiling is emerging as a promising technique to assist in diagnosis and research.[6]

This rapidly changing landscape calls for periodic stops to make sense of the current status of the field. In this review, the authors detail morphologic features of glioblastomas, including those of diagnostically significant subtypes, followed by

[a] Laboratory of Pathology, National Cancer Institute, National Institutes of Health, Building 10, Room 2S235 Bethesda, MD 20892, USA; [b] Division of Neuropathology, University of Pittsburgh Medical Center, Room S701 Scaife Hall, 3550 Terrrace Street, Pittsburgh, PA 15261 USA
* Corresponding author.
E-mail address: kenneth.aldape@nih.gov

Neurosurg Clin N Am 32 (2021) 149–158
https://doi.org/10.1016/j.nec.2021.01.001
1042-3680/21/© 2021 Elsevier Inc. All rights reserved.

commentaries on the immunohistochemical and intraoperative evaluations of these tumors. A summary of the current understanding of the molecular bases and classification of glioblastomas ensues. The final section discusses the use of DNA methylation profiling as a tool to advance research and diagnosis of CNS tumors, in general, and glioblastomas, in particular.

MORPHOLOGIC FEATURES OF GLIOBLASTOMAS

Glioblastomas are hypercellular proliferations of atypical glial cells, which diffusely infiltrate brain parenchyma (**Fig. 1**A). The neoplastic cells are pleomorphic, but most characteristically have enlarged hyperchromatic nuclei with clumped chromatin and irregular outlines and variable amounts of cytoplasm from which emanate thick and stout fibrillary processes. Normal CNS astrocytes, on the other hand, even when in a reactive state, have in comparison a smaller and regular elongated nucleus with evenly distributed chromatin, in addition to a cytoplasm with fine and long fibrillary processes. Reactive astrocytes also keep a regular distance from each other, whereas glioblastoma cells heap up disorderly. Glial fibrillary acidic protein (GFAP) immunostains exquisitely highlight these differences (**Fig. 1**B, C).

The variability of individual neoplastic cell morphology is illustrated by the occurrence and occasional predominance of foamy cells,[7] gemistocytic cells (having an abundant eosinophilic cytoplasm), multinucleated giant cells, and cells with metaplastic differentiation.[8] However, the pleomorphism can be less conspicuous in certain tumors, in particular, small cell glioblastomas and others that present with marked oligodendroglial-like features.[9] These neoplasms show a monomorphic proliferation of oval bland nuclei, indistinguishable from anaplastic oligodendrogliomas on morphologic grounds, the differentiation from which rests on molecular testing.

Glioblastomas, as diffuse glial neoplasms, have the capability of widely infiltrating brain parenchyma without effort. There tends to be a higher concentration of neoplastic cells in the center of the tumor, with gradually reducing cellularity toward the periphery. However, neoplastic glial cells cannot easily breach histologic barriers. The intrinsic confinement of the proliferation is the basis for the rarity of metastatic disease-neoplastic cells have trouble penetrating vessels - and for unique and diagnostically helpful phenomena, such as the formation of secondary structures,[10] clusters of neoplastic cells percolating around vessels

neurons, and the "edges" of brain parenchyma, that is, subpial and ependymal surfaces (**Fig. 1**D).

Mitotic activity is invariably brisk and a required criterion for high-grade glial neoplasms but can be remarkably variable depending on the area of the tumor. A pHH3 immunostain is helpful in expediting the identification of mitoses in difficult cases. Ki-67 immunostains likewise show an elevated proliferative rate, ranging from 15% to 40%, which is higher in areas with increased mitotic activity.

Current official 2016 WHO criteria for assigning a *glioblastoma, WHO grade 4* diagnosis to a diffuse glioma still require the presence of either microvascular proliferation or necrosis on histologic assessment.[3] These criteria will not be necessary for assigning a grade 4 in the next edition if specific molecular features are identified (*TERT* or *EGFR* genetic alterations, or the combination of gain of chromosome 7 and loss of chromosome 10).[5]

Microvascular proliferation occurs as a response of endothelial cells to stimulating factors originating from neoplastic cells to produce angiogenesis and is observed as vascular structures with multiple layers, often forming glomeruloid structures, with increased mitotic activity[11] (**Fig. 1**E). In markedly hypercellular tumors, neoplastic cells can obscure the vascular structures on hematoxylin and eosin (H&E) -stained slides. A GFAP immunostain helps delineate hyperplastic vessels as clearings in a background of intensely staining glioma cells (**Fig. 1**F). There is regional variation to microvascular proliferation, which is more pronounced at the tumor edges and areas close to necrosis, where ischemic neoplastic cells more profusely release stimulating factors. These regions correspond to regions of contrast ring enhancement on MRI, and thus, the presence of microvascular proliferation within a hypercellular glial neoplasm on a biopsy sent for intraoperative consultation is a reliable surrogate that representative tissue from a high-grade tumor has been sampled.

Necrosis in glioblastomas is characteristically of the palisading type,[12] whereby tumor cells are arranged radially in a picket fence-like distribution around a central area of necrosis (**Fig. 1**G). However, as per current WHO recommendations, any type of tumor cell necrosis can be used to meet the criteria. On the other hand, care must be exercised in evaluating specimens where necrosis may have been the result of treatment, especially radiotherapy.

The pleomorphism of glioblastomas has over time allowed the identification and further classification of specific subtypes with unique biologic

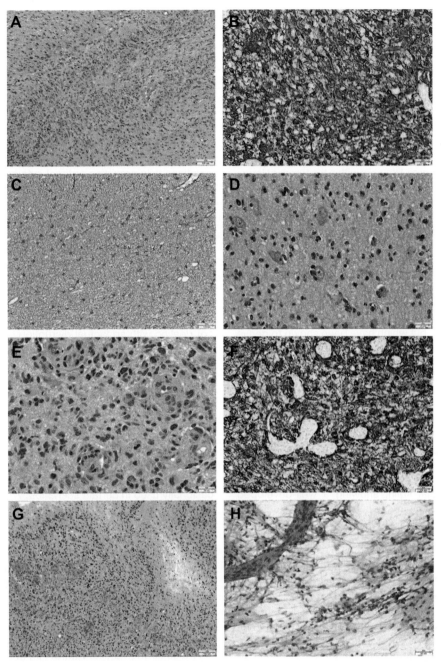

Fig. 1. Morphology of glioblastomas and immunohistochemical stains. (*A*) Hypercellular GBM cells infiltrating brain parenchyma and Virchow-Robin spaces (H&E, original magnification ×100). (*B*) GFAP immunostain highlights cluttered neoplastic GBM cells with strong cytoplasmic and thick fibrillary staining (GFAP, original magnification ×200). (*C*) GFAP immunostain in reactive brain decorates evenly spaced reactive astrocytes (GFAP, original magnification ×100). (*D*) Infiltrating GBM cells forming secondary structures around neurons and blood vessels (H&E, original magnification ×400). (*E*) Glomeruloid microvascular proliferation in a GBM (H&E, original magnification ×400). (*F*) GFAP immunostain in GBM shows negative (unstained) outlines of proliferating endothelial cells in the background of proliferating neoplastic cells (GFAP, original magnification ×200). (*G*) Necrosis in GBM is frequently of the palisading type (H&E, original magnification ×100). (*H*) Smear preparations of GBM specimens show atypical cells with irregular enlarged nuclei and fibrillary processes, associated with proliferating vessels (H&E smear preparation, original magnification ×200).

behaviors and molecular profiles. Giant cell glio-blastomas show extremely large, bizarre cells with multiple nuclei, in addition to smaller spindled cells and focal ill-defined rosettes, in a background rich in reticulin (**Fig. 2**A). They tend to have a more circumscribed architecture, with increased resectability and consequently slightly improved prognosis.[13,14]

Glioblastomas with a primitive neuroectodermal tumor (PNET) component present delimited nests of neoplastic cells differentiated into neuronal, medulloblastoma-like cells within the tumor at large, even showing Homer-Wright rosettes at times, and are associated with abnormalities in *MYCN* (**Fig. 2**B). Epithelioid glioblastomas (**Fig. 2**C) are characterized by discohesive rounded epithelioid cells with eccentric nuclei and abundant eosino-philic cytoplasm, sharing molecular features with pleomorphic xanthoastrocytomas (*BRAF* V600E mutation in about half of cases).[15]

Gliosarcomas are tumors with biphasic cells that can either present a glial or spindled sarcomatous morphology, but which have been shown to derive from the same precursor[16] (**Fig. 2**D). The firm mesenchymal component and the capability to invade the skull are red herrings for a meningioma or metastasis and sometimes pose a radiologic and gross diagnostic challenge. Sarcomatous areas can differentiate into bone, cartilage, and muscle, but the glial component can also take on epithelial features (squamous or adenoid). The sarcomatous component is rich in collagen and reticulin, which can be explored microscopically with a special stain, showing a well-developed intensely staining network around spindle cells.

INTRAOPERATIVE CONSULTATION

The radiologic differential diagnosis of a ring-enhancing CNS lesion, the usual initial presentation for glioblastomas, is broad and includes both neoplasms that require completely different treatment approaches, such as CNS lymphomas and metastases, and numerous nonneoplastic conditions, ranging from infectious diseases to vascular and demyelinating lesions. The intraoperative consultation of a lesional biopsy is thus a critical first step in the workup of a suspected glioblastoma case. Its main purposes are to confirm the diagnosis and to ensure sufficient material has been obtained for the full molecular characterization of the neoplasm, which will guide subsequent therapy.

The ideal biopsy specimen should be representative of the higher-grade area of the tumor, showing unequivocal morphologic features of a high-grade neoplasm (necrosis or microvascular proliferation) and potentially having a high viable tumor cell cellularity, yielding the maximum amount of genetic material for molecular testing.

Various tissue assessment techniques can be used individually or in combination during an intraoperative consultation and include touch and smear preparations and frozen sections. Different services have preferred methods dictated primarily by prior experience. However, for small biopsies of a suspected high-grade glioma, smear preparations offer the advantages of maximal tissue preservation while providing optimal cytologic detail.

Interpretation of smear preparations reliably distinguish gliomas from the main differential diagnoses. Smear preparations of glioblastomas show a predominant population of atypical cells with enlarged elongated nuclei, inconspicuous nucleoli, and a variably sized cytoplasm that characteristically displays fine fibrillary processes (**Fig. 1**H). The smear background is also finely fibrillary. Processes oriented perpendicular to the direction of the smearing offer stronger evidence that one is not dealing with artifactual disruption of the cytoplasm of other potential tumor cell types. Mitotic figures are occasionally identified, further boosting confidence in a correct diagnosis.

IMMUNOHISTOCHEMICAL EVALUATION

A limited number of immunohistochemical stains are helpful for the initial characterization of diffuse gliomas and include GFAP, IDH1 R132H, ATRX, p53, EGFR, and Ki-67. Olig2 and pHH3 can be occasionally used in certain scenarios. When appropriate, immunostains for the histone H3 K27M mutation and various H3 G34 mutations are also available, as is a *BRAF* V600E stain for epithelioid glioblastomas.

GFAP is expected to diffusely and strongly stain neoplastic cells in glioblastomas, highlighting the thick glial protein content extending into stout abnormal processes that nevertheless recapitulate the astrocytic nature of the cells (see **Fig. 1**B). The abundant cytoplasm of gemistocytic cells also strongly stains with GFAP. In cytoplasm-poor variants of glioblastoma, and in cases where there is partial loss of GFAP expression in neoplastic cells, such as in gliosarcomas, an immunostain for Olig2 can be helpful in further establishing the glial nature of the neoplasm.[17] GFAP is also helpful in the evaluation of microvascular proliferation when equivocal on H&E, as negative outlines of endothelial cells starkly contrast with strongly staining neoplastic cells.

The IDH1 R132H immunostain stains the abnormal protein product resulting from the specific *IDH1* R132H mutation and is thus negative

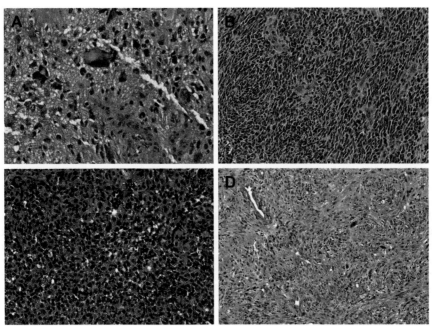

Fig. 2. Morphology of glioblastoma subtypes. (*A*) Giant cell glioblastoma shows bizarre markedly enlarged "monstrocellular" neoplastic cells (H&E, original magnification ×400). (*B*) Glioblastoma with PNET features is characterized by primitive hyperchromatic cells mimicking medulloblastoma (H&E, original magnification ×100). (*C*) Epithelioid glioblastoma is composed of cells with abundant eosinophilic cytoplasm (H&E, original magnification ×100). (*D*) Gliosarcoma shows a prominent spindle cell component admixed with pleomorphic glial cells (H&E, original magnification ×200).

in IDH-mutant gliomas harboring alternative mutations in *IDH1* or *IDH2*. In the initial evaluation of glioblastomas, it helps suggest, coupled with a retained nuclear expression of ATRX, the IDH-wildtype nature of the neoplasm. In patients younger than 55 years or with a prior history of lower-grade glioma, particularly with loss of ATRX expression, the possibility of an IDH-mutant glioma with a noncanonical *IDH1* or *IDH2* mutation must be confirmed with molecular testing. In the right clinical context, immunostains that work with the same principle as IDH1 R132H, to detect a particular mutation, are available for H3 K27M, H3 G34R, and H3 G34V, as is a *BRAF* V600E immunostain when considering an epithelioid glioblastoma.

ATRX retained nuclear positivity is expected in IDH-wildtype glioblastomas, whereas it is lost in IDH-mutant diffuse astrocytomas of any grade, as a result of truncating mutations in ATRX determining loss of protein expression. As for any negative stain, it is crucial to evaluate for the presence of proper internal positive controls in the examined tissue, most frequently by looking for intact nuclear staining in endothelial cells.

The immunostain for p53 shows variable weak positivity in normal brain parenchymal components and in neoplastic cells that do not harbor p53 mutations. In *TP53*-mutated glial neoplasms, 2 abnormal staining patterns are possible. In 1 pattern, a subset of clonally expanded neoplastic cells shows strong intense staining, corresponding to the accumulation of an abnormal protein product, which results from a missense mutation. In the second pattern (null pattern), neoplastic cells have a complete absence of p53 staining, a consequence of the lack of protein expression owing to biallelic truncating (null) mutations. Although diagnostically helpful, especially taken together with staining patterns of other immunostains, the immunohistochemical evaluation of p53 is not completely concordant with the ultimate molecular *TP53* status and therefore does not substitute the latter.

The same can be said of the EGFR immunostain, which can help suggest the presence of *EGFR* amplification when strongly and diffusely positive in the cytoplasm of neoplastic glioblastoma cells, but too frequently shows weak to moderate staining otherwise. The best use of the EGFR immunostain is to evaluate for the presence of individual infiltrating cells in hypocellular samples of recurrent tumors that are known to be EGFR amplified, in a way similar to the use of the IDH1 R132H mutant for recurrences of an IDH-mutant diffuse glioma.

The Ki-67 immunostain is used to establish the proliferative rate, which ranges from 15% to 40% in most glioblastomas and is higher in areas with increased mitotic activity. A pHH3 immunostain decorates mitotic figures and is useful in the occasional equivocal case whereby the morphology of the neoplastic cells or the processing of the sample make mitoses harder to identify.

MOLECULAR FEATURES AND WORKUP

Since the advent of next-generation sequencing (NGS), several custom molecular panels have been developed that cover clinically relevant genetic alterations identified in CNS tumors.[18] These panels include sequencing of DNA to detect frequent point mutations, as well as RNA to capture common fusions.[19] As the knowledge of the genetic landscape of glioblastomas develops further and the technologies become cheaper and more widely available, the panels also evolve in coverage and breadth.

Although the current state of the genetic sequencing technology maturity justifies, from a cost perspective, that panels cover hundreds of genes, at a minimum, an NGS panel for a purported glioblastoma should include evaluation of the following genes: IDH1, IDH2, ATRX, TP53, PTEN, TERT, and EGFR (including structural alterations). Assessment of the methylation status of MGMT is also considered standard of care but is typically carried out as a separate assay or can be extrapolated from DNA methylation profiling data. In dealing with epithelioid glioblastomas, evaluation for the presence of the BRAF V600E mutation can be sought by either molecular testing or immunohistochemistry.

The 2016 WHO classification of brain tumors admits glioblastomas into IDH-wildtype and IDH-mutant subtypes based on the mutation status of the genes that codify isocitrate dehydrogenases 1 and 2 (IDH1 and IDH2). IDH-wildtype status is associated with primary glioblastomas, which arise in older patients with a grade 4 morphology at presentation and display a more aggressive biological behavior. Conversely, IDH-mutant glioblastomas were described as a secondary evolution of more indolent lower-grade diffuse and/or anaplastic astrocytomas in younger patients (55 years is the usual threshold) and therefore have a better prognosis. These subtypes are in essence indistinguishable on morphologic grounds, except for subtle but unreliable signs (for example, IDH-mutant tumors have a tendency to show a relative admixture of more well-differentiated astrocytic neoplastic cells). Nevertheless, IDH-wildtype and IDH-mutant glioblastomas represent entirely different tumor classes from a molecular standpoint, and future editions of the WHO classification of brain tumors will reflect that understanding by restricting the glioblastoma designation exclusively to those tumors with an IDH-wildtype status.[4] Going forward, IDH-mutant glioblastomas will likely receive the alternate designation of astrocytoma, IDH-mutant WHO grade 4. Along the same line of reasoning, cases of IDH-wildtype grade 2 and 3 astrocytomas, rarely observed in practice, which correspond biologically either to undersampled or not yet fully morphologically developed IDH-wildtype glioblastomas, will be flat out called glioblastomas, regardless of whether necrosis and microvascular proliferation, signatures of a grade 4 morphology, are present. For the remainder of the discussion in this section, the term glioblastoma will be used interchangeably with IDH-wildtype glioblastoma.

Mutations in TP53 and ATRX are molecular signatures of IDH-mutant gliomas, but are rare in glioblastomas. They correlate inversely with the presence of TERT mutations.[20] The TERT gene encodes one of the components of the enzyme telomerase, essential for keeping chromosomal telomere lengths from shortening, a mechanism that allows cells to avoid undergoing apoptosis as they age and divide. Noncoding mutations in the TERT promoter region lead to an overactive telomerase that overshoots this protective mechanism and permits cells to survive and divide indefinitely. The TERT promoter mutations c.-124C > T and c.-146C > T are signature molecular alterations in glioblastomas, present in up to 90% of cases, and can be used as one of the definitional molecular criteria for this class of tumors.[21] Because TERT promoter mutations can also be found in other CNS tumors that are part of the differential diagnosis of glioblastomas, judicious integrated molecular and histologic workup must be followed.

The DNA repair enzyme O-6-methylguanine-DNA methyltransferase (MGMT) protects DNA from damage caused by alkylating agents, including temozolomide, a key chemotherapeutic agent in the treatment of glioblastomas. Glioblastomas holding high levels of methylation (silencing) of the MGMT gene promoter, which correspond to up to 40% of the total, have not only an improved response to temozolomide but also a better prognosis.[22] MGMT methylation is thus considered both a predictive and a prognostic marker and a key component of the molecular workup of glioblastomas.[23] Epidermal growth factor receptor (EGFR) amplification is found in 40% of glioblastomas[24] and is one of the molecular criteria that authorizes a grade 4 designation to morphologically lower-grade gliomas.[5] Of all *EGFR* amplified glioblastomas, about half additionally carry a rearrangement that generates *EGFRvIII*, a variant purported to give rise to a worse prognosis.[24] *EGFR* is not only diagnostically relevant but also represents a potential therapeutic target. Other than EGFR, several proteins involved in the RTK/PI3K/PTEN/AKT/mTOR pathway have been implicated in glioblastomas. *PTEN* mutations are found in up to 40% of cases, *PDGFRA* in 15%, and *NF1* in 20%, whereas occasional cases (<10%) have amplification of *MET* or *PI3K*, or fusions involving *FGFR1* or *FGFR3*.[25] Another pathway frequently altered in glioblastomas is the CDKN2A/CDK4/RB protein pathway, which occurs in up to 80% of tumors, predominantly owing to alterations in CDKN2A and CDK4 (RB1 mutations are rare in glioblastomas but more common in IDH-mutant gliomas). CDKN2A, in particular, is also involved in the p53 pathway. Although the *TP53* gene itself is infrequently mutated in glioblastomas, other proteins of the p53 pathway are implicated in up to 90% of them.[26] These proteins include MDM2, a protein that degrades p53 and is thus tumorigenic when overexpressed, which can occur in more than 50% of cases,[27] and the abovementioned CDKN2A, a tumor suppressor protein that inhibits MDM2.

Genetic alterations identified as a result of running molecular panels should be integrated with clinical, morphologic, and immunohistochemical findings into a final molecular diagnosis, whereby the pathologist exercises the best judgment to reconcile all findings and provides his opinion as how to best interpret the findings.

DNA METHYLATION CLASSIFICATION

Recently, there has been a breakthrough improvement in the characterization of CNS tumors with the development of an artificial intelligence classifier based on DNA methylation profiling.[6] The system has been shown to represent a fast, reliable, and reproducible means to subclassify CNS tumors.

The method is DNA based and works well with low amounts extracted from frozen or formalin-fixed, paraffin-embedded tissue, including old, archived specimens. A streamlined benchwork of a few days can be summarized in a few steps. First, the bisulfite conversion of previously extracted DNA is followed by hybridization of the sample to a standardized microarray chip containing complementary probes to approximately 850,000 genome-wide sites of interest. Then, a scanner reads the chip in a couple of hours and

generates a small data file (idat extension) containing normalized methylation levels for all sites of interest. These computer files can be stored indefinitely and occupy little space compared with NGS or imaging data (the average size is a few megabytes).

The classifier was developed using a reference cohort of more than 2000 samples of various types of CNS tumors, including almost all WHO-defined entities. Initially, the methylation data generated from the samples were presented to an artificial intelligence system, which used unsupervised statistical techniques to create clusters of samples with similar methylation profiles, defining methylation "classes." Such computer-defined classes have a dimensionality incomprehensible to the human brain and eye but closely correlate with tumor entities defined by morphologic or molecular features. For example, IDH-wildtype glioblastomas samples have a similar methylation signature and are clustered together by the system (**Fig. 3**A) in a clearly separate class from clusters of IDH-mutant gliomas, which themselves have unique methylation signatures.

Reference samples were then used to train a random forest algorithm to assign a single methylation class to every presented sample methylation profile (idat file), the actual DNA methylation-based tumor classifier. New original samples of methylation profiling, when run on the classifier, receive a class determination together with a confidence score, depending on how close the methylation signature of the sample matches the expected signature of the class. The classifier was validated by running a cohort of an additional 1155 original tumors, including rare and challenging tumors, almost 90% of which were correctly diagnosed, some of which were in conflict with the original pathologic report but substantiated by additional workup.

The DNA methylation classifier can be continuously refined by expanding the reference cohort used to train the algorithm, a process facilitated by the easy exchange of the standardized small idat files. Refinement includes not only subclassification of defined tumor groups but also delineation of new classes. Several tumors to which the classifier fails to assign a methylation class correspond to potentially unrecognized entities that have a unique methylation signature. One such entity is *anaplastic astrocytoma with piloid features*, identified and defined after the methylation analysis of a cohort of pilocytic astrocytomas with high-grade features, which showed that the cohort clustered together with a profile different from existing reference classes.[28] Methylation profiling analyses also speed up identification of clinical

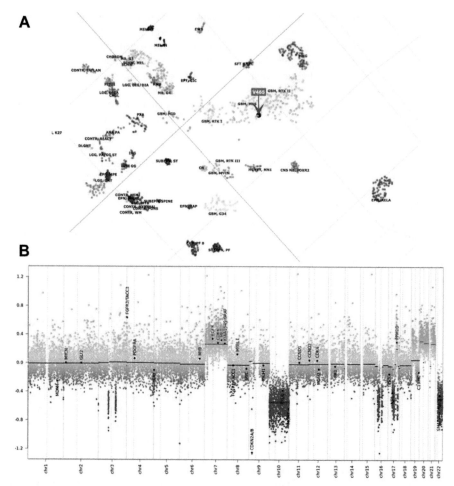

Fig. 3. DNA methylation profiling. (*A*) t-SNE representation of methylation classes defined by the CNS tumor classifier. The interrogated neoplasm (V465) matched to the methylation class "glioblastoma, mesenchymal" (GBM, MES). (*B*) Genome-wide plotting of methylation levels showing detection of copy number variation. This GBM had copy number gains of chromosomes 7, 20, and 21, and copy number losses of chromosomes 10 and 22. There are additionally partial losses in regions of chromosomes 3, 16, and 17.

and molecular subgroups within well-established morphologic entities, with potential prognostic or therapeutic significance.[29] For glioblastomas, there are initiatives to identify methylation subclasses predictive of specific molecular alterations and potential prognostic implications. In particular, glioblastomas harboring FGFR3-TACC3 fusions define a subcluster within the broader glioblastoma, IDH wildtype methylation class (Aldape, 2020).

Methylation signatures have been shown to be specific for cell of origin and to be retained even when neoplastic cells dedifferentiate or metastasize. Methylation data with no match in the CNS tumor classifier can be run on multiple classifiers for further tumor characterization. For example, a "beta-version" of a sarcoma classifier can be used to evaluate skull or dural-based tumors that

invade the brain, or a metastatic tumor can be run on specific organ system classifiers for a potential match. The ultimate methylation classifier would be one trained with samples of any human organ system and be capable of solving any metastatic tumor of unknown origin or markedly undifferentiated neoplasms.

A bonus feature of DNA methylation profiling is that the high density of probes allows the graphical genome-wide visualization of methylation levels to serve as a surrogate for copy number variation testing (**Fig. 3**B). Relative gains or losses of entire or partial chromosomes can be easily identified relative to the baseline average methylation levels, allowing for example, the assessment for the complete loss of chromosome arms 1p and 19q in oligodendrogliomas. More specific "zooming in" of regions of interest can determine the likelihood of the presence of individual gene amplifications, such as of *EGFR*, or losses of heterozygosity in clinically relevant chromosomal regions, for example, 9p21 (containing *CDKN2A*). Furthermore, queries of specific sites can establish with confidence methylation levels of individual genes. In particular, methylation levels of the MGMT promoter region are easily extracted from methylation profiling data and can avoid the extra cost of the additional molecular test for that purpose.

Most histologically diagnosed glioblastomas are readily diagnosed by histopathology. However, the methylation classifier can be helpful to conform the diagnosis in specific cases and rule out related entities that can mimic glioblastoma on histopathology (for example, anaplastic ependymoma, anaplastic pleomorphic xanthoastrocytoma). Currently, several methylation subclasses of glioblastoma are recognized (GBM_MYCN, GBM_RTK_I, GBM_RTK_II, GBM_RTK_III, GBM_MES, GBM_MID). To date, the clinical relevance of these subclasses remains to be determined. Additional molecular features that are helpful include the copy number changes +7/−10 as well as TERT promoter mutation, both of which are observed in most adult IDH-wildtype glioblastomas. High-level amplification of EGFR, which is not present in all glioblastomas, is helpful when present. An additional advantage of DNA methylation is in the setting of an undersampled IDH-wildtype diffuse glioma, where the requisite histologic hallmarks of glioblastoma are not present. In this setting, the finding of a glioblastoma subtype on the classifier, along with one or more of the genomic alterations noted above, can lead to a diagnosis of "molecular glioblastomas" (or more formally, diffuse astrocytoma with molecular features of glioblastoma, grade 4). Pediatric glioblastomas represent distinct molecular subtypes (they are enriched in RTK_III and GBM-MID), and methylation can be quite helpful in the setting of a pediatric high-grade tumor to conform the diagnosis.

Finally, idat files derived from methylation profiling are relatively small and easy to share, allowing for the consolidation of larger numbers of training sets to develop better classifiers. Archived methylation profiled cases can then be effortlessly revisited.

SUMMARY

In summary, glioblastomas have evolved in concept and definition over time from a neoplasm diagnosed solely on morphologic grounds to an entity with strictly defined molecular features. In the era of personalized cancer genomics and targeted molecular treatments, obtaining a precise molecular diagnosis is of utmost importance.

The optimal workup of a potential case of glioblastoma involves a stepwise approach, which includes early diagnosis at the time of intraoperative consultation while using minimal amount of tissue, obtention of viable tumor in sufficient quantity for molecular studies, workup with classic histologic techniques and immunohistochemistry, and the application of various molecular tests and techniques, which include NGS and DNA methylation profiling.

As the understanding of the biology and molecular aspects of glioblastomas continues to evolve, reevaluations of definitions and classifications of this class of tumors will be periodically necessary.

DISCLOSURE

The authors have nothing to disclose.

REFERENCES

1. Ostrom QT, Patil N, Cioffi G, et al. CBTRUS statistical report: primary brain and other central nervous system tumors diagnosed in the United States in 2013-2017. Neuro Oncol 2020;22:iv1–96.
2. Parsons DW, Jones S, Zhang X, et al. An integrated genomic analysis of human glioblastoma multiforme. Science 2008;321(5897):1807–12.
3. Louis DN, Ohgaki H, Wiestler OD, et al. WHO classification of tumours of the central nervous system revised. 4th edition. Lyon: IARC; 2016.
4. Louis DN, Wesseling P, Aldape K, et al. cIMPACT-NOW update 6: new entity and diagnostic principle recommendations of the cIMPACT-Utrecht meeting on future CNS tumor classification and grading. Brain Pathol 2020;30(4):844–56.
5. Brat DJ, Aldape K, Colman H, et al. cIMPACT-NOW update 3: recommended diagnostic criteria for "Diffuse astrocytic glioma, IDH-wildtype, with molecular features of glioblastoma, WHO grade IV. Acta Neuropathol 2018;136(5):805–10.
6. Capper D, Jones DTW, Sill M, et al. DNA methylation-based classification of central nervous system tumours. Nature 2018;555(7697):469–74.
7. Rosenblum MK, Erlandson RA, Budzilovich GN. The lipid-rich epithelioid glioblastoma. Am J Surg Pathol 1991;15(10):925–34.
8. Mørk SJ, Rubinstein LJ, Kepes JJ, et al. Patterns of epithelial metaplasia in malignant gliomas. II. Squamous differentiation of epithelial-like formations in gliosarcomas and glioblastomas. J Neuropathol Exp Neurol 1988;47(2):101–18.
9. Perry A, Aldape KD, George DH, et al. Small cell astrocytoma: an aggressive variant that is

clinicopathologically and genetically distinct from anaplastic oligodendroglioma. Cancer 2004; 101(10):2318–26.

10. Scherer HJ. The forms of growth in gliomas and their practical significance. Brain 1940;63:1–35.

11. Haddad SF, Moore SA, Schelper RL, et al. Vascular smooth muscle hyperplasia underlies the formation of glomeruloid vascular structures of glioblastoma multiforme. J Neuropathol Exp Neurol 1992;51(5): 488–92.

12. Rong Y, Durden DL, Van Meir EG, et al. 'Pseudopalisading' necrosis in glioblastoma: a familiar morphologic feature that links vascular pathology, hypoxia, and angiogenesis. J Neuropathol Exp Neurol 2006; 65(6):529–39.

13. Margetts JC, Kalyan-Raman UP. Giant-celled glioblastoma of brain. A clinico-pathological and radiological study of ten cases (including immunohistochemistry and ultrastructure). Cancer 1989;63(3):524–31.

14. Kozak KR, Moody JS. Giant cell glioblastoma: a glioblastoma subtype with distinct epidemiology and superior prognosis. Neuro Oncol 2009;11(6): 833–41.

15. Kleinschmidt-DeMasters BK, Aisner DL, Birks DK, et al. Epithelioid GBMs show a high percentage of BRAF V600E mutation. Am J Surg Pathol 2013; 37(5):685–98.

16. Reis RM, Könü-Leblebicioglu D, Lopes JM, et al. Genetic profile of gliosarcomas. Am J Pathol 2000; 156(2):425–32.

17. Ishizawa K, Komori T, Shimada S, et al. Olig2 and CD99 are useful negative markers for the diagnosis of brain tumors. Clin Neuropathol 2008;27(3): 118–28.

18. Nikiforova MN, Wald AI, Melan MA, et al. Targeted next-generation sequencing panel (GlioSeq) provides comprehensive genetic profiling of central nervous system tumors. Neuro Oncol 2016;18(3): 379–87.

19. Woo HY, Na K, Yoo J, et al. Glioblastomas harboring gene fusions detected by next-generation sequencing. Brain Tumor Pathol 2020;37(4):136–44.

20. Nonoguchi N, Ohta T, Oh JE, et al. TERT promoter mutations in primary and secondary glioblastomas. Acta Neuropathol 2013;126(6):931–7.

21. Killela PJ, Reitman ZJ, Jiao Y, et al. TERT promoter mutations occur frequently in gliomas and a subset of tumors derived from cells with low rates of self-renewal. Proc Natl Acad Sci U S A 2013;110(15): 6021–6.

22. Stupp R, Hegi ME, Mason WP, et al. Effects of radiotherapy with concomitant and adjuvant temozolomide versus radiotherapy alone on survival in glioblastoma in a randomised phase III study: 5-year analysis of the EORTC-NCIC trial. Lancet Oncol 2009;10(5):459–66.

23. Wick W, Weller M, van den Bent M, et al. MGMT testing–the challenges for biomarker-based glioma treatment. Nat Rev Neurol 2014;10(7):372–85.

24. Brennan CW, Verhaak RG, McKenna A, et al. The somatic genomic landscape of glioblastoma. Cell 2013;155(2):462–77.

25. Verhaak RG, Hoadley KA, Purdom E, et al. Integrated genomic analysis identifies clinically relevant subtypes of glioblastoma characterized by abnormalities in PDGFRA, IDH1, EGFR, and NF1. Cancer Cell 2010;17(1):98–110.

26. McLendon R, Friedman A, Bigner D, et al. Comprehensive genomic characterization defines human glioblastoma genes and core pathways. Nature 2008;455(7216):1061–8.

27. Biernat W, Kleihues P, Yonekawa Y, et al. Amplification and overexpression of MDM2 in primary (de novo) glioblastomas. J Neuropathol Exp Neurol 1997;56(2):180–5.

28. Reinhardt A, Stichel D, Schrimpf D, et al. Anaplastic astrocytoma with piloid features, a novel molecular class of IDH wildtype glioma with recurrent MAPK pathway, CDKN2A/B and ATRX alterations. Acta Neuropathol 2018;136(2):273–91.

29. Deng MY, Sill M, Chiang J, et al. Molecularly defined diffuse leptomeningeal glioneuronal tumor (DLGNT) comprises two subgroups with distinct clinical and genetic features. Acta Neuropathol 2018;136: 239–53.

Metabolic Vulnerabilities in Brain Cancer

Danielle Morrow, BS[a,1], Jenna Minami, BS[a,1], David A. Nathanson, PhD[a,b,*]

KEYWORDS

- Metabolism • GBM • Tumor microenvironment • Oncogene

KEY POINTS

- Rewired metabolism in glioblastoma (GBM) is a result of both tumor-intrinsic (genotype) and tumor-extrinsic (tumor microenvironment) factors.
- Choosing the appropriate model system for GBM is important when studying metabolism, because each system has its own benefits and limitations.
- GBM metabolism is complex; therefore, it is important to take a comprehensive, multimodel system and multiomics approach when identifying metabolic vulnerabilities and therapeutic targets.

INTRODUCTION

Rewired cellular metabolism is a hallmark of cancer. Like most malignancies, glioblastomas (GBMs) exhibit altered metabolism to support a variety of bioenergetic and biosynthetic demands for tumor growth, invasion, and drug resistance.[1–3] Changes in glycolytic flux, oxidative phosphorylation (OXPHOS), the pentose phosphate pathway (PPP), fatty acid biosynthesis and oxidation, and nucleic acid biosynthesis are observed in GBMs to help drive tumorigenesis. Although the mechanistic underpinnings of metabolic rewiring in GBM are still being elucidated, evidence in GBMs and other cancers supports that augmented oncogenic signaling—emanating from mutations in oncogenic divers and/or loss of tumor suppressors—can rewire cellular metabolism. In addition to tumor-intrinsic drivers of metabolism, the tumor microenvironment (TME) also can have an impact on cancer cell metabolism via changes in nutrient availability and/or interactions with non-tumor cells. This may be relevant particularly for GBM tumors, which exist within a complex milieu of normal brain and immune cells as well as the tightly regulated metabolic environment due to the presence of the blood-brain barrier (BBB). Thus, an understanding of how both intrinsic and extrinsic factors modulate metabolism is becoming increasingly important for identifying more effective targets and therapeutics for GBMs. This review outlines the dynamic nature of GBM metabolism and highlights how both molecular alterations and as well as the TME regulate metabolic remodeling in GBM (**Fig. 1**). The challenges of studying metabolic interactions in the TME and how the TME can act as a double-edged sword when considering potential therapies for GBM also are discussed.

THE INFLUENCE OF NATURE AND NURTURE ON METABOLISM IN GBM
Glycolysis

A defining feature of many cancers, including GBM, is increased aerobic glycolysis.[4] Despite being a less efficient source of adenosine triphosphate (ATP) relative to OXPHOS, glycolysis enables rapid production of metabolic intermediates for macromolecular biosynthesis and improving the capacity to reduce damaging reactive oxygen species (ROS).[4] GBM cells display a dependency on glycolysis for growth and survival.[5,6] The enhanced glycolytic phenotype

[a] Department of Molecular and Medical Pharmacology, University of California Los Angeles; [b] David Geffen School of Medicine, University of California Los Angeles
[1] Present address: UCLA CHS 23-234, 650 Charles E. Young Drive South, Los Angeles, CA 90036.
* Corresponding author. UCLA CHS 23-234, 650 Charles E. Young Drive South, Los Angeles, CA 90036.
E-mail address: dnathanson@mednet.ucla.edu

Neurosurg Clin N Am 32 (2021) 159–169
https://doi.org/10.1016/j.nec.2020.12.006

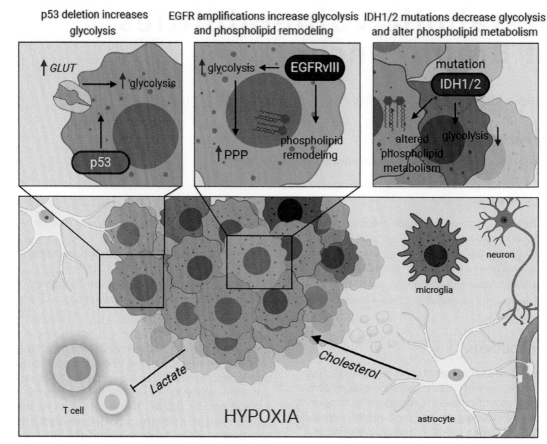

Fig. 1. Examples of metabolic remodeling in GBM. Genetic alterations rewire metabolism in GBM—EGFR amplifications and mutations can increase glycolysis and PPP activity (upper middle)—furthermore, EGFRvIII has been shown to induce phospholipid remodeling. Loss of p53 increases glycolysis by activating GLUTs (upper left). IDH1/2 mutations decrease glycolysis by reducing LDH expression. 2-hydroxyglutarate (2HG), the metabolic byproduct produced by mutant IDH1/2, also can alter epigenetic modifications (upper right). Finally, GBM metabolism is both rewired by and can rewire the TME. GBMs can uptake astrocyte-derived cholesterol to meet increased metabolic demands and can release lactate into the environment to suppress immune cells. The acidic and hypoxic TME also can promote aerobic glycolysis, tumor invasion, and resistance to certain therapeutics (bottom).

observed in GBM tumors is, at least in part, driven by various recurring oncogenic mutations. For example, a defining feature of GBM is the up-regulation and constitutive activation of the receptor tyrosine kinase epidermal growth factor receptor (EGFR), which is highly correlated with decreased patient prognosis and occurs in approximately 60% of GBM tumors.[3] The most frequent activating mutation in EGFR found in GBM—a ligand independent variant, termed *EGFRvIII*—can drive glycolysis via c-MYC activation, which can drive glycolytic gene expression, specifically increasing the expression of glucose transporter (GLUT) 1 and GLUT3, hexokinase 2, and pyruvate dehydrogenase kinase 1.[7–10] Moreover, hyperactivated EGFR signaling in GBM also can promote heightened glucose metabolism via regulating the plasma membrane localization of GLUT1 and GLUT3.[3] Targeting EGFR-driven glucose metabolism, consequently, can engage

the intrinsic apoptotic machinery in primary GBM cells,[3] emphasizing the importance of this relationship for GBM growth and viability.

Mutations in the tumor suppressor, TP53, are another common feature of GBM tumors.[11] Although not directly shown in GBM, loss of function mutations in TP53 can increase aerobic glycolysis via altered regulation of the GLUT genes GLUT1 and GLUT4.[9] Critically, cytoplasmic p53 in GBM has been shown to connect EGFR-driven glucose metabolism to apoptosis, indicating dependencies in the cross-talk between oncogenic signaling and metabolism.[3] Heightened glycolysis, however, is not universal to all GBMs. A defining feature of low-grade GBMs, isocitrate dehydrogenase (IDH) 1 mutations, inhibit glucose uptake by reducing expression of lactate dehydrogenase (LDH) A, which converts glucose to lactate. As a result, mutations in IDH1 in GBM gliomaspheres were shown to result in reduced glucose uptake compared with IDH wild-type gliomasphere as well as reduced uptake of the glucose analog fluorodeoxyglucose (^{18}F-FDG) in vivo.[12,13]

THE PENTOSE PHOSPHATE PATHWAY

Many cancers up-regulate flux through the PPP to drive the synthesis of nucleotides for DNA replication and repair as well as the production of reducing equivalents (eg, NADPH) to support redox homeostasis and lipid biosynthesis.[14–16] Entry into the PPP proceeds via the conversion of glucose-6 phosphate by glucose-6-phosphate dehydrogenase into 6-phosphogluconolactone and, via additional enzymatic steps, ultimately producing ribulose-5-phosphate, CO_2, and NADPH.[14] Through the oxidative branch of this pathway, glucose is converted to NADPH and ribonucleotides.[14] Nucleotide biosynthesis is critical to support rapidly proliferating cells, and de novo biosynthesis of both purines and pyrimidines has been observed to be altered in cancers.[14] A recent study found that low levels of nucleobase-containing metabolites were strongly associated with sensitivity to radiation therapy[17] in GBM and that supplementing GBM cells with exogenous nucleotides protected them from radiation by promoting repair of double-stranded breaks. The protective effects of these nucleotides were found to be due to purines, because de novo purine biosynthesis can generate guanosine triphosphate (GTP), which thus promotes tRNA and rRNA synthesis.[17] Together, these findings suggest that modulating purine biosynthesis through targeting the nonoxidative branch of the PPP may radiosensitize GBM. It also has been shown in GBM that the rate-limiting enzyme for de novo guanine nucleotide biosynthesis, inosine monosphate dehydrogenase (IMPDH2)), is up-regulated and results in increased de novo GTP biosynthesis.[18] Contrary to normal primary glial cells, which can utilize the salvage pathway, inhibition of IMPDH2 in GBM cells reduced nucleotide synthesis and proliferation.[18] Finally, the combination of targeting both de novo biosynthesis and nucleotide salvage can impair primary GBM cell growth and survival significantly.[19–21]

OXIDATIVE PHOSPHORYLATION

In many cancers, OXPHOS is up-regulated even in the presence of increased glycolysis.[22] OXPHOS produces ATP via the transfer of electrons from nicotinamide adenine dinucleotide (NADH) or Flavin adenine dinucleotide ($FADH_2$) to oxygen via electron carriers in the inner mitochondrial membrane, known as the electron transport chain. This process produces a proton gradient that enables ATP synthesis via phosphorylation of ADP.[22] There are multiple protumorigenic consequences of increased OXPHOS, including the production of ROS, which can increase proliferation, survival signaling, and genomic instability.[23] Additionally, the ability of tumor cells to utilize both glycolysis and OXPHOS confers metabolic flexibility that may contribute to therapeutic resistance.[24] Importantly, the ability of cells to utilize OXPHOS may be impacted not only by respiratory capacity but also by oxygen availability within the TME.[25] In vivo analysis of GBM tumor metabolism via isotopically labeled nutrient infusion identified that molecularly diverse GBMs utilize both glycolysis and mitochondrial glucose oxidation.[26] Importantly, multiple studies have demonstrated that OXPHOS represents a targetable vulnerability in GBM cells. For example, IMP2 was shown to be both highly expressed and a critical regulator of OXPHOS in GBM. Consequently, ablation of IMP2 or treatment with the complex I inhibitor rotenone could inhibit GBM cell growth.[27] Moreover, a recent study demonstrated that the ATP synthase inhibitor, Gboxin, could reduce in vitro and in vivo proliferation of primary GBM cells, presumably as a consequence of impaired energy production.[28]

Cancers can utilize multiple bioenergetic substrates for OXPHOS, including fatty acids, ketone bodies, glutamate, and acetate.[29] The ability to alternate between these substrates based on nutrient availability may provide these tumors with a metabolic advantage. Studies conducted by Mashimo and colleagues[30] revealed that, in GBM patient-derived xenograft (PDX) models, acetate, a widely available nutrient in the brain, served as a critical bioenergetic substrate in the microenvironment for human GBM. Six GBM PDX models received infusions of 13C-labelled acetate and glucose, and 13C-nuclear magnetic resonance analysis revealed that GBMs exhibited a shift toward acetate oxidation to acetyl–coenzyme A (CoA). They also found that levels of acetyl-CoA synthetase 2 (ACCS2), an enzyme that converts acetate to acetyl-CoA, was high in GBM PDX tumors, and that ACSS2 expression was inversely correlated with GBM patient survival.[30] Astrocytes have the capability to utilize acetate under limited glucose conditions, including diabetic hypoglycemia[31]; therefore, the capacity to metabolize acetate may result from the astroglial lineage of GBM.[30] Further research is needed to elucidate the role of molecular heterogeneity and TME on oxidative capacity.

GLUTAMINE METABOLISM

Glutamine serves as a source of nitrogen and carbon for the biosynthesis of nucleotides and amino acids as well as a potential fuel source for the TCA.[32] In normal brain tissue, glutamate can be taken up by astrocytes via astrocytic glutamate transporters and subsequently synthesized to glutamine.[33,34] Glutamine then is transported to neurons, where it is converted back to glutamate for synaptic transmission through a process that is termed, *glutamine-glutamate cycle*.[35,36] The glutamine/glutamate-rich brain microenvironment enables brain tumors to make synaptic connections with glutamatergic neurons and reprogram glutamine metabolism to enable growth.[37–39] Glutamine metabolism was found to be increased in human GBM xenografts compared with surrounding brain tissue.[26] Under glutamine-starved conditions, GBM cells either can convert glutamate into glutamine via up-regulation of glutamine synthetase or uptake astrocyte-derived glutamine via ASCT2.[40] In vivo isotope-tracing studies have identified that human GBM cell lines and PDXs preferentially utilize glucose over glutamine to supply TCA cycle intermediates,[26,30] with glucose-derived carbons supporting glutamine synthesis from glutamate.[40,41] The findings from these studies suggest that GBMs do not utilize glutamine as a major fuel for the TCA cycle; however, other studies conducted in vitro have suggested that primary glioma cell lines do require glutamine to support oxidative metabolism.[42] The discrepancy between these findings highlights the differences between the in vitro and in vivo microenvironment and raises the question of whether in vitro nutrient dependencies are metabolic adaptations to the nonphysiological nutrient contentration in media.[43,44]

The role of glutamine in GBM has also been shown to be dictated by the presence of genetic alterations in glutamine metabolism. IDH1 and IDH2 mutations catalyze the production of the oncometabolite D-2-hydroxyglutarate (2HG) from α-ketoglutarate.[45] 2HG inhibits DNA and histone demethylases, resulting in the inhibition of cell differentiation. In vivo studies of patient-derived chondrosarcoma IDH1-mutant xenografts revealed that glutamine is a primary carbon source for 2HG.[44,46,47] The role of 2HG, however, has yet to be fully elucidated in the brain TME, and recent studies point to interactions between 2HG and the immune cell milieu of the TME.[48] In vivo syngeneic mouse models of IDH1-mutant GBM have shown that 2HG decreases CXCL10 expression, resulting in a reduction of T-cell accumulation at the tumor site.[49] Further in vivo studies are required to understand the extent to which production of this oncometabolite may lead to immune cell evasion and cancer progression.

LIPID METABOLISM

Rapidly proliferating tumor cells require increased biosynthesis and uptake of fatty acids to form new cellular membranes during cell division, support increased post-translation modification of signaling molecules, and serve as energy stores.[44] The brain is a distinctly unique microenvironment when it comes to lipid metabolism. Lipid molecules are key components of the brain's structure and comprise approximately 50% of the brain's dry weight.[50–52] Several recent studies have provided evidence that fatty acids, including essential fatty acids obtained from the diet, can cross the BBB and be taken up by neurons via fatty acid transporters.[51] Unlike fatty acids, all cholesterol obtained in the central nervous system must be formed in situ, because the brain cannot access dietary or hepatic cholesterol due to the BBB.[53,54] Although both neurons and astrocytes can make cholesterol de novo, the major input of cholesterol into the brain originates from in situ synthesis in the endoplasmic reticulum of astrocytes.[55] Neurons and astrocytes both produce oxysterols as a product of cholesterol metabolism, which acts as an endogenous ligand for liver X receptors (LXRs). LXR activation decreases excess cellular cholesterol and, by promoting efflux through sterol transporters,[56] maintains cholesterol homeostasis within the brain. Previous studies have shown that GBM cells display dysregulated cholesterol metabolism and accumulate astrocyte-derived cholesterol from the brain microenvironment.[57] GBM cells also were found to suppress LXR ligand synthesis—treatment of GBM with LXR agonists killed GBM cell lines in vitro, while sparing normal human astrocytes.[57]

GBM cells also contain higher levels of cholesterol esters (CEs) and triacylglycerides (TAGs) than normal surrounding brain tissue.[58] Several studies have documented an increased number of lipid droplets in GBM cells, which are composed of CEs and TAGs, as a characteristic feature of GBM tumor cells in vivo.[59] Recently, it was shown that monounsaturated fatty acids increase lipid droplet formation and fatty acid oxidation in GBM, which also was associated with increased rates of glycolysis and cell proliferation.[60] A key characteristic of astrocytes is the formation of lipid droplets, which act as a buffer for neurons experiencing high stress. Studies have shown that stressed neurons induce astrocyte lipid droplet formation by shuttling their oxidized fatty acids to neighboring astrocytes[61]—the ability for GBMs to synthesize lipid droplets again may hint to their astroglial lineage; yet, future studies are necessary to connect cell of origin to metabolic phenotype.

Several genetic alterations common to GBM have been implicated in lipid metabolic reprograming in cancer. It has been shown that EGFR activates the transcription factor SREBP-1, a master regulator of lipid metabolism.[62] Consequently, inhibition of fatty acid synthesis rendered EGFRvIII, and not EGFR wild-type GBM, sensitive to cell death, indicating an EGFRvIII-dependent lipid metabolic vulnerability.[62] In breast cancer cells, mutant P53 was shown to bind to and activate SREBPs, leading to enhancement of the mevalonate pathway to up-regulate cholesterol biosynthesis and increase proliferation.[63] EGFRvIII signaling has been shown to induce phospholipid remodeling via LPCAT1 by saturating phosphatidylcholine lipid species. The LPCAT1-mediated shift toward saturated phospholipids also regulates EGFRvIII signaling by controlling the amount of EGFRvIII on the plasma membrane[61] and targeting LPCAT1 caused EGFRvIII to dissociate from cellular membranes, inducing massive tumor death.[61] Aberrant phospholipid metabolism also was identified via in situ matrix-assisted laser desorption/ionization imaging of patient-derived orthotopic IDH1-mutant GBM xenografts compared with IDH1Wildtype (IDH1WT) tumors.[64,65] Comprehensive metabolic profiling comparing low-grade astrocytoma and GBM patient-derived tumors revealed a shift from fatty acid synthesis to catabolism in GBM, with fatty acid β-oxidation being a key node differentiating GBM from low-grade astrocytoma.[66] Fatty acid β-oxidation can serve both anapleurotic and catapleurotic roles and is thought to provide metabolic plasticity in GBM, allowing these cells to accommodate to its harsh microenvironment.

HYPOXIA

Numerous microenvironmental factors may have an impact on tumor metabolism. It has been hypothesized that the TME dictates intertumoral metabolic heterogeneity.[67] A consequence of overwhelming the vascular supply in the brain, hypoxia has been shown to correlate with tumor aggressiveness and poor patient prognosis.[68,69] Hypoxia inducible factor (HIF) transcription factors are regulators of the adaptive response to hypoxia that frequently are up-regulated in GBM.[68] The transcription factor HIF-1α is activated during hypoxia, leading to the activation of enzymes that stimulate glycolytic flux to lactate efflux into the extracellular matrix.[70] Export of lactate acidifies the tumor environment, which can induce local protumorigenic inflammatory responses[70] and enhance tumor cell invasion,[68] further highlighting the interactions between GBM and the TME. Finally, stabilization of HIF-1α could also could lead to decreased cell proliferation.[71,72] Although counterintuitive, a hypoxic TME could result in a problematic population of cells that can survive under hypoxic stress and overcome common cancer therapeutics. Given that most cancer drugs are designed to target rapidly proliferating cells, tumor cells in a hypoxic niche may evade these therapeutics by demonstrating decreased proliferation. Low oxygen tension also results in an acidic environment, which can inhibit drug uptake rates via diffusion due to polarization of the cell membrane.[73] This key factor may be lost or overlooked in cell culture, however, because cells often are cultured under normoxic conditions.[74] In vitro studies have shown that hypoxia alters the GBM metabolome by transcriptional regulation of key metabolic enzymes.[75] Among the observed alterations are increased glycolysis and biosynthesis of macromolecules and nucleotide cofactor NAD and NADP biosynthesis as well as the oncometabolite 2-hydroxyglutarate.[75] Additionally, hypoxia induces a decrease in TCA cycle intermediates and altered cholesterol, glycerolipid, and sphingolipid metabolism. Engel and colleagues[71] recently demonstrated that modulating serine availability under conditions mirroring the GBM microenvironment sensitized GBM cells to hypoxia-induced cell death by increased ROS.

TUMOR MICROENVIRONMENT INFLUENCE ON GLIOBLASTOMA METABOLISM: IMPLICATIONS FOR EXPERIMENTAL AND TRANSLATIONAL STUDIES

The unique features of the brain TME pose a difficult challenge when studying GBM and other primary brain cancers. The brain consumes 25% of the body's glucose and 20% of its oxygen and is composed largely of lipids.[51,76] Moreover, recent evidence supports that cancer cells, including GBM, can shift their metabolic flux in response to nutrient availability in the TME.[66,77,78] Although the impact of physical environmental factors on cell metabolism is beginning to be appreciated,[43,79,80] an understanding of nutrient availability within the GBM TME remains largely understudied.

Although advances in methodologies have provided researchers much insight into cancer biology, deploying these experiments in the appropriate model system remains crucial. Investigations of TME-tumor metabolic interactions remain sparse due to the lack of model systems that appropriately recapitulate the brain microenvironment. There often are trade-offs between the physiologic relevance of a given model and its tractability for experiments—orthotopic xenograft models can recapitulate GBM progression in the brain; however, these models are inherently complex and most likely lack an immune system.

In contrast, in vitro culture models are experimentally tractable but rely on studying cells in a context that is vastly different metabolic environment from that of the TME.

The presence of intratumoral heterogeneity renders in vitro modeling of GBM exceptionally challenging when studying metabolism.[81–84] Additionally, cell culture media does not accurately recapitulate nutrient levels within the TME.[44] Classic synthetic cell culture media contains glucose, amino acids, vitamins, and salts that largely do not reflect those of human plasma or cerebral spinal fluid and lack additional components, such as lipids and nucleotide precursors.[85,86] Investigations into the effect of Dulbecco's Modified Eagle Medium (DMEM)/F12 media on neuronal activity found that the supraphysiologic levels of calcium (2–3 times higher than brain concentrations) impaired synaptic activity and reduced synaptic communication and action potential firing.[87] Disruptions to glucose homeostasis is known to disrupt brain physiology, and levels of glucose in DMEM and neurobasal media are approximately 2-times to 5-times higher than glucose levels in the brain of hyperglycemic patients.[88] Three-dimensional organoids grown from GBM cells and biopsies have become an increasingly popular method for modeling GBM in vitro—although organoid culture maintains regional heterogeneity and tissue architecture of the brain TME, it still lacks physiologic nutrient levels because the media used for organoid culture may not be representative of the nutrient milieu found in tumors in vivo.[89] In vitro models also may select against tumors that are auxotrophic for particular nutrients found in the TME but not found in cell culture media,[86,90] potentially leaving these tumors underrepresented and understudied. Although in vivo models may better represent the complexity and heterogeneity of cells within the brain TME, when using mouse models to study metabolism, multiple factors, such as strain, diet, sex, age, and environment stressors, should be considered, because these could affect tumor metabolism.[90,91]

Both biochemical and genetic experiments support the notion that the TME has an impact on metabolism. As discussed previously, stable-isotope tracing experiments have shown that tricarboxylic acid (TCA) cycle substrates can be utilized differently between in vivo and in vitro conditions. For example, Davidson and colleagues[43] showed that in 2-dimensional culture models of lung cancer, glutamine is the primary carbon substrate for the TCA cycle; however, experiments performed in lung tumors in vivo suggest that tumors favor the use of glucose for TCA cycle intermediates.[43,92] Similarly, GBM cells in culture appear to be dependent on glutamine for TCA cycle anapleurosis[40]; however, experiments performed in vivo suggest that GBM tumors utilize other TCA cycle substrates and are even glutamine autonomous.[40] Moreover, cancer cells in human plasma-like media drastically altered the metabolism of cells compared with that in traditional media and inhibited de novo pyrimidine synthesis.[85] At concentrations present in human plasma, uric acid, a metabolite not found in traditional cell culture media, was found an endogenous inhibitor of uridine monophosphate synthase, which catalyzes the last 2 steps in de novo pyrimidine synthesis.[85] Finally, recent genetic experiments have identified vast differences in metabolic pathway utilization between in vitro culture models (RNAi) and in vivo tumor models—RNA interference and clustered regularly interspaced short palindromic repeats (CRISPR) screens performed to identify essential metabolic enzymes share little overlap in the essential enzymes these screens identified between model systems.[93,94] Collectively, these studies highlight how a model environment can shape specific nutrient consumption and utilization, which may have profound implications on assessment of a metabolic dependency of a tumor.

THERAPEUTIC OPPORTUNITIES: UNRAVELING METABOLIC DEPENDENCIES IN GLIOBLASTOMA

Metabolic reprogramming arises as a consequence of interactions between the altered intrinsic characteristics of the tumor and the unique tissue context that fuels aggressive proliferation. Metabolic interactions between the tumor and microenvironment present a double-edged sword and can both fuel and hinder GBM. Nutrients obtained from the microenvironment can regulate signaling pathways through nutrient sensors, such as mTORC1 and AMPK, which support the metabolic demands of the tumor.[95] Cancer cells also can compete with infiltrating immune cells for nutrients that are limited in the TME, and secretion of metabolic byproducts can create an immunosuppressive niche that limits antitumor immune responses.[96] Likewise, interactions between oncogenic alterations and the microenvironment can select for favorable metabolic dependencies, which can present a therapeutic opportunity. EGFR presents a promising molecularly targeted metabolic therapy. In their article, Mai and colleagues[3] discovered a subset of GBMs termed, metabolic responders, that exhibit EGFR-driven glucose utilization. ^{18}F-FDG PET scans revealed that GBMs classified as metabolic responders had decreased glucose metabolism after EGFR inhibition; although EGFR inhibition alone did not cause significant cell death, it primed the cells for apoptosis,[3] creating an opportunity for synthetic lethality. Molecular therapies targeting mutant IDH also has become an attractive and promising therapeutic strategy, because it reduces the tumorigenic properties of 2HG. Phase I studies of 2 mutant IDH1 inhibitors (AG-881 and AG-120) showed favorable safety and efficacy in patients with IDH-mutated gliomas,[97] and ivosidenib (AG-120) has been approved by the Food and Drug Administration as a first-line treatment of IDH1-mutant acute myeloid leukemia.[98] Several lines of evidence suggest that indirect targeting of mutant IDH through its metabolic vulnerabilities also could prove beneficial. Patients with IDH-mutant GBMs seem to have a better prognosis than those with IDH wild-type GBM; however, it is not clear whether this is due to 2HG-mediated vulnerabilities or to the histology between these 2 tumor types.[49] 2HG has been shown to decrease the glycolytic capacity[12,13]; therefore, targeting energy production may decrease tumor growth and proliferation in IDH-mutant GBM.

Metabolic dependencies in gliomas arise as a consequence of many factors, including tumor genotype, cell line lineage, and environmental context; therefore, studies that consider these factors in isolation may not identify translatable therapeutic targets.[64] Relying solely on in vivo models to identify metabolic targets is impractical; however, current in vitro models do not fully recapitulate the physiologic microenvironment of tumors. Aspects of the physical and biochemical environment can alter therapeutic response, and differences in nutrient utilization between tumor and tissue could present targetable liabilities in cancer. The ketogenic diet (KD) has been used for more than 90 years as a treatment of drug-resistant seizures in children and adults with epilepsy.[62] This diet relies on fat as the main source of energy, and a drastic decrease in carbohydrate intake to induce ketosis[63]—although the normal brain can utilize ketones as an alternate energy source, it has been shown that certain GBMs do not have the metabolic flexibility to do so, and glucose depletion through the KD could deprive GBMs of their main energy supply.[99,100] Despite the potential of utilizing the KD to treat GBM, the practical application of this therapy has been limited in clinical studies, because patient compliance to the KD is difficult due to severely limited carbohydrate intake.[63] In the setting of dietary therapy for GBM, clinicians specialized in nutrition should be included in the neuro-oncology team. Treatment through dietary alterations may be effective particularly for patients with highly glycolytic GBMs and could be implemented as a monotherapy or in conjunction with antiglycolytic drugs, molecular therapies, or radiation and chemotherapies.

As proposed previously, a comprehensive analysis would require studies that integrate both in vitro and in vivo patient-derived cell line models, studies in patients, and ultimately clinical trials.[64] A systems biology approach that integrates multiple data types and contextual information may yield novel vulnerabilities that are missed when examining single molecular features in isolation. Although progress has been made in deciphering the metabolic network of GBM, there is still much to be learned about how both genetic aspects in the environmental context of the brain TME determine metabolic vulnerabilities. Applying a comprehensive analysis will allow unraveling the intricacies of the multi-faceted metabolic interactions in GBM.

CLINICS CARE POINTS

- Both intermolecular heterogeneity and intramolecular heterogeneity in GBM tumors complicate the efficacy of single-target therapies and may contribute to therapeutic resistance.

- Targeting specific metabolic pathways, including lipid synthesis, glycolysis, and nucleotide metabolism, has shown efficacy in several GBM studies.

- Tumor metabolism is impacted by multiple factors of the TME, including tumor-cell/immune interactions, the BBB, hypoxia, and nutrient availability, necessitating the investigation of tumor metabolism in various physiologic settings.

DISCLOSURE

This work was funded by National Institutes of Health (NIH) R01 CA227089 (D.A.N). D.H.M was supported by the Department of Defense U.S. Army Medical Research and Development Command Congressionally Directed Medical Research Programs Fiscal Year 2019 Peer Reviewed Cancer Research Program Horizon Award CA191084. The authors declare the following competing financial interests: D.A.N. is a co-founder of Trethera Corporation, Katmai Pharmaceuticals, and is a shareholder of Sofie Biosciences.

REFERENCES

1. Venneti S, Thompson CB. Metabolic programming in brain tumors. Annu Rev Pathol Mech Dis 2017;12(1): 515–45.

2. Pavlova NN, Thompson CB. The emerging hall-marks of cancer metabolism. Cell Metab 2016; 23(1):27–47.

3. Mai W, Laura G, Veerle WD, et al. Cytoplasmic p53 couples oncogene-driven glucose metabolism to apoptosis and is a therapeutic target in glioblastoma. Nat Med 2017;23(11):1342–51.

4. Vander Heiden MG, Cantley LC, Thompson CB. Understanding the Warburg effect: the metabolic requirements of cell proliferation. Science 2009; 324(5930):1029–33.

5. Wolf Amparo, Agnihotri Sameer, Micallef Johann, et al. Hexokinase 2 is a key mediator of aerobic glycolysis and promotes tumor growth in human glioblastoma multiforme. J Exp Med 2011;208(2): 313–26.

6. Flavahan WA, Wu Q, Hitomi M, et al. Brain tumor initiating cells adapt to restricted nutrition through preferential glucose uptake. Nat Neurosci 2013;16(10): 1373–82.

7. Babic I, Anderson ES, Tanaka K, et al. EGFR mutation-induced alternative splicing of Max contributes to growth of glycolytic tumors in brain cancer. Cell Metab 2013;17(6):1000–8.

8. Guardiola S, Varese M, Sanchez-Navarro M, et al. A third shot at EGFR: New opportunities in cancer therapy. Trends Pharmacol Sci 2019;40(12): 941–55.

9. Levine AJ, Puzio-Kutre AM. The control of the metabolic switch in cancers by oncogenes and tumor suppressor genes. Science 2010;330(6009): 1340–4.

10. Amelio I, Mara M, Varvara P, et al. (2018) p53 mutants cooperate with HIF-1 in transcriptional regulation of extracellular matrix components to promote tumor progression. Proc Natl Acad Sci U S A 2018; 115(46):E10869–78.

11. Brennan CW, Verhaak RG, McKenna A, et al, TCGA Research Network. The somatic genomic landscape of glioblastoma. Cell 2013;155(2):462–77.

12. Garrett M, Sperry J, Braas D, et al. Metabolic characterization of isocitrate dehydrogenase (IDH) mutant and IDH wildtype gliomaspheres uncovers cell type-specific vulnerabilities. Cancer Metab 2018; 6:4.

13. Kim D, Kim S, Kim H, et al. IDH1 mutation is associated with low FDG uptake in cerebral gliomas. J Nucl Med 2017;58:1281.

14. Patra KC, Hay N. The pentose phosphate pathway and cancer. Trends Biochem Sci 2014;39(8): 347–54.

15. Bensaad K, Atsushi T, Mary AS, et al. TIGAR, a p53-inducible regulator of glycolysis and apoptosis. Cell. 2006;126(1):107–20.

16. Ying H, Kimmelman AC, Lyssiotis CA, et al. Oncogenic kras maintains pancreatic tumors through regulation of anabolic glucose metabolism. Cell 2012;149(3):656–70.

17. Zhou W, Yao Y, Wahl D. Purine metabolism regulates DNA repair and therapy resistance in glioblastoma. Nat Commun 2020;11(1):3811.

18. Kofuji S, Akiyoshi H, Alexander OE, et al. IMP dehydrogenase-2 drives aberrant nucleolar activity and promotes tumorigenesis in glioblastoma. Nat Cell Biol 2019;21(8):1003–14.

19. Tarrado-Castellarnau M, Atauri P, Cascante M. Oncogenic regulation of tumor metabolic reprogramming. Oncotarget 2016;7:62726–53. Available at: https://www.oncotarget.com/article/10911/.

20. Laks Dan R, Lisa Ta, Crisman Thomas J, et al. (2016). Inhibition of nucleotide synthesis targets brain tumor stem cells in a subset of glioblastoma. Mol Cancer Ther 2016;15(6):1271–8.

21. Guo Deliang, Hildebrandt Isabel J, Prins Robert M. The AMPK agonist AICAR inhibits the growth of EGFRvIII-expressing glioblastomas by inhibiting lipogenesis. Proc Natl Acad Sci U S A 2009; 106(31):12932–7.

22. Ashton TM, McKenna WG, Kunz-Schughart LA, et al. Oxidative phosphorylation as an emerging target in cancer therapy. Clin Cancer Res 2018; 24(11):2482–90.

23. Liou GY, Storz P. Reactive oxygen species in cancer. Free Radic Res 2010;44(5):479–96.

24. McGuirk S, Audet-Delage Y, St-Pierre J. Metabolic fitness and plasticity in cancer progression. Trends Cancer 2020;6(1):49–61.

25. Vaupel P, Mayer A. Availability, not respiratory capacity governs oxygen consumption of solid tumors. Int J Biochem Cell Biol 2012;44:1477–81.

26. Marin-Valencia I, Yang C, Mashimo T, et al. Analysis of tumor metabolism reveals mitochondrial glucose oxidation in genetically diverse human glioblastomas in the mouse brain in vivo. Cell Metab 2012;15:827–37.

27. Janiszewska M, Suvà ML, Riggi N, et al. Imp2 controls oxidative phosphorylation and is crucial for preserving glioblastoma cancer stem cells. Genes Dev 2012;26(17):1926–44.

28. Molina JR, Sun Y, Protopopova M, et al. An inhibitor of oxidative phosphorylation exploits cancer vulnerability. Nat Med 2018;24: 1036–1046.

29. Mafeezzini C, Calvo-Garrido J, Wredenberg A, et al. Metabolic regulation of neurodifferentiation in the adult brain. Cell Mol Life Sci 2020;77:2483–6.

30. Mashimo T, Pichumani K, Vemireddy V, et al. Acetate is a bioenergetic substrate for human glioblastoma and brain metastases. Cell 2014;159: 1603–14.

31. Jiang L, Gulanski BI, De Feyter HM, et al. Increased brain uptake and oxidation of acetate

in heavy drinkers. J Clin Invest 2013;123(4): 1605–14.

32. DeBerardinis RJ, Mancuso A, Daikhin E, et al. Beyond aerobic glycolysis: transformed cells can engage in glutamine metabolism that exceeds the requirement for protein and nucleotide synthesis. Proc Natl Acad Sci U S A 2007;104:19345–50.

33. Sequerra EB, Goyal R, Castro PA, et al. NMDA receptor signaling is important for neural tube formation and for preventing antiepileptic drug-induced neural tube defects. J Neurosci 2018;38(20): 4762–73.

34. Hamberger A, Nystrom B, Larsson S, et al. Amino acids in the neuronal microenvironment of focal human epileptic lesions. Epilepsy Res 1991;9(1):32–43.

35. Hertz L. The glutamate-glutamine (GABA) cycle: importance of late postnatal development and potential reciprocal interactions between biosynthesis and degradation. Front Endocrinol (Lausanne) 2013;4:59.

36. Daikhin Y, Yudkoff M. Compartmentation of brain glutamate metabolism in neurons and glia. J Nutr 2000;130:1026–31.

37. Venkatesh HS, Morishita W, Geraghty AC, et al. Electrical and synaptic integration of glioma into neural circuits. Nature 2019;573. 549-545.

38. Venkataramani V, Ivanov Tanev D, Kuner T. Glutamatergic synaptic input to glioma cells drives brain tumour progression. Nature 2019;573:532–8.

39. Sidoryk M, Matyja E, Dybel A, et al. Increase expression of glutamine transporter SNAT3 is a marker of malignant gliomas. Neuroreport 2004; 15(4):575–8.

40. Tardito S, Anaïs O, Shafiq UA, et al. Glutamine synthetase activity fuels nucleotide biosynthesis and supports growth of glutamine-restricted glioblastoma. Nat Cell Biol 2015; 17:1556–68.

41. Cheng T, Sudderth J, Yang C, et al. Pyruvate carboxylase is required for glutamine-independent growth of tumor cells. Proc Natl Acad Sci U S A 2001;108(21):8674–9.

42. Oizel K, Chauvin C, Oliver L, et al. Efficient mitochondrial glutamine targeting prevails over glioblastoma metabolic plasticity. Clin Cancer Res 2017;23(20):6292–304.

43. Davidson SM, Papagiannakopoulos T, Olenchock BA, et al. Environment impacts the metabolic dependencies of Ras-driven non-small cell lung cancer. Cell Metab 2016;23:517–28.

44. Lagziel S, Gottlieb E, Sholomi T. Mind your media. Nat Metab 2020;2(12):1369–72.

45. Zhou W, Wahl DR. Metabolic abnormalities in glioblastoma and metabolic strategies to overcome treatment resistance. Cancers 2019;11(9):1231.

46. Salamanca-Cardona L, Shah H, Poot AJ, et al. In vivo imaging of glutamine metabolism to the oncometabolite 2-Hydroxyglutarate in IDH1/2 mutant tumors. Cell Metab 2017;26(6):830–41.e3.

47. Baenke F, Peck B, Miess H, et al. Hooked on fat: the role of lipid synthesis in cancer metabolism and tumor development. Dis Model Mech 2013;(6):1353–63.

48. Zhang L, Sorensen MD, Kristensen BW, et al. D-2-hydroxyglutarate is an intercellular mediator in IDH-mutant gliomas inhibiting complement and T cells. Clin Cancer Res 2018;24(21):5381–91.

49. Kohanbash G, Carrera DA, Shrivastav S, et al. Isocitrate dehydrogenase mutations suppress STAT1 and CD8+ T cell accumulation in gliomas. J Clin Invest 2017;127(4):1425–37.

50. O'Brien JS, Sampson EL. Lipid Composition of the normal human brain: gray matter, white matter, and myelin. J Lipid Res 1965;6(4):537–44.

51. Bruce KD, Zsombok A, Eckel RH. Lipid processing in the brain: a key regulator of systemic metabolism. Front. Endocrinol 2017; 8:60.

52. Bazinet RP, Laye S. Polyunsaturated fatty acids and their metabolites in brain function and disease. Nat Rev Neurosci 2014;15(12):771–85.

53. Dietschy JM, Turley SD. Cholesterol metabolism in the brain. Curr Opin Lipidol 2001;12(2):105–12.

54. Dietschy JM. Central nervous system: cholesterol turnover, brain development and neurodegeneration. Biol Chem 2009;390(4):287–93.

55. Petrov AM, Kasimov MR, Zefirov AL. Brain cholesterol metabolism and its defects: linkage to neurodegenerative diseases and synaptic dysfunction. ActaNaturae 2016;8(1):58–73.

56. Mouzat K, Chudinova A, Polge A, et al. Regulation of brain cholesterol: what role do liver x receptors play in neurodegenerative diseases? Int J Mol Sci 2019;20(16):3858.

57. Villa GR, Jonathan JH, Ciro Z, et al. An LXR–cholesterol axis creates a metabolic co-dependency for brain cancers. Cancer Cell 2016; 30:683–93.

58. Tugnoli V, Tosi MR, Tinti A, et al. Characterization of lipids from human brain tissues by multinuclear magnetic resonance spectroscopy. Biopolymers 2001;62(6):297–306.

59. Wu Z, Geng F, Cheng X, et al. Lipid droplets maintain energy homeostasis and glioblastoma growth via autophagic release of stored fatty acids. iScience 2020;23(10):101569.

60. Taïb B, Aboussalah AM, Moniruzzaman M, et al. Lipid accumulation and oxidation in glioblastoma multiforme. Sci Rep 2019;9:19593.

61. Ioannou M, Jackson J, Sheu S-H, et al. Neuron-astrocyte metabolic coupling during neuronal stimulation protects against fatty acid toxicity. BioRxiv 2018;177(6):1361–662.

62. Guo D, Prins RM, Dang J, et al. EGFR signaling through an Akt-SREBP-1-dependent, rapamycin-resistant pathway sensitizes glioblastomas to antilipogenic therapy. Sci Signal 2009;2(101):ra82.

63. Freed-Pastor WA, Mizuno H, Zhao X, et al. Mutant p53 disrupts mammary tissue architecture via the mevalonate pathway. Cell 2012;148:244–58.

64. Bi J, Chowdhry S, Wu S, et al. Altered cellular metabolism in gliomas – an emerging landscape of actionable co-dependency targets. Nat Rev Cancer 2020;20:57–70.

65. Fack F, Tardito S, Hochart G, et al. Altered metabolic landscape in IDH-mutant gliomas affects phospholipid, energy, and oxidative stress pathways. EMBO Mol Med 2017;9(12):1681–95.

66. Kant S, Pravin K, Antony P, et al. Enhanced fatty acid oxidation provides glioblastoma cells metabolic plasticity to accommodate to its dynamic nutrient microenvironment. Cell Death Dis 2020; 11:253.

67. Strickaert A, Saiselet M, Dom G, et al. Cancer heterogeneity is not compatible with one unique cancer cell metabolic map. Oncogene 2017;36(19):2637–42.

68. Monteiro AR, Hill R, Pilkington GJ, et al. The role of hypoxia in glioblastoma invasion. Cells 2017;6(4):45.

69. Velásquez C, Mansouri S, Gutiérrez O, et al. Hypoxia can induce migration of glioblastoma cells through a methylation-dependent control of ODZ1 gene expression. Front Oncol 2019;9:1036.

70. Agnihotri S, Zadeh G. Metabolic reprogramming in glioblastoma: the influence of cancer metabolism on epigenetics and unanswered questions. Neuro Oncol 2016;18(2):160–72.

71. Engel AJ, Lorenz NI, Klann K, et al. Serine-dependent redox homeostasis regulates glioblastoma cell survival. Br J Cancer 2020;122:1391–8.

72. Muz B, de la Puenta P, Azab F, et al. The role of hypoxia in cancer progression, angiogenesis, metastasis, and resistance to therapy. Hypoxia (Auckl) 2015;3:83–92.

73. Jing K, Yang F, Shao C, et al. Role of hypoxia in cancer therapy by regulating the tumor microenvironment. Mol Cancer 2019;18:157.

74. Bhattacharya S, Calar K, de la Puenta P. Mimicking tumor hypoxia and tumor-immune interactions employing three-dimensional in vitro models. J Exp Clin Cancer Res 2020;39:75.

75. Kucharzewska Paulina, Christianson Helena, Belting Mattias. Global profiling of metabolic adaptation to hypoxic stress in human glioblastoma cells. PLoS one 2015;10:e0116740.

76. Belanger M, Allamn I, Magistretti PJ. Brain energy metabolism: focus on astrocyte-neuron metabolic cooperation. Cell Metab 2011;14(6):724–38.

77. Sullivan MR, Mattaini KR, Dennstedt EA, et al. Increased serine synthesis provides an advantage for tumors arising in tissues where serine levels are limiting. Cell Metab 2019;30:1410–21.

78. Newman AC, Maddocks ODK. Serine and functional metabolites in cancer. Trends Cell Biol 2017;27(9):645.

79. DeNicola GM, Cantley LC. Cancer's fuel choice: new flavors for a picky eater. Mol Cell 2015;60: 514–23.

80. Mayers JR, Torrence ME, Danai LV, et al. Tissue of origin dictates branched-chain amino acid metabolism in mutant Kras-driven cancers. Science 2016;353:1161–5.

81. Ignatova TN, Kukekov VG, Laywell ED, et al. Human cortical glial tumors contain neural stem-like cells expressing astroglial and neuronal markers in vitro. Glia 2002;39(3):193–206.

82. Hemmati HD, Nakano I, Lazareff JA, et al. Cancerous stem cells can arise from pediatric brain tumors. Proc Natl acad sci U S A 2003;100(25): 15178–83.

83. Signh SK, Hawkins C, Clarke ID, et al. Identification of human brain tumour initiating cells. Nature 2004; 432:396–401.

84. Campos LS. Neurospheres: insights into neural stem cell biology. J Neurosci Res 2004. https://doi.org/10.1002/jnr.20333.

85. Cantor JR, Abu-Remaileh M, Kanarek N, et al. Physiologic medium rewires cellular metabolism and reveals uric acid as an endogenous inhibitor of UMP synthase. Cell 2017;169(2):258–72.

86. Ackerman T, Tardito S. Cell culture medium formulation and its implications in cancer metabolism. Trends Cancer 2019;5(6):329–32.

87. Bardy C, van den Hurk M, Eames T, et al. Neuronal medium that supports basic synaptic functions and activity of human neurons in vitro. Proc Natl acad sci U S A 2015;112(20):2725–34.

88. Gruetter R, Novotny EJ, Boulware SD, et al. Direct measurement of brain glucose concentrations in humans by 13C NMR spectroscopy. Proc Natl Sci U S A 1992;89(3):1109–12.

89. Hubert CG, Rivera M, Spangler LC, et al. A three-dimensional organoid culture system derived from human glioblastomas recapitulates the hypoxic gradients and cancer stem cell heterogeneity of tumors found in vivo. Cancer Res 2016;76(8): 2465–77.

90. Muir A, Danai LV, Vander Heiden MG. Microenvironmental regulation of cancer cell metabolism: implications for experimental design and translational studies. Dis Model Mech 2018;11:dmm035758.

91. Alquier T, Poitout V. Considerations and guidelines for mouse metabolic phenotyping in diabetes research. Diabetologia 2017;61:526–38.

92. Sellers K, Fox MP, Bousamra M 2nd, et al. Pyruvate carboxylase is critical for non-small-cell lung cancer proliferation. J Clin Invest 2015;125(2):687–98.

93. Yau EH, Kummetha IR, Lichinchi G, et al. Genome-wide CRISPR screen for essential cell growth mediators in mutant KRAS colorectal cancers. Cancer Res 2017;77(22):6330–9.

94. Alvarez SW, Sviderskiy VO, Terzi EM, et al. NFS1 undergoes positive selection in lung tumours and protects cells from ferroptosis. Nature 2017;551: 639–43.

95. Chhipa RR, Fan Q, Anderson J, et al. AMP kinase promotes glioblastoma bioenergetics and tumour growth. Nat Cell Biol 2018;20(7):823–35.

96. Buck MD, Sowell RT, Kaech SM, et al. Metabolic Instructions of Immunity. Cell 2017;169(4):570–86.

97. Mellinghoff IK, Cloughesy TF, Wen PY, et al. "A phase I, open label, perioperative study of AG-120 and AG-881 in recurrent IDH1 mutant, low-grade glioma: Results from cohort 1". Journal of Clinical Oncology 2019 37:15_suppl, 2003-2003.

98. Roboz, Gail J et al. "Ivosidenib induces deep durable remissions in patients with newly diagnosed IDH1-mutant acute myeloid leukemia." Blood vol. 135,7 (2020): 463-471. doi:10.1182/blood. 2019002140.

99. Klein P, Tyrlikova I, Zuccoli G, et al. Treatment of glioblastoma multiforme with "classic" 4:1 ketogenic diet total meal replacement. Cancer Metab 8, 24 (2020). https://doi.org/10.1186/s40170-020-00230-9.

100. Mukherjee P, Augur ZM, Li M, et al. Therapeutic benefit of combining calorie-restricted ketogenic diet and glutamine targeting in late-stage experimental glioblastoma. Commun Biol 2, 200 (2019). https://doi.org/10.1038/s42003-019-0455-x.

The Role of Mismatch Repair in Glioblastoma Multiforme Treatment Response and Resistance

Nalin Leelatian, MD, PhD[a], Christopher S. Hong, MD[b], Ranjit S. Bindra, MD, PhD[c],*

KEYWORDS

- GBM • MMR • MGMT • TMZ • Alkylators • MSI • TMB

KEY POINTS

- Alkylating agents are diverse with the regard to the lesions they induce, and this is important for how 06-methylguanine methyltransferase status affects drug sensitivity.
- Mismatch repair (MMR) mutations drive resistance to specific alkylating agents and often arise in subsets of recurrent glioblastoma multiforme.
- MMR mutations induce microsatellite instability (MSI) and increased tumor mutational burden (TMB), and there are multiple approaches to measure these phenotypes in pathology specimens.
- Although the link between MSI/TMB and immunotherapy response has been established for many cancers, it is poorly understood in GBM, and further studies are needed.

INTRODUCTION

Mismatch repair (MMR) is a highly conserved DNA repair pathway that is critical for the maintenance of genomic integrity. This pathway targets base substitution and insertion-deletion mismatches, which primarily arise from replication errors that escape DNA polymerase proof-reading function.[1] As such, MMR is thought to increase the overall fidelity of replication by up to 1000-fold, and loss of this pathway induces a strong mutator phenotype characterized by microsatellite instability (MSI).[2,3] MMR is particularly important in glioblastoma multiforme (GBM) for at least 3 reasons: (1) key proteins within this DNA repair pathway mediate the sensitivity to alkylating agents that are commonly used in glioma, including temozolomide (TMZ), specifically in tumors that lack expression of O⁶-methylguanine methyltransferase (MGMT); (2) defects in MMR drive TMZ resistance in subsets of recurrent GBM; and (3) MMR-induced MSI is an important predictor of the response to immunotherapy in many cancers, including possibly GBM. Here, the authors review key concepts in the molecular mechanisms of MMR in response to alkylation damage, approaches to detect MMR status in the clinic, and the clinical relevance of this pathway in GBM treatment response and resistance.

OVERVIEW OF THE MISMATCH REPAIR PATHWAY AND ITS RELEVANCE TO GLIOBLASTOMA MULTIFORME

Research on MMR has a rich history in which numerous seminal discoveries in molecular biology were made, which fueled the DNA repair field and led to the elucidation of many key DNA

[a] Department of Pathology, Yale School of Medicine, 310 Cedar Street LH 108, New Haven, CT 06510, USA;
[b] Department of Neurosurgery, Yale School of Medicine, 333 Cedar Street Tompkins 4, New Haven, CT 06510, USA; [c] Department of Therapeutic Radiology, Yale School of Medicine, 333 Cedar Street Hunter 2, New Haven, CT 06510, USA
* Corresponding author.
E-mail address: Ranjit.bindra@yale.edu

Neurosurg Clin N Am 32 (2021) 171–180
https://doi.org/10.1016/j.nec.2020.12.009
1042-3680/21/© 2020 Elsevier Inc. All rights reserved.

damage response (DDR) pathways in mammalian cells. As such, a comprehensive review of this pathway is beyond the scope of this article, but key historical findings and their relevance to GBM are briefly summarized here, and readers are directed to additional references for a more detailed description of MMR pathway intricacies.[4]

The MMR system was initially discovered in seminal, elegant research studies in *Escherichia coli*, which led to the 2015 Nobel Prize in Chemistry.[5] There are 8 MMR proteins in humans: MSH2, MSH3, MSH5, MSH6, MLH1, PMS1, MLH3, and PMS2. MSH2 and MSH6 heterodimers recognize single-base mismatches and dinucleotide distortions, whereas MSH2 and MSH3 process larger insertion-deletion loops ($\sim$1–14 bps).[6] Following lesion recognition, MLH1 and PMS2 heterodimers degrade the mutant sequence and trigger resynthesis. As will be discussed later, MSH6 mutations are found in subsets of recurrent GBM following alkylator exposure. The functions of the other MMR proteins are reviewed elsewhere.[4]

Alkylating chemotherapies are commonly used in the treatment of newly diagnosed and recurrent gliomas, including TMZ, procarbazine, ACNU (nimustine), BCNU (carmustine), and CCNU (lomustine) (reviewed extensively in[7]). TMZ and procarbazine are monofunctional methylating agents in the triazene class, and they primarily induce 3 lesions: 7-methylguanine (7meG), 3-methyladenine (3meA), and O^6-methylguanine (O^6meG). ACNU, BCNU, and CCNU are chloroethylating nitrosoureas that essentially act as bifunctional methylating agents, and they induce lesions on both DNA strands, including interstrand crosslinks. VAL-083 is a bifunctional alkylator in clinical development for GBM, which also induces more complex DNA damage.[8] Bendamustine, although not commonly used in GBM, is another example of a bifunctional alkylator that is CNS-penetrant.[9] The structures of these molecules are shown in **Fig. 1**.

The lesions described earlier are addressed by multiple DNA repair pathways in cells, but it is the O^6meG lesion that is relevant to both MMR and GBM. O^6meG lesions are repaired by the protein MGMT, which was first described in the early 1980s.[10–12] Around this time, it was discovered that some cancer cell lines were hypersensitive to monofunctional alkylating agents such as MNNG and MNU, which correlated with the inability to resolve O^6meG lesions.[13,14] These cells, initially called Mex- and Mer-cells, were subsequently found to be deficient in MGMT functional activity.[15] It was not until the 1990s that researchers discovered MGMT expression is suppressed via promoter silencing.[16–21] In parallel,

emerging data at the time also revealed loss of functional MGMT activity in subsets of gliomas,[22] which subsequently was confirmed to occur via MGMT promoter silencing.[23] Of note, the MGMT dependence applies largely to monofunctional alkylators, which induce lesions at the O^6 position of guanine without crosslinks, as the latter typically cannot be addressed by MGMT. Our group recently profiled mono- versus bifunctional alkylator activity in isogenic MGMT-proficient and -deficient cell line pairs, which confirmed that the MGMT dependence is only relevant for monofunctional alkylating agents.[24]

Regarding the mechanistic basis for monofunctional alkylator sensitivity in MGMT-deficient cells, the Mitra, Masker, and Essigman laboratories were the first to demonstrate that O^6meG mispairs with thymine (T) during replication.[25–27] O^6meG:T mismatches are detected by MMR,[28] which removes the T in the nascent strand, but once again a T is incorporated during the repair process. These "futile cycles" are thought to trigger apoptosis[29–31] and thus contribute to the exquisite levels of alkylators sensitivity seen in MGMT-deficient cells. This model is further supported by findings that MMR defects confer monofunctional alkylator resistance.[28,32] Importantly, MMR loss does not affect the sensitivity to bifunctional alkylators,[33] which mirrors MGMT independence for these agents as noted earlier. The authors and other investigators have also proposed an alternate or partially overlapping mechanistic basis for monofunctional alkylator sensitivity in MGMT-deficient cells, in which unrepaired O^6meG lesions activate the ATM- and Rad3-Related (ATR) axis of the DDR.[24,34–36] It was found that treatment with ATR inhibitors induces exquisite synergy with TMZ, specifically in MGMT-deficient cells. However, this synergistic interaction was abolished in the setting of defective MMR, which suggests a link between MMR and ATR signaling in MGMT-deficient cells treated with monofunctional alkylators.[24]

The basic science findings presented earlier provide critical insights into the patterns of therapeutic efficacy and resistance for agents that are currently being used to treat newly diagnosed and recurrent GBM. Building on early studies of clinical data suggesting a correlation between MGMT expression and the response to alkylating agents in glioma,[37,38] Hegi and colleagues[39] demonstrated that MGMT methylation status is an independent predictor for TMZ response in GBM. This study was based on data from the prospective phase II trial testing radiation therapy (RT) with concurrent and adjuvant TMZ,[40] which formed the basis for the landmark phase III Stupp

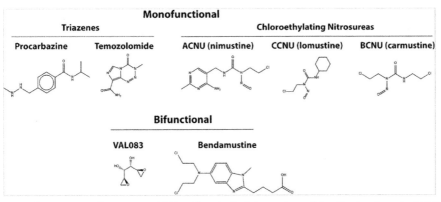

Fig. 1. Classes and structures of mono- and bifunctional alkylators relevant for the treatment of GBM.

trial.[41] Hegi and colleagues[42] subsequently demonstrated that the benefit of adding concurrent and adjuvant TMZ to RT for GBM is restricted to patients with MGMT promoter silencing, based on data from the Stupp trial. The unique spectra of DNA damage induced by mono- versus bifunctional alkylators also likely explains the enhanced efficacy of lomustine and TMZ combination therapy compared with TMZ alone in newly diagnosed GBM.[43–45] Finally, MMR mutations are found in patients with recurrent GBM who develop TMZ resistance, which again can be explained by the link between MMR and alkylation damage repair presented earlier.

DETECTION OF MISMATCH REPAIR STATUS IN CLINIC

Clinical assessment of MMR protein expression is performed on formalin-fixed paraffin-embedded tissue using a cost-effective immunohistochemistry (IHC) technique, with a panel that generally includes antibodies that target MLH1, PMS2, MSH2, and MSH6. IHC for MMR proteins is routinely performed as part of the clinical stratification to determine therapeutic approaches in other cancers outside of the brain, such as colon cancer. This technique also enables screening for patients who may have Lynch syndrome, which is characterized by germline mutations in MMR genes, as these patients are susceptible to developing other malignancies.[46] An additional key advantage of IHC assessment of MMR proteins is that the protein targets can be evaluated individually, which can guide subsequent germline testing of specific genes if indicated.

As presented earlier, MSH2/MSH6 and MLH1/PMS2 form 2 distinct heterodimeric complexes that are recruited in a stepwise fashion to the mismatched bases, and thus different patterns of protein loss can predict the most likely inactivated genes. Tumors with MLH1 loss usually show concurrent absence of PMS2 protein expression, as the stability of PMS2 depends on complex formation with MLH1.[47] In cases with loss of both MLH1 and PMS2, it is prudent to further determine if the loss is due to a sporadic or germline alteration. The former usually correlates with *BRAF* V600E mutations and/or *MLH1* promoter silencing, and the latter most commonly occurs via *MLH1* gene mutations.[48] In contrast, tumors with isolated PMS2 loss are highly suspicious for Lynch syndrome due to a *PMS2* mutation. Likewise, tumors with defective MSH2 frequently show concurrent loss of MSH6 immunoreactivity. This dual deficiency, as well as isolated MSH6 loss, highly suggests Lynch syndrome due to *MSH2* mutation or much less frequently *MSH6* mutation.[48] In gliomas, loss of MSH6 has been shown to be associated with prior exposure to alkylation therapy and tumor progression,[49,50] whereas defective MMR expression is uncommon in therapy-naïve gliomas, with the exception of the rare cases with germline mutation susceptibility.

Loss of MMR protein expression is defined as complete absence of nuclear immunoreactivity to one or more of the MMR proteins, whereas intact MMR expression is characterized by presence of some or diffuse nuclear staining in tumor cells.[51,52] This interpretation scheme, however, disregards 2 critical parameters: (1) intratumor heterogeneity and (2) expression levels of MMR proteins. Intratumor MMR protein expression heterogeneity has been observed in colon cancer,[53,54] as well as noncolonic malignancies including gliomas.[55] Its significance, however, is currently not well understood and may differ between different types of malignancies. Critically, a clearly defined MMR IHC interpretation guideline is currently lacking for tumors with clearly heterogeneous MMR protein expression. In addition, reduced expression of MMR proteins has been observed in recurrent gliomas[56] and seems to be associated with therapy resistance.[57] These findings emphasize the need to incorporate quantitative measures, to capture both cellular diversity and per-cell expression level, in assessing MMR status in tumors.

As discussed earlier, MMR-deficient tumors lack the ability to repair base pair mismatches that occur during DNA replication, and thus these tumors are characterized by widespread genomic mutations. Microsatellites are short nucleotide repeats that are susceptible to mutational accumulation secondary to lack of effective DNA repair mechanisms. MMR-deficient tumors are associated with accumulation of mutations in microsatellites, resulting in MSI. The basis for MSI detection involves polymerase chain reaction–based amplification of microsatellite loci, followed by analysis of fragment lengths.[58] The National Cancer Institute workshop has proposed a standardized analysis of 5 microsatellite loci as follows: 2 loci of mononucleotide repeats (BAT-25 and BAT-26) and 3 loci of dinucleotide repeats (D2S123, D5S346, and D17S250).[59] Tumors with at least 2 unstable loci are termed MSI-high (MSI-H), those with 1 unstable locus are called MSI-low (MSI-L), and MSI-stable (MSS) tumors are those that show stability of all 5 loci. However, MSI-L and MSS tumors are often regarded by many, as being in the same category as their distinction highly depends on the number of microsatellite loci tested and because their clinical prognosis is generally similar.[60,61]

The choice of microsatellite loci tested affects the sensitivity of MSI detection.[58,62] Specifically, dinucleotide repeats are less sensitive and less specific than mononucleotide microsatellites for the detection of MSI tumors.[2,63] More recent studies that implemented next-generation sequencing (NGS) showed that mononucleotide microsatellites were the predominantly affected sites.[60] Many groups have proposed examination of only mononucleotide repeats as a more sensitive and specific approach for MSI detection.[62,64–66] Of note, some alternative panels of microsatellite loci can effectively distinguish the controversial MSI-L tumors into either MSS or MSI-H categories.[67] Importantly, the available approved MSI tests are predominantly optimized for specific cancer types.[68] Although a pan-cancer approach has been proposed,[69] cancer-specific MSI panels might yield a better insight into clinical outcomes and responses to therapy, as mutational susceptibility of distinct microsatellites might be mechanism dependent and differ across tumor types.

In general, MMR protein IHC and MSI testing are complimentary, as deficient MMR protein expression usually corresponds to MSI.[70,71] They are prognostic and predictive biomarkers for responses to immune checkpoint inhibitor therapy in colon cancer, as well as screening markers for potential identification of patients with Lynch syndrome. However, unlike colon cancer, MMR protein expression status in gliomas does not accurately predict the stability status of microsatellites using standard assays.[72,73] In addition, MSI in gliomas are observed at a higher frequency in recurrent/residual tumors than therapy naïve gliomas.[74] These findings may indicate alternative mechanisms by which gliomas obtain MSI and possibly indicate clonal selection and/or evolution in response to alkylation therapy.[73]

Tumor mutational burden (TMB) likely reflects the overall tumor genomic stability and the efficiency of tumor DNA repair mechanisms, including MMR pathway.[75,76] Currently, NGS technology is generally used to assess TMB, although there is variation in the targeted regions that are used for assessment (eg, whole genome, whole exome, or targeted panels). TMB is a promising emerging biomarker that has been shown to effectively predict clinical response to immune checkpoint inhibitors in many cancer types, potentially related to immune recognition of neoantigens.[77–81] Although TMB in gliomas are not as high as many other malignancies,[82–84] it seems to be associated with tumor grade, MMR status, and is more prevalent in tumors with prior exposure to therapy.[49,84,85] Therefore, TMB assessment can be a promising complementary strategy to evaluate baseline genomic stability and to predict responses to immune-mediated and alkylation therapies in gliomas.

The current standard clinical test for predicting responsiveness to alkylation treatment in gliomas only includes MGMT promoter methylation status. As previously discussed, MMR- and MGMT-driven DNA repair mechanisms are intricately connected and can potentially affect microsatellite stability and TMB. Therefore, evaluation of MGMT promoter methylation profiles, in parallel with MMR/MSI status and TMB, can potentially reveal a subset of patients with glioma that may benefit from immune checkpoint inhibition as an adjunct or alternative treatment modality to alkylation therapy. Of note, the current analytical criteria for these tests either were not specifically designed for evaluation of gliomas or categorized the tumors in a semi-quantitative fashion, which frequently failed to provide clarity for clinical prognostics and management. Therefore, it would be critical to define quantitative, glioma-specific criteria, and cut-offs for all these assays for future therapeutic and clinical trial purposes.[86] A summary of

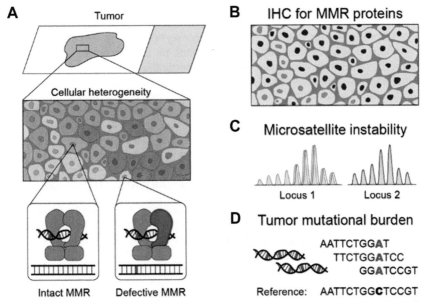

Fig. 2. Current approaches for detecting MMR status in the clinic. (*A*) Microscopic examination of tumors often reveals cellularity diversity, which comprises a mix of tumor cells with distinct morphologic and molecular profiles, including heterogeneous DNA mismatch repair status. (*B*) Routine immunohistochemistry (IHC) analysis can readily assess the integrity of MRR molecules at the protein level, and emerging evidence has revealed intratumor heterogeneity of MMR proteins between single tumor cells. (*C*) DNA microsatellite instability (MSI) and (*D*) tumor mutational burden (TMB) can also reflect MMR status in many tumor types. However, MSI and TMB are generally evaluated using bulk tumor tissue for which intratumor diversity cannot be directly assessed.

current approaches for detecting MMR status in the clinic is presented in **Fig. 2**.

MISMATCH REPAIR STATUS AND IMMUNOTHERAPY RESPONSE

Gene expression analyses of MMR-deficient tumors with MSI demonstrated upregulation of immune-mediated pathways and greater immune infiltration seen on histopathology,[87,88] which is likely secondary to immune response to tumor-related neoantigens.[4] As such, these tumors were thought to be excellent candidates for checkpoint immunotherapies, including blockade of CTLA4, PD-1, or PD-L1. This led to several clinical trials demonstrating the efficacy of pembrolizumab, an anti-PD-1 monoclonal antibody, in colorectal and other cancers with deficient MMR and high MSI,[79,89] prompting the first tissue-agnostic drug approval of pembrolizumab by the US Food and Drug Administration for patients with cancer.

Although MMR deficiency in gliomas has not strongly correlated with MSI,[50,73,90] it has been associated with a hypermutation phenotype, characterized by high TMB.[90,91] The latter may be secondary to de novo constitutional defects in DNA polymerase and MMR genes or an acquired resistance secondary to MMR deficiency that develops after treatment with standard alkylating agents, most commonly TMZ.[73,92] Clinically, the potential for immunotherapy to target MMR-deficient gliomas with high neoantigen load was first described in 2 pediatric siblings with rare germline MMR gene mutations resulting in biallelic MMR deficiency, who demonstrated dramatic clinical and radiographic responses to the anti-PD-1 monoclonal antibody, nivolumab.[76] Additional case studies have redemonstrated the efficacy of immunotherapy in patients with germline MMR mutations and high TMB in the absence of prior treatment.[93–95]

However, the clinical efficacy of checkpoint inhibition has not been clearly recapitulated in case series of recurrent high-grade gliomas,[96] and larger clinical trials have also not shown a clear benefit. Neoadjuvant PD-1/PD-L1 blockade in patients undergoing surgery for recurrent GBM showed modest or no survival benefits with pembrolizumab[97] and nivolumab,[98] respectively, compared with adjuvant therapy, although these studies did not compare checkpoint blockade with standard therapies. The Keynote-028 clinical trial, which evaluated pembrolizumab across 20 different cancers including GBM, found limited efficacy among patients with GBM with an objective response rate of 8% and median overall survival of 14.4 months.[99] However, none of the patients with GBM exhibited positive PD-L1 IHC or elevated TMB, whereas greater objective response rates were observed in other studied tumors with elevations in these indices. CheckMate 143 was the first phase III randomized clinical trial to evaluate PD-1 inhibitor therapy for GBM, in which nivolumab was compared with bevacizumab in patients with initial recurrent GBM after standard radiation and TMZ therapy.[100] At a median follow-up of 9.5 months, median overall survival was similar between both groups, but a higher objective response rate was observed in the bevacizumab group. Likewise, in a phase II clinical trial, pembrolizumab as a monotherapy or in combination with bevacizumab failed to show survival benefits in patients with recurrent GBM.[101]

More recent studies have been designed to consider MMR deficiency and/or high TMB as biomarkers for checkpoint inhibition in gliomas. A small case series of 4 patients with recurrent gliomas exhibiting MMR deficiency and/or high TMB did not exhibit any survival benefit with checkpoint inhibition.[102] Likewise, a larger single-center prospective study of 13 patients failed to find any objective response with pembrolizumab in recurrent high-grade gliomas, all having progressed through prior chemotherapy, and exhibited MMR deficiency.[103] Notably in this study, MMR deficiency was defined as partial or complete loss of MMR protein expression; this was a different definition compared with what is clinically used for other cancer types including colon cancer, which requires a complete loss of at least one MMR protein. The lack of uniform criteria for MMR and TMB evaluation specific to gliomas may have in part led to the variable observed efficacy of immune checkpoint inhibition in previous trials. Of note, an additional phase II trial is underway, studying the efficacy of ipilimumab and nivolumab, in patients with recurrent GBM and high TMB (NCT04145115).

Based on these previous trials, checkpoint inhibition does not seem as clinically effective in gliomas acquiring MMR deficiency after TMZ therapy, compared with gliomas with inherited MMR defects. Despite high TMB, the development of subclonal neoantigen populations, and thus inadequate immune exposure after TMZ therapy, has been proposed as a possible mechanism of immunotherapy resistance.[73] Indeed, in chemotherapy-driven hypermutated systemic tumors, those with subclonal populations of neoantigens did not respond well to immune checkpoint blockade, whereas responders demonstrated high TMB and high clonal neoantigen burden, particularly in lower stage cancers.[104] These data raise the possibility that primary MMR deficiency may be a more optimal biomarker for checkpoint blockade in gliomas and may be particularly relevant for chemotherapy-naïve GBM as well as lower grade gliomas.[105] The results of forthcoming clinical trials as well as molecular subanalyses of responders to checkpoint blockade in completed trials may help elucidate MMR deficiency and/or TMB status as biomarkers for glioma immunotherapy. Importantly, glioma-specific criteria for MMR defects and TMB cut-offs, especially ones that integrate cellular expression levels and capture intratumor clonal diversity, are critical for future trials to appropriately assess the efficacy of immune checkpoint inhibitors as adjunct and/or alternative therapeutic modalities in gliomas.

SUMMARY AND FUTURE DIRECTIONS

In conclusion, MMR plays a critical role in response to alkylating chemotherapies, although it is important to consider the unique DNA damage spectra and DNA repair pathways when considering the impact on antitumor efficacy. Furthermore, efforts to combine DDR inhibitors with DNA damaging agents such as TMZ should incorporate the potential effects of MMR loss on efficacy, particularly in recurrent disease, where MMR mutations have been described. Inherited or intrinsic loss of MMR in GBMs seem to confer marked sensitivity to immunotherapy-based strategies, although efficacy in the setting of acquired MMR loss is less clear. However, glioma-specific criteria for MMR defects and TMB cut-offs, which capture intratumoral diversity, may provide additional insights into the improving immunotherapy efficacy in GBM. These findings suggest we have much to learn about the interplay between MMR and the response to novel DDR inhibitor- and immunotherapy-based therapeutic strategies, and thus we await to see what the future holds for research in this area.

CLINICS CARE POINTS

- Loss of MGMT only predicts for sensitivity to specific alkylators, based on the type of damage that is induced.

- MMR mutations confer resistance to monofunctional alkylators such as TMZ but not others such as lomustine.

- MMR mutations arise after TMZ resistance and induce MSI/TMB, although whether this is a true biomarker for immunotherapy response has yet to be established.

- In contrast, intrinsic/inherited MMR mutations are associated with immunotherapy response.

- Better molecular markers for MSI/TMB/MMR status are needed specifically for GBM.

DISCLOSURE

The authors have nothing to disclose.

REFERENCES

1. Hsieh P, Yamane K. DNA mismatch repair: Molecular mechanism, cancer, and ageing. Mech Ageing Dev 2008;129(7–8):391–407.
2. Umar A, Boland CR, Terdiman JP, et al. Revised Bethesda guidelines for hereditary nonpolyposis colorectal cancer (lynch syndrome) and microsatellite instability. J Natl Cancer Inst 2004;96(4):261–8.
3. Kolodner R. Biochemistry and genetics of eukaryotic mismatch repair. Genes Dev 1996;10(12):1433–42.
4. Pećina-Šlaus N, Kafka A, Salamon I, et al. Mismatch repair pathway, genome stability and cancer. Front Mol Biosciences 2020;7:122.
5. Modrich P. Mechanisms in E. coli and human mismatch repair (nobel lecture). Angew Chem Int Ed Engl 2016;55(30):8490–501.
6. Dowen JM, Putnam CD, Kolodner RD. Functional studies and homology modeling of Msh2-Msh3 predict that mispair recognition involves DNA bending and strand separation. Mol Cell Biol 2010;30(13):3321–8.
7. Fu D, Calvo JA, Samson LD. Balancing repair and tolerance of DNA damage caused by alkylating agents. Nat Rev Cancer 2012;12(2):104–20.
8. O'Brien B, de Groot J, Kamiya-Matsuoka C, et al. Abstract CT115: Phase II study of dianhydrogalactitol (VAL-083) in patients with MGMT-unmethylated, bevacizumab-naïve recurrent glioblastoma. Cancer Res 2019;79(13 Supplement):CT115.
9. Chamberlain MC, Colman H, Kim BT, et al. Salvage therapy with bendamustine for temozolomide refractory recurrent anaplastic gliomas: a prospective phase II trial. J Neurooncol 2017;131(3):507–16.
10. Karran P, Lindahl T, Griffin B. Adaptive response to alkylating agents involves alteration in situ of O6-methylguanine residues in DNA. Nature 1979;280(5717):76–7.
11. Foote RS, Mitra S, Pal BC. Demethylation of O6-methylguanine in a synthetic DNA polymer by an inducible activity in Escherichia coli. Biochem Biophys Res Commun 1980;97(2):654–9.
12. Olsson M, Lindahl T. Repair of alkylated DNA in Escherichia coli. Methyl group transfer from O6-methylguanine to a protein cysteine residue. J Biol Chem 1980;255(22):10569–71.
13. Sklar R, Strauss B. Removal of O6-methylguanine from DNA of normal and xeroderma pigmentosum-derived lymphoblastoid lines. Nature 1981;289(5796):417–20.
14. Day RS 3rd, Ziolkowski CH, Scudiero DA, et al. Defective repair of alkylated DNA by human tumour and SV40-transformed human cell strains. Nature 1980;288(5792):724–7.
15. Yarosh DB, Foote RS, Mitra S, et al. Repair of O6-methylguanine in DNA by demethylation is lacking in Mer- human tumor cell strains. Carcinogenesis 1983;4(2):199–205.
16. von Wronski MA, Harris LC, Tano K, et al. Cytosine methylation and suppression of O6-methylguanine-DNA methyltransferase expression in human rhabdomyosarcoma cell lines and xenografts. Oncol Res 1992;4(4–5):167–74.
17. He XM, Ostrowski LE, von Wronski MA, et al. Expression of O6-methylguanine-DNA methyltransferase in six human medulloblastoma cell lines. Cancer Res 1992;52(5):1144–8.
18. Ostrowski LE, von Wronski MA, Bigner SH, et al. Expression of O6-methylguanine-DNA methyltransferase in malignant human glioma cell lines. Carcinogenesis 1991;12(9):1739–44.
19. Pieper RO, Futscher BW, Dong Q, et al. Comparison of O-6-methylguanine DNA methyltransferase (MGMT) mRNA levels in Mer+ and Mer- human tumor cell lines containing the MGMT gene by the polymerase chain reaction technique. Cancer Commun 1990;2(1):13–20.
20. Harris LC, Potter PM, Tano K, et al. Characterization of the promoter region of the human O6-methylguanine-DNA methyltransferase gene. Nucleic Acids Res 1991;19(22):6163–7.
21. Esteller M, Hamilton SR, Burger PC, et al. Inactivation of the DNA Repair Gene O[6]-Methylguanine-DNA Methyltransferase by Promoter Hypermethylation is a Common Event in Primary Human Neoplasia. Cancer Res 1999;59(4):793–7.
22. Citron M, Decker R, Chen S, et al. O6-methylguanine-DNA methyltransferase in human normal and tumor tissue from brain, lung, and ovary. Cancer Res 1991;51(16):4131–4.
23. Costello JF, Futscher BW, Tano K, et al. Graded methylation in the promoter and body of the O6-methylguanine DNA methyltransferase (MGMT) gene correlates with MGMT expression in human glioma cells. J Biol Chem 1994;269(25):17228–37.
24. Jackson CB, Noorbakhsh SI, Sundaram RK, et al. Temozolomide Sensitizes MGMT-Deficient Tumor Cells to ATR Inhibitors. Cancer Res 2019;79(17):4331–8.
25. Dodson LA, Foote RS, Mitra S, et al. Mutagenesis of bacteriophage T7 in vitro by incorporation of O6-methylguanine during DNA synthesis. Proc Natl Acad Sci U S A 1982;79(23):7440–4.
26. Loechler EL, Green CL, Essigmann JM. In vivo mutagenesis by O6-methylguanine built into a unique site in a viral genome. Proc Natl Acad Sci U S A 1984;81(20):6271–5.

27. Snow ET, Foote RS, Mitra S. Base-pairing properties of O6-methylguanine in template DNA during in vitro DNA replication. J Biol Chem 1984;259(13):8095–100.

28. Branch P, Hampson R, Karran P. DNA Mismatch Binding Defects, DNA damage tolerance, and mutator phenotypes in human colorectal carcinoma cell lines. Cancer Res 1995;55(11):2304–9.

29. Ochs K, Kaina B. Apoptosis induced by DNA damage O6-methylguanine is Bcl-2 and caspase-9/3 regulated and Fas/caspase-8 independent. Cancer Res 2000;60(20):5815–24.

30. Karran P, Hampson R. Genomic instability and tolerance to alkylating agents. Cancer Surv 1996; 28:69–85.

31. D'Atri S, Tentori L, Lacal PM, et al. Involvement of the mismatch repair system in temozolomide-induced apoptosis. Mol Pharmacol 1998;54(2):334–41.

32. Pepponi R, Marra G, Fuggetta MP, et al. The effect of O6-alkylguanine-DNA alkyltransferase and mismatch repair activities on the sensitivity of human melanoma cells to temozolomide, 1,3-bis(2-chloroethyl)1-nitrosourea, and cisplatin. J Pharmacol Exp Ther 2003;304(2):661–8.

33. Liu L, Markowitz S, Gerson SL. Mismatch repair mutations override alkyltransferase in conferring resistance to temozolomide but not to 1,3-bis(2-chloroethyl)nitrosourea. Cancer Res 1996;56(23):5375–9.

34. Ito M, Ohba S, Gaensler K, et al. Early Chk1 phosphorylation is driven by temozolomide-induced, DNA double strand break- and mismatch repair-independent DNA damage. PLoS One 2013;8(5): e62351.

35. Eich M, Roos WP, Nikolova T, et al. Contribution of ATM and ATR to the resistance of glioblastoma and malignant melanoma cells to the methylating anti-cancer drug temozolomide. Mol Cancer Ther 2013;12(11):2529–40.

36. Caporali S, Falcinelli S, Starace G, et al. DNA damage induced by temozolomide signals to both ATM and ATR: role of the mismatch repair system. Mol Pharmacol 2004;66(3):478–91.

37. Esteller M, Garcia-Foncillas J, Andion E, et al. Inactivation of the DNA-repair gene MGMT and the clinical response of gliomas to alkylating agents. N Engl J Med 2000;343(19):1350–4.

38. Friedman HS, McLendon RE, Kerby T, et al. DNA mismatch repair and O6-alkylguanine-DNA alkyltransferase analysis and response to Temodal in newly diagnosed malignant glioma. J Clin Oncol 1998;16(12):3851–7.

39. Hegi ME, Diserens AC, Godard S, et al. Clinical trial substantiates the predictive value of O-6-methylguanine-DNA methyltransferase promoter methylation in glioblastoma patients treated with temozolomide. Clin Cancer Res 2004;10(6):1871–4.

40. Stupp R, Dietrich PY, Ostermann Kraljevic S, et al. Promising survival for patients with newly diagnosed glioblastoma multiforme treated with concomitant radiation plus temozolomide followed by adjuvant temozolomide. J Clin Oncol 2002; 20(5):1375–82.

41. Stupp R, Mason WP, van den Bent MJ, et al. Radiotherapy plus concomitant and adjuvant temozolomide for glioblastoma. N Engl J Med 2005; 352(10):987–96.

42. Hegi ME, Diserens AC, Gorlia T, et al. MGMT gene silencing and benefit from temozolomide in glioblastoma. N Engl J Med 2005;352(10): 997–1003.

43. Herrlinger U, Tzaridis T, Mack F, et al. Lomustine-temozolomide combination therapy versus standard temozolomide therapy in patients with newly diagnosed glioblastoma with methylated MGMT promoter (CeTeG/NOA-09): a randomised, open-label, phase 3 trial. Lancet 2019;393(10172): 678–88.

44. Herrlinger U, Rieger J, Koch D, et al. Phase II trial of lomustine plus temozolomide chemotherapy in addition to radiotherapy in newly diagnosed glioblastoma: UKT-03. J Clin Oncol 2006;24(27): 4412–7.

45. Glas M, Happold C, Rieger J, et al. Long-term survival of patients with glioblastoma treated with radiotherapy and lomustine plus temozolomide. J Clin Oncol 2009;27(8):1257–61.

46. Dominguez-Valentin M, Sampson JR, Seppälä TT, et al. Cancer risks by gene, age, and gender in 6350 carriers of pathogenic mismatch repair variants: findings from the Prospective Lynch Syndrome Database. Genet Med 2020;22(1):15–25.

47. Takahashi M, Shimodaira H, Andreutti-Zaugg C, et al. Functional Analysis of Human MLH1 Variants Using Yeast and In vitro Mismatch Repair Assays. Cancer Res 2007;67(10):4595–604.

48. Chen W, Frankel WL. A practical guide to biomarkers for the evaluation of colorectal cancer. Mod Pathol 2019;32(Suppl 1):1–15.

49. Cahill DP, Levine KK, Betensky RA, et al. Loss of the mismatch repair protein MSH6 in human glioblastomas is associated with tumor progression during temozolomide treatment. Clin Cancer Res 2007;13(7):2038–45.

50. Yip S, Miao J, Cahill DP, et al. MSH6 mutations arise in glioblastomas during temozolomide therapy and mediate temozolomide resistance. Clin Cancer Res 2009;15(14):4622–9.

51. Rodriguez-Bigas MA, Boland CR, Hamilton SR, et al. A National Cancer Institute Workshop on Hereditary Nonpolyposis Colorectal Cancer Syndrome: meeting highlights and Bethesda guidelines. J Natl Cancer Inst 1997;89(23):1758–62.

52. McCarthy AJ, Capo-Chichi JM, Spence T, et al. Heterogenous loss of mismatch repair (MMR) protein expression: a challenge for immunohistochemical

interpretation and microsatellite instability (MSI) evaluation. J Pathol Clin Res 2019;5(2):115–29.

53. Watson N, Grieu F, Morris M, et al. Heterogeneous staining for mismatch repair proteins during population-based prescreening for hereditary nonpolyposis colorectal cancer. J Mol Diagn 2007;9(4):472–8.

54. Kheirelseid EA, Miller N, Chang KH, et al. Mismatch repair protein expression in colorectal cancer. J Gastrointest Oncol 2013;4(4):397–408.

55. McCord M, Steffens A, Javier R, et al. The efficacy of DNA mismatch repair enzyme immunohistochemistry as a screening test for hypermutated gliomas. Acta Neuropathol Commun 2020;8(1):15.

56. Felsberg J, Thon N, Eigenbrod S, et al. Promoter methylation and expression of MGMT and the DNA mismatch repair genes MLH1, MSH2, MSH6 and PMS2 in paired primary and recurrent glioblastomas. Int J Cancer 2011;129(3):659–70.

57. McFaline-Figueroa JL, Braun CJ, Stanciu M, et al. Minor changes in expression of the mismatch repair protein MSH2 exert a major impact on glioblastoma response to temozolomide. Cancer Res 2015;75(15):3127–38.

58. Baudrin LG, Deleuze JF, How-Kit A. Molecular and computational methods for the detection of microsatellite instability in cancer. Front Oncol 2018;8:621.

59. How-Kit CR, Thibodeau SN, Hamilton SR, et al. A National Cancer Institute Workshop on Microsatellite Instability for cancer detection and familial predisposition: development of international criteria for the determination of microsatellite instability in colorectal cancer. Cancer Res 1998;58(22):5248–57.

60. Hause RJ, Pritchard CC, Shendure J, et al. Classification and characterization of microsatellite instability across 18 cancer types. Nat Med 2016;22(11):1342–50.

61. Samadder NJ, Vierkant RA, Tillmans LS, et al. Associations between colorectal cancer molecular markers and pathways with clinicopathologic features in older women. Gastroenterology 2013;145(2):348–56.e1-2.

62. Hatch SB, Lightfoot HM, Garwacki CP, et al. Microsatellite instability testing in colorectal carcinoma: choice of markers affects sensitivity of detection of mismatch repair-deficient tumors. Clin Cancer Res 2005;11(6):2180–7.

63. Cicek MS, Lindor NM, Gallinger S, et al. Quality assessment and correlation of microsatellite instability and immunohistochemical markers among population- and clinic-based colorectal tumors results from the Colon Cancer Family Registry. J Mol Diagn 2011;13(3):271–81.

64. Bianchi F, Galizia E, Catalani R, et al. CAT25 is a mononucleotide marker to identify HNPCC patients. J Mol Diagn 2009;11(3):248–52.

65. Findeisen P, Kloor M, Merx S, et al. T25 repeat in the 3' untranslated region of the CASP2 gene: a sensitive and specific marker for microsatellite instability in colorectal cancer. Cancer Res 2005;65(18):8072–8.

66. Buhard O, Lagrange A, Guilloux A, et al. HSP110 T17 simplifies and improves the microsatellite instability testing in patients with colorectal cancer. J Med Genet 2016;53(6):377–84.

67. Murphy KM, Zhang S, Geiger T, et al. Comparison of the microsatellite instability analysis system and the Bethesda panel for the determination of microsatellite instability in colorectal cancers. J Mol Diagn 2006;8(3):305–11.

68. Xicola RM, Llor X, Pons E, et al. Performance of different microsatellite marker panels for detection of mismatch repair-deficient colorectal tumors. J Natl Cancer Inst 2007;99(3):244–52.

69. Waalkes A, Smith N, Penewit K, et al. Accurate pan-cancer molecular diagnosis of microsatellite instability by single-molecule molecular inversion probe capture and high-throughput sequencing. Clin Chem 2018;64(6):950–8.

70. Gibson J, Lacy J, Matloff E, et al. Microsatellite instability testing in colorectal carcinoma: a practical guide. Clin Gastroenterol Hepatol 2014;12(2):171.e1.

71. Lindor NM, Burgart LJ, Leontovich O, et al. Immunohistochemistry versus microsatellite instability testing in phenotyping colorectal tumors. J Clin Oncol 2002;20(4):1043–8.

72. Rodriguez-Hernandez I, Garcia JL, Santos-Briz A, et al. Integrated analysis of mismatch repair system in malignant astrocytomas. PLoS One 2013;8(9):e76401.

73. Touat M, Li YY, Boynton AN, et al. Mechanisms and therapeutic implications of hypermutation in gliomas. Nature 2020;580(7804):517–23.

74. Martinez R, Schackert HK, Plaschke J, et al. Molecular mechanisms associated with chromosomal and microsatellite instability in sporadic glioblastoma multiforme. Oncology 2004;66(5):395–403.

75. Wang L, Ge J, Lan Y, et al. Tumor mutational burden is associated with poor outcomes in diffuse glioma. BMC Cancer 2020;20(1):213.

76. Bouffet E, Larouche V, Campbell BB, et al. Immune checkpoint inhibition for hypermutant glioblastoma multiforme resulting from germline biallelic mismatch repair deficiency. J Clin Oncol 2016;34(19):2206–11.

77. Snyder A, Makarov V, Merghoub T, et al. Genetic basis for clinical response to CTLA-4 blockade in melanoma. N Engl J Med 2014;371(23):2189–99.

78. Rizvi NA, Hellmann MD, Snyder A, et al. Cancer immunology. Mutational landscape determines sensitivity to PD-1 blockade in non-small cell lung cancer. Science 2015;348(6230):124–8.

79. Le DT, Uram JN, Wang H, et al. PD-1 blockade in tumors with mismatch-repair deficiency. N Engl J Med 2015;372(26):2509–20.

80. Mandal R, Samstein RM, Lee KW, et al. Genetic diversity of tumors with mismatch repair deficiency influences anti-PD-1 immunotherapy response. Science 2019;364(6439):485–91.

81. Luksza M, Riaz N, Makarov V, et al. A neoantigen fitness model predicts tumour response to checkpoint blockade immunotherapy. Nature 2017; 551(7681):517–20.

82. Alexandrov LB, Nik-Zainal S, Wedge DC, et al. Signatures of mutational processes in human cancer. Nature 2013;500(7463):415–21.

83. Grobner SN, Worst BC, Weischenfeldt J, et al. The landscape of genomic alterations across childhood cancers. Nature 2018;555(7696):321–7.

84. Campbell BB, Light N, Fabrizio D, et al. Comprehensive analysis of hypermutation in human cancer. Cell 2017;171(5):1042.e10.

85. Hodges TR, Ott M, Xiu J, et al. Mutational burden, immune checkpoint expression, and mismatch repair in glioma: implications for immune checkpoint immunotherapy. Neuro Oncol 2017;19(8):1047–57.

86. Buttner R, Longshore JW, López-Ríos F, et al. Implementing TMB measurement in clinical practice: considerations on assay requirements. ESMO Open 2019;4(1):e000442.

87. Greenson JK, Bonner JD, Ben-Yzhak O, et al. Phenotype of microsatellite unstable colorectal carcinomas: Well-differentiated and focally mucinous tumors and the absence of dirty necrosis correlate with microsatellite instability. Am J Surg Pathol 2003;27(5):563–70.

88. Liu S, Gönen M, Stadler ZK, et al. Cellular localization of PD-L1 expression in mismatch-repair-deficient and proficient colorectal carcinomas. Mod Pathol 2019;32(1):110–21.

89. Marabelle A, Le DT, Ascierto PA, et al. Efficacy of pembrolizumab in patients with noncolorectal high microsatellite instability/mismatch repair-deficient cancer: results from the phase II KEYNOTE-158 Study. J Clin Oncol 2020;38(1):1–10.

90. Indraccolo S, Lombardi G, Fassan M, et al. Genetic, Epigenetic, and Immunologic Profiling of MMR-Deficient Relapsed Glioblastoma. Clin Cancer Res 2019;25(6):1828–37.

91. Wang J, Cazzato E, Ladewig E, et al. Clonal evolution of glioblastoma under therapy. Nat Genet 2016;48(7):768–76.

92. Sa JK, Choi SW, Zhao J, et al. Hypermutagenesis in untreated adult gliomas due to inherited mismatch mutations. Int J Cancer 2019;144(12):3023–30.

93. AlHarbi M, Ali Mobark N, AlMubarak L, et al. Durable response to nivolumab in a pediatric patient with refractory glioblastoma and constitutional biallelic mismatch repair deficiency. Oncologist 2018; 23(12):1401–6.

94. Larouche V, Atkinson J, Albrecht S, et al. Sustained complete response of recurrent glioblastoma to combined checkpoint inhibition in a young patient with constitutional mismatch repair deficiency. Pediatr Blood Cancer 2018;65(12):e27389.

95. Pavelka Z, Zitterbart K, Nosková H, et al. Effective immunotherapy of glioblastoma in an adolescent with constitutional mismatch repair-deficiency syndrome. Klin Onkol 2019;32(1):70–4.

96. Kurz SC, Cabrera LP, Hastie D, et al. PD-1 inhibition has only limited clinical benefit in patients with recurrent high-grade glioma. Neurology 2018;91(14):e1355–9.

97. Cloughesy TF, Mochizuki AY, Orpilla JR, et al. Neoadjuvant anti-PD-1 immunotherapy promotes a survival benefit with intratumoral and systemic immune responses in recurrent glioblastoma. Nat Med 2019;25(3):477–86.

98. Schalper KA, Rodriguez-Ruiz ME, Diez-Valle R, et al. Neoadjuvant nivolumab modifies the tumor immune microenvironment in resectable glioblastoma. Nat Med 2019;25(3):470–6.

99. Ott PA, Bang YJ, Piha-Paul SA, et al. T-cell-inflamed gene-expression profile, programmed death ligand 1 expression, and tumor mutational burden predict efficacy in patients treated with pembrolizumab across 20 cancers: KEYNOTE-028. J Clin Oncol 2019;37(4):318–27.

100. Reardon DA, Brandes AA, Omuro A, et al. Effect of Nivolumab vs Bevacizumab in Patients With Recurrent Glioblastoma: The CheckMate 143 Phase 3 Randomized Clinical Trial. JAMA Oncol 2020;6(7):1003–10.

101. Reardon DA, Nayak L, Peters KB, et al. Phase II study of pembrolizumab or pembrolizumab plus bevacizumab for recurrent glioblastoma (rGBM) patients. J Clin Oncol 2018;36(15_suppl):2006.

102. Ahmad H, Fadul CE, Schiff D, et al. Checkpoint inhibitor failure in hypermutated and mismatch repair-mutated recurrent high-grade gliomas. Neurooncol Pract 2019;6(6):424–7.

103. Lombardi G, Barresi V, Indraccolo S, et al. Pembrolizumab activity in recurrent high-grade gliomas with partial or complete loss of mismatch repair protein expression: a monocentric, observational and prospective pilot study. Cancers (Basel) 2020;12(8).

104. McGranahan N, Furness AJ, Rosenthal R, et al. Clonal neoantigens elicit T cell immunoreactivity and sensitivity to immune checkpoint blockade. Science 2016;351(6280):1463–9.

105. Ulgen E, Can Ö, Bilguvar K, et al. Whole exome sequencing-based analysis to identify DNA damage repair deficiency as a major contributor to gliomagenesis in adult diffuse gliomas. J Neurosurg 2019;1–12. https://doi.org/10.3171/2019.1.JNS182938.

Pediatric Gliomas
Molecular Landscape and Emerging Targets

Sophie M. Peeters, MD[a], Yagmur Muftuoglu, MD, PhD[a], Brian Na, MD[b],
David J. Daniels, MD, PhD[c], Anthony C. Wang, MD[a],*

KEYWORDS

- Targeted therapy • Molecular genetics • Pediatric glioma • Histone mutation
- Diffuse midline glioma • Next-generation sequencing

KEY POINTS

- Molecular genetic characterization of pediatric gliomas identifies oncogenic pathways and potential therapeutic targets.
- The MAPK and PI3K pathways are highly active in pediatric glioma biology.
- Mechanisms of oncogenesis unique to pediatric forms of glioma may lead to unique therapeutic opportunities.
- Genetic alterations identified through next-generation exome sequencing have yielded targeted therapeutics currently in clinical trials.
- Adequate drug penetration, sensitivity of brain tissue to treatment-associated toxicities, and a multiplicity of mechanisms of resistance present significant challenges to effective treatment.

CURRENT TREATMENT STRATEGIES AND PROGNOSIS
Pediatric Low-Grade Gliomas

Pediatric low-grade gliomas (pLGGs) are the most common brain tumors in children.[1,2] PLGGs generally are slow growing and devoid of malignant features. Anatomic location appears to correlate with genetic landscape. These tumors are clinically and genetically distinct from the low-grade gliomas seen in adults and must be treated as such. PLGGs broadly include all World Health Organization (WHO) grade I and grade II gliomas: pilocytic astrocytoma (PA), dysembryoplastic neuroepithelial tumor (DNET), ganglioglioma (GG), pleomorphic xanthoastrocytoma (PXA), subependymal giant cell astrocytoma (SEGA), and diffuse astrocytoma (DA), among others.

PLGGs generally portend a favorable prognosis and often can be cured by surgical resection alone.[3] PAs are the most benign of pLGGs, with 10-year overall survival rates of 96% and recurrence rates of 10% to 20%.[4,5] Where complete surgical resection is not possible, however, treatment of these tumors can be lengthy and complex, with risks of tumor progression, malignant transformation, and non-negligible treatment-related neurologic deficits, visual impairment, and endocrine dysfunction.[3,5]

Surgical resection is the mainstay of treatment in pLGGs, undertaken when feasible and safe to perform with curative intent.[5] Debulking procedures are reserved most frequently for symptomatic relief. When considering systemic therapies and radiation treatment, a balance must be maintained

Funding: None.
[a] Department of Neurosurgery, University of California Los Angeles, 300 Stein Plaza, Suite #520, Los Angeles, CA 90095, USA; [b] Department of Pediatrics, Division of Hematology/Oncology, University of California Los Angeles, 200 UCLA Medical Plaza, Suite 265, Los Angeles, CA 90095, USA; [c] Department of Neurosurgery, Mayo Clinic, 200 1st St SW, Rochester, MN 55905, USA
* Corresponding author. 300 Stein Plaza, Suite #520; Los Angeles, CA 90095.
E-mail address: ACWang@mednet.ucla.edu

Neurosurg Clin N Am 32 (2021) 181–190
https://doi.org/10.1016/j.nec.2020.12.001
1042-3680/21/

between the likelihood of tumor control, and minimizing long-term treatment-related morbidity because pLGGs typically are slow-growing, rarely undergo malignant transformation, and portend a long overall survival.[6] Four scenarios typically are encountered in pLGG: (1) tumors in surgically accessible locations (most of which are cured by resection alone); (2) tumors in high-consequence locations hostile to surgical resection; (3) Neurofibromatosis type 1 (NF1) patients with optic pathway gliomas, which typically are observed and are managed surgically only after significant symptomatic tumor progression refractory to other treatment modalities; and (4) tuberous sclerosis (TS) patients with SEGAs, for which mechanistic target of rapamycin (mTOR) inhibitors and surgery yield excellent results.[1,3]

A majority of pLGGs harbor a single driver alteration within a cluster of commonly altered genes and alterations. A majority of sporadic pLGG cases carry *KIAA1549:BRAF* and *BRAF*[V600E] gene mutations[7]; however, chemotherapies utilized for pLGG patients are limited to traditional agents, and targeted molecular therapies are only in their nascency.[3,5] Radiotherapy generally offers improved progression-free survival for many pLGG types but potentially at the cost of worsening overall survival.[3] Importantly, radiotherapy is avoided in the setting of germline cancer predisposition syndromes, such as NF1, and in very young patients (<3 years old) due to an extremely high risk of endocrine dysfunction, neurologic deficits, developmental delay, impaired vision, and radiation-induced malignancies.[2]

Pediatric High-Grade Gliomas

Pediatric high-grade gliomas (pHGGs) often are divided into diffuse midline glioma (DMG), essentially all H3K27M mutants,[8,9] and the non-brainstem pHGGs, which include H3G34R/V gliomas (**Fig. 1**).[10,11] Although histopathologic features are similar, the malignant gliomas seen in children are distinct from those seen in adult patients in many important ways. Whereas the classical adult forms of glioblastoma most frequently are diseases of copy number alteration, pHGGs frequently carry somatic point mutations. pHGGs often involve chromothripsis and a hypermutator phenotype, referring to combinations of multiple somatic and potentially germline mutations involved in DNA repair.[12] Next generation sequencing (NGS) has identified some overlap between WHO low-grade and high-grade gliomas in terms of genetic alterations, and the prognostic value of WHO grading in pediatric glioma potentially is diminished, in favor of molecular genetic characterization.[13–17] Two main subtypes of pHGG are marked by somatic *H3-3A* gene mutations.[18–20]

The H3G34R/V glioma subtype displays distinct characteristics that differentiate it from the better-characterized DMGs. H3G34R/V gliomas occur most typically in adolescent children and young adults, whereas DMG presents most commonly in early childhood. H3G34R/V gliomas typically are supratentorial and lobar in location, in contrast with the midline DMGs that occur in rhombencephalic and diencephalic structures. Concurrent *TP53* and *ATRX/DAXX* alterations are frequent in H3G34R/V gliomas and are thought to contribute to its CpG island promotor hypomethylated phenotype, whereas concurrent *TP53* mutations also accompany DMGs but without the same perturbations in chromatin remodeling, alternative lengthening of telomeres, or CpG island promotor methylation.[18–20]

Extent of resection is correlated directly to prognosis in pHGG[21]; however, as in adult glioblastoma, radiotherapy, with or without alkylating chemotherapy agents, remains the primary treatment modalities in pHGGs.[10,11,22] Advances in treatment have been few—none of the 68 clinical trials in DMG between 1984 and 2014 has conferred any survival benefits relative to radiation alone.[1,10,23] Chemotherapy agents commonly employed in young children to treat pHGG include vincristine, carboplatin, temozolomide, and thiotepa,[2,22] although evidence for survival benefit is scant. Therefore, pHGGs remain a devastating diagnosis with a poor overall prognosis, with an estimated 2-year survival of less than 20%.[10,12,24] DMGs in particular carry a median survival of less than 1 year.[4,10,11,22,25–27] The gain-of-function oncogenic p53 protein has a significant effect on 5-year progression-free survival in pHGG—44% with low mutant p53 expression compared with 17% with high p53 expression.[6,12] Specific to pHGG cases, other factors contributing to treatment challenges include a population of slow-cycling stem cells and new mutations gained on evolution toward recurrence.[28]

MOLECULAR LANDSCAPES WITH PROMISING THERAPIES
mTOR Pathway Inhibition for Subependymal Giant Cell Astrocytoma in Tuberous Sclerosis

Two germline disorders are associated strongly with the development of pLGGs. The intracranial manifestations of TS, including SEGAs, are thought to arise from germline *TSC1* or *TSC2* gene mutations, sometimes compounded by somatic Phosphoinositide 3-kinase/Protein kinase

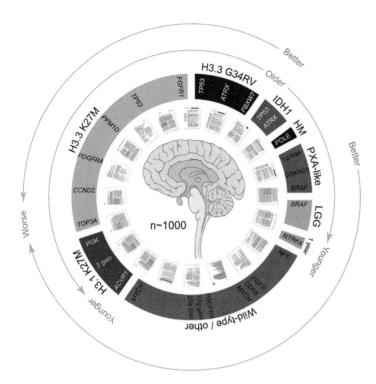

Fig. 1. Molecular patterns and clinical features of pediatric glioma subtypes It has become increasingly apparent that pHGG differ from their adult counterparts, with molecular profiling studies carried out over the last 6–7 years having incrementally identified key genetic and epigenetic differences in pHGG associated with distinct ages of onset, anatomical distribution, clinical outcome, and histopathological and radiological features. The outer ring represents relative frequencies of the pediatric gliomas with most common molecular genetic alterations associated with each subgroup. Subgroups are arranged and labelled by median age at presentation and overall survival prognosis. Original data from the German Cancer Research Center in Heidelberg aligned with published data from other studies. (*From* Mackay A, et. al. Pediatric High-Grade and Diffuse Intrinsic Pontine Glioma. Cancer Cell. 32(4):520-537.e5. https://doi.org/10.1016/j.ccell.2017.08.017; with permission.)

B/mTOR (PI3K/Akt/mTOR) pathway mutations (**Fig. 2**).[29] Patients with TS are at increased risk of developing SEGAs in early childhood, thought to result from loss of heterozygosity in the same chromosomal region containing the *TSC1* or *TSC2* mutation.

Despite the name, SEGAs should not be confused with astrocytomas. Rather, they are distinct entities with a unique molecular genetic pathogenesis and serve as a paragon for targeted molecular therapy. Everolimus, an mTOR inhibitor, and rapamycin have demonstrated seizure control benefit and reduction in tumor volume in TS patients with SEGAs (see **Fig. 2**).[1,3,30–32]

mTOR Pathway Inhibition for Low-Grade Glioma in NF1

Twenty percent of NF1 patients manifest hypothalamic/optic pathway pLGGs.[33] The *NF1* gene encodes neurofibromin, a Ras-Guanosine triphosphate (GTP)ase–activating protein that regulates Mitogen-activated protein kinase/ extracellular receptor kinase (MAPK/ERK) activity through Ras. When mutated, Ras regulation is disrupted, causing constitutive activation of both MAPK and PI3K pathways, thus leading to tumorigenesis (see **Fig. 2**).[34] Histologically, these tumors appear consistent with PAs; however, in NF1 patients, these hypothalamic/optic pathway PAs demonstrate a less aggressive

natural history than sporadic hypothalamic/optic pathway PAs.[35]

NF1-deficient malignant gliomas have shown initial responsiveness to mitogen-activated kinase kinase (MEK or MAP2K) inhibitors, such as selumetinib[36]; however, only a partial response has been observed in NF1-associated pLGGs.[37] Promising findings have been mentioned from preclinical studies with Akt-mediated or MEK-mediated mTOR inhibition.[38]

Targeting Mitogen-Activated Protein Kinase (MAPK) Signaling in BRAF-Mutant Glioma

MAPK signaling is known to affect cell proliferation, differentiation, migration, and cell death. Recently, 2 large, whole-genome sequencing studies identified genomic alterations in MAPK pathways to be the most common molecular characteristic in pLGGs.[5,39,40] Almost all PAs harbor a single-hit somatic mutation involving the MAPK signaling pathway without any additional mutations—a single-pathway disease.[41] *BRAF*, an early transducer in the MAPK pathway, is the most frequently mutated gene in PAs; 90% of cerebellar PAs and 50% of supratentorial PAs have a noted alteration in the *BRAF* gene.[5,42]

The most common point mutation in PAs is the *BRAF*[V600E] mutation, identified in 17% of pLGGs.[43] This mutation seems to demonstrate some

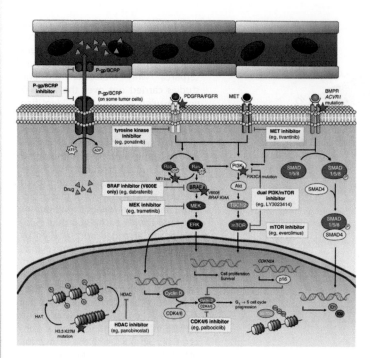

Fig. 2. Schematic of key pathways in pediatric glioma, including the frequent efflux of drugs from CNS tissue by efflux proteins, such as P-glycoprotein (P-gp) and breast cancer resistance protein. ACVR1, activin A receptor type 1; Akt, protein kinase B; BMPR, bone morphogenetic protein receptor; G1, gap 1 phase; HAT, histone acetyltransferase; ID1/2, inhibitor of DNA binding 1/2; MET, MET RTK; p16, cyclin-dependent kinase inhibitor 2A (protein); Ras, Ras family GTPase; S, synthesis phase; SETD2, SET domain containing 2; SMAD1/5/8, mothers against decapentaplegic homolog 1/5/8; SMAD4, mothers against decapentaplegic homolog 4. (*From* Miklja Z, Pasternak A, Stallard S, et al. Molecular profiling and targeted therapy in pediatric gliomas: review and consensus recommendations. *Neuro Oncol.* February 2019. https://doi.org/10.1093/neuonc/noz022 [81]; with permission. (Figure 1 in original).)

specificity to tumor location and is present in approximately 20% of extracerebellar PAs versus only 2% of posterior fossa PAs.[44] *BRAF*[V600] mutations are not limited to PAs, and are, in fact, more common among other forms of pLGG, although they are seen sparsely among low-grade gliomas in adults.[40] Certain pediatric tumors are far more likely to carry *BRAF* alterations; *BRAF*[V600] mutations have been found in an estimated 66% of PXAs,[44] 18% to 58% of GGs,[44–46] 30% of DNETs,[45] and 44% of desmoplastic infantile GGs/astrocytomas.[47]

PLGG patients harboring *BRAF*[V600] mutations are likely to have a worse prognosis than those with wild-type *BRAF*, particularly in the setting of a concurrent *CDKN2A* deletion.[43] Although common in adults, malignant transformation is rare in pLGG. Among secondary pHGG, a majority have been found to harbor this particular combination of genetic alterations.[48] *CDKN2A* deletion was identified in 25% of pLGGs with the *BRAF*[V600E] mutation, 60% of PXAs, and 16.7% of GGs.[43] The downstream effects include unopposed MAPK pathway activation and dysregulation of neuroglial cell proliferation via the mTOR pathway (see **Fig. 2**).[49]

Much clinical effort has focused on targeting *BRAF* mutations. Clinical trials of the first-generation BRAF inhibitor dabrafenib reported up to 44% responsiveness in pLGGs,[50] with subsequent studies echoing these results.[1,3,51] On the other hand, sorafenib, a multikinase inhibitor with impact on the activity of both wild-type BRAF and *BRAF*[V600E], caused rapid tumor progression

due to paradoxic ERK activation.[52] Unfortunately, most of these therapies have not been as effective against *BRAF*[V600E] tumors as with the *KIAA1549:BRAF* fusion tumors, and novel targeted drugs effective for both are required. Importantly, MAPK reactivation by Ras-independent activation of MEK and ERK or from EGFR signaling has resulted in eventual resistance to BRAF inhibitors.[53] Combinations of a BRAF inhibitor with MEK, EGFR, ERK, and EGFR inhibition are strategies that have begun testing in the clinical setting to prevent BRAF escape.

The second most common point mutation in supratentorial PAs involves *FGFR1* mutations.[39] These gene alterations appear to be common in gliomas of the nonastrocytic lineage, such as DNET and oligodendroglioma.[1,49,54] FGFR1 dysfunction triggers unregulated activation of both the PI3K and MAPK/ERK pathways.[1,49,54] Similarly, *ROS1* and anaplastic lymphoma kinase (ALK) fusions also result in constitutive activation of Ras/MAPK, PI3K, and Janus kinase (JAK)/ signal transducer and activator of transcription proteins (STAT) pathways.[42] These alterations are seen mostly in infants and younger children, for both pLGGs and pHGGs.[42]

Immunotherapy

A comprehensive review of immunomodulatory therapies for pHGGs is beyond the scope of this topic. Particular examples of molecular genetic targets of immunotherapy, however, serve to highlight the potential for future development. Chheda and colleagues demonstrated that cloned T-cell receptors could bind a presented antigen encompassing the H3K27M mutant peptide[55] and, in the corresponding peptide vaccine trial, identified a selective systemic expansion of H3K27M-reactive cytotoxic T lymphocytes in response to vaccination.[56]

EMERGING TARGETS AND THERAPIES UNDER INVESTIGATION

In developing targeted molecular therapies, 3 general approaches are common: (1) identification of patient populations who may benefit from existing targeted pharmaceuticals; (2) creating targeted therapies based on the molecular genetic profile of a particular patient population; and (3) individualizing treatment regimens to target molecular genetic findings specific to a patient's tumor.

Histone Alterations and Inhibitors of Histone Deacetylases

In pHGGs, mutations are estimated to involve histone modification or chromatin remodeling even more frequently than cell-cycle regulation and receptor tyrosine kinase (RTK)/Ras/PI3K signaling (see **Fig. 1**).[12] The H3K27M H3.3 (*H3-3A*) and H3.1 (*HIST1H3A/B/C*) are mutually exclusive events that result in loss of H3K27M trimethylation and hyperacetylation of the epigenome[10,24] and, ultimately, a variety of post-translational epigenetic alterations. H3.1K27M mutants tend to occur only in the brainstem and frequently are associated with *ACVR1* mutations (see **Fig. 1**). H3.3K27M mutants are found both in the pons or other midline intracranial locations, including the thalamus, and frequently co-occur with *TP53* and *FGFR1* mutations (see **Fig. 1**).[4,42]

One mechanism of oncogenesis appears to involve a shift of the downstream kinase to its active conformation and subsequent increased activity of bromodomain and extraterminal (BET) protein BRD4 which, in turn, activates an acetyltransferase, known as cyclic AMP response element–binding protein (CREB), and stimulates DMG super enhancer-driven oncogenes.[12,25]

The second described oncogenic mechanism is inhibition of 2 (PRC2) by sequestering enhancer of zeste homolog 2 (EZH2), thus interrupting histone H3 methylation and impacting downstream gene regulation.[1,26,57,58] The extent of PRC2 inhibition appears to depend on the concentration of H3K27M,[57] although PRC2 remains inhibited even after dissociation from chromatin.[57] This results in a significant decrease in global trimethylation of wild-type

H3K27 and ultimately in unregulated proliferation of DMG cells.[10,57,59] At the same time, unusually high acetylation occurs at certain repetitive elements in the chromatin, boosting gene expression and stimulating, among many other possible foci, MYC-driven immune evasion.[24]

Several drugs targeting these epigenetic changes have been proposed, specifically that alter histone trimethylation, acetylation, or phosphorylation. Various mechanisms have been explored, including inhibition of H327 demethylase and methyltransferase to target trimethylation, inhibition of histone deacetylase (HDAC) and BET to target acetylation, and inhibition of phosphatase-related enzymes to target phosphorylation.[60] A phase I clinical trial describes achieving in vivo inhibition of H3K27M-mutant gliomatosis with panobinostat, an HDAC inhibitor (see **Fig. 2**).[22,61] This class of drugs (including vorinostat, entinostat, and valproic acid) currently is part of multiple phase I clinical trials, as monotherapy and in combination with other drugs, and via various delivery modalities to address systemic toxicity.[1,11]

Additional epigenetic therapies in early stages of development include a histone H3K27 demethylase inhibitor, EZH2 inhibitors, and CBP or BET bromodomain inhibitors.[1,25] Gene editing studies using cell culture of pediatric gliomas also has revealed that both K27M and G34R mutations cause gliomagenesis by inducing genes in the NOTCH pathway, raising the possibility of gamma secretase inhibitor targets among these tumors.[62]

In contrast to H3K27M DMGs, H3G34R/V gliomas are even less understood, and mechanisms of oncogenicity remain largely unknown. Early studies identify N-MYC up-regulation, H3K36 hypomethylation, and dysregulated telomere lengthening.[1,10,13,54] H3G34 R/V tumors also often harbor ATRX/DAXX mutations, which encode proteins that form part of a chromatin-remodeling complex that is essential for histone H3.3 incorporation into telomeres and heterochromatin.[4,6,10,42]

Growth Factor Mutations and Kinase Inhibitors

The remaining pHGGs with wild-type *BRAF*, *IDH*, and *H3-3A* demonstrate significant intratumoral heterogeneity, implicating many potential oncogene drivers.[4,28] Pharmacologic ACVR1 inhibitors are being investigated as a potential DMG therapy (see **Fig. 2**).[63] The *ACVR1* gene encodes a bone morphogenic protein type I receptor and initially was identified as part of fibrodysplasia ossificans progressive syndrome, although it does not predispose to cancer in that disease.[64] The BMP pathway plays an important role in regulating differentiation and proliferation of astrocytic cells.[63] The mutation is found only in a minority of DMGs and likely is not an independent oncogenic driver.[10,12,64,65] The *ACVR1* mutation is associated with younger age, increased survival, and *HIST1H3B*, *PIK3CA*, and *PIK3R1* mutations (see **Fig. 1**).[12,13,64] The latter 2, along with mutations in growth factor receptor genes (ie, Platelet Derived Growth Factor Receptor Alpha (*PDGFRA*), *EGFR*, *FGFR*, and *ACVR1*), altered *PTEN* promoter methylation, and overexpression of *YB1*, all are known to act through amplification of cell proliferation via the RTK/Ras/PI3K pathway (see **Fig. 2**).[2,4,6,10,64]

Fusion Proteins and Other Potential Targets

The most common somatic alterations seen in infants appear to be gene fusion events. Many of the fusion genes involved in pHGGs appear to affect the MAPK pathway, and some are targetable by existing drugs. Among these, neurotrophic tyrosine kinase (*NTRK*)*1/2/3* fusion events appear to be extremely common,[12,39,40] as are *ALK*, *ROS1*, and mesenchymal epithelial transition factor (*MET*) gene fusions.[66] *RTK* gene fusions in infant gliomas of differing histologies have been reported.[67–76] Additionally, studies have found *MYBL1* amplification and/or rearrangement (41% of DAs) and *MYB-QKI* fusion (87% of angiocentric gliomas) to have a predilection for astrocytic pLGGs.[1,49,54] Alterations in the *MYB* gene lead to structural changes, possibly driving oncogenesis, although the mechanism is not fully understood.[13] Certain DAs exhibit concomitant *BRAF* alterations.

Mutations in transcription regulators, such as MYC amplification, have been described and lend themselves to a poor prognosis.[1,2,10,12] The *PPM1D* gene, often overexpressed in medulloblastoma, has been found to affect a gain-of-function in DMG that attenuates activity of p53 and DNA damage protein *CHK2*.[10,13,77,78] Other genes contributing to p53 function with mutation potential include *CHK2* and *ATM*.[13] *TP53* mutations are more common in DMG but also can occur in hemispheric pHGG (see **Fig. 1**).[64] Finally, 59% of pHGG carry mutations leading to cell-cycle dysregulation, including *TP53* and G1 checkpoint regulators (*CCND*1, *CCND*2, and *CCND*3; *CDK4*; and *CDK6*) (see **Fig. 2**).[2,12,64]

Second-generation ALK inhibitors (ceritinib, alectinib, brigatinib, and ensartinib) have exhibited favorable efficacy and safety profiles, with lorlatinib having the best intracranial activity.[2] Other ongoing clinical trials for pHGGs include TRK inhibitors (larotrectinib),[2,12,68] with promising results so far in mouse models without additional mutations required, and PDGFRA inhibitors (crenolanib and dasatinib), the latter also being investigated in combination with c-MET (a MET proto-oncogene) and ALK inhibitor crizotinib (see **Fig. 2**).[1,2,77,79] Increased sensitivity to palbociclib, a CDK4/6 inhibitor, was observed in H3K27M versus wild-type tumors.[80]

CLINICAL CHALLENGES AND FUTURE DIRECTIONS

- Low-grade gliomas in children pose the unique challenge of balancing the opportunity for long-term tumor control with protection from treatment-induced morbidity in the highly sensitive central nervous system.
- Higher-grade gliomas in children pose perhaps the greatest challenge in pediatric oncology today. Therapeutic options are limited due to toxicity and morbidity. Molecular heterogeneity and intrinsic mechanisms of treatment resistance result in universal recurrence. The relative scarcity of these tumors makes developing therapies difficult to assess through clinical trials.
- Molecular genetic profiling of pediatric gliomas has identified valuable prognostic information, has confounded previously held assertions regarding the biology of these entities, and has identified targeted therapy options.
- Radiotherapy generally should be avoided in patients younger than 3 years of age as well as in patients with genomic tumor predisposition, such as NF1, due to high risk of developmental delay, neurologic deficits, vision impairment, endocrine dysfunction, and radiation-induced malignancies.
- It is recommended to analyze each brain tumor sample for the presence of a BRAF alteration because there are promising therapies on the horizon against this oncogenic driver.

SUMMARY

The clinical impact of prior investigational therapy trials in pediatric glioma has been limited. The standard of care for many of these tumors remains unchanged over decades, with stagnant survival outcomes. Molecular genetic characterization of pediatric gliomas already, in a short amount of time, has revealed new potential therapeutic targets, many of which already are under investigation in clinical trials. Although understanding of the exact mechanisms linking genetic and epigenetic alterations in pediatric gliomas has only begun to scratch the surface, tremendous progress has been made in the past decade. Lessons learned from NGS efforts include the existence of significant intratumoral and intertumoral heterogeneity and the value of employing combined targeted therapies to simultaneously affect multiple prominent oncogenic pathways. Furthermore, transition to an integrated histopathologic-molecular genetic approach to pediatric glioma characterization is likely to alter the therapies offered to patients. Improved understanding of cellular mechanisms and gene expression regulation will guide investigatory efforts to identify the most effective, and least toxic, therapies for these devastating pathologies.

CLINICS CARE POINTS

- Low-grade gliomas in children pose the unique challenge of balancing the opportunity for long-term tumor control with protection from treatment-induced morbidity in the highly sensitive central nervous system.

- Molecular genetic profiling of pediatric gliomas has identified valuable prognostic information, has confounded previously held assertions regarding the biology of these entities, and has identified targeted therapy options.

- Higher-grade gliomas in children pose perhaps the greatest challenge in pediatric oncology today. Therapeutic options are limited due to toxicity and morbidity. Molecular heterogeneity and intrinsic mechanisms of treatment resistance result in universal recurrence. The relative scarcity of these tumors makes developing therapies difficult to assess through clinical trials.

- It is recommended to analyze each brain tumor sample for the presence of a BRAF alteration because there are promising therapies on the horizon against this oncogenic driver.

- Radiotherapy generally should be avoided in patients younger than 3 years of age as well as in patients with genomic tumor predisposition, such as NF1, due to high risk of developmental delay, neurologic deficits, vision impairment, endocrine dysfunction, and radiation-induced malignancies.

DISCLOSURE

The authors have no conflicts relevant to this manuscript to disclose. The authors of this article have no financial conflict of interest to disclose.

REFERENCES

1. Filbin MG, Sturm D. Gliomas in Children. Semin Neurol 2018;38(1):121–30.

2. Ceglie G, Vinci M, Carai A, et al. Infantile/Congenital High-Grade Gliomas: Molecular Features and Therapeutic Perspectives. Diagnostics (Basel) 2020; 10(9). https://doi.org/10.3390/diagnostics10090648.

3. Guerreiro Stucklin AS, Tabori U, Grotzer MA. The changing landscape of pediatric low-grade gliomas: clinical challenges and emerging therapies. Neuropediatrics 2016;47(2):70–83.

4. Firme MR, Marra MA. The molecular landscape of pediatric brain tumors in the next-generation sequencing era. Curr Neurol Neurosci Rep 2014;14(9):474.

5. Aichmüller CF, Iskar M, Jones DTW, et al. Pilocytic astrocytoma demethylation and transcriptional landscapes link bZIP transcription factors to immune response. Neuro Oncol 2020;22(9):1327–38.

6. Braunstein S, Raleigh D, Bindra R, et al. Pediatric high-grade glioma: current molecular landscape and therapeutic approaches. J Neurooncol 2017; 134(3):541–9.

7. Ryall S, Zapotocky M, Fukuoka K, et al. Integrated molecular and clinical analysis of 1,000 pediatric low-grade gliomas. Cancer Cell 2020;37(4): 569–83.e5.

8. Castel D, Kergrohen T, Tauziède-Espariat A, et al. Histone H3 wild-type DIPG/DMG overexpressing EZHIP extend the spectrum diffuse midline gliomas with PRC2 inhibition beyond H3-K27M mutation. Acta Neuropathol 2020;139(6):1109–13.

9. Castel D, Philippe C, Calmon R, et al. Histone H3F3A and HIST1H3B K27M mutations define two subgroups of diffuse intrinsic pontine gliomas with different prognosis and phenotypes. Acta Neuropathol 2015;130(6):815–27.

10. Buczkowicz P, Hawkins C. Pathology, Molecular Genetics, and Epigenetics of Diffuse Intrinsic Pontine Glioma. Front Oncol 2015;5:147.

11. Clymer J, Kieran MW. The integration of biology into the treatment of diffuse intrinsic pontine glioma: a review of the North American clinical trial perspective. Front Oncol 2018;8:169.

12. Wu G, Diaz AK, Paugh BS, et al. The genomic landscape of diffuse intrinsic pontine glioma and pediatric non-brainstem high-grade glioma. Nat Genet 2014;46(5):444–50.

13. Northcott PA, Pfister SM, Jones DTW. Next-generation (epi)genetic drivers of childhood brain tumours and the outlook for targeted therapies. Lancet Oncol 2015;16(6):e293–302.

14. Varlet P, Le Teuff G, Le Deley M-C, et al. WHO grade has no prognostic value in the pediatric high-grade glioma included in the HERBY trial. Neuro Oncol 2020;22(1):116–27.

15. Capper D, Jones DTW, Sill M, et al. DNA methylation-based classification of central nervous system tumours. Nature 2018;555(7697):469–74.

16. Mackay A, Burford A, Carvalho D, et al. Integrated molecular meta-analysis of 1,000 pediatric high-

grade and diffuse intrinsic pontine glioma. Cancer Cell 2017;32(4):520–37.e5.

17. Masui K, Mischel PS, Reifenberger G. Chapter 6 - Molecular classification of gliomas. In: Berger MS, Weller M, editors. Handbook of clinical neurology, vol. 134. Gliomas. Elsevier; 2016. p. 97–120.

18. Schwartzentruber J, Korshunov A, Liu X-Y, et al. Driver mutations in histone H3.3 and chromatin re-modelling genes in paediatric glioblastoma. Nature 2012;482(7384):226–31.

19. Sturm D, Witt H, Hovestadt V, et al. Hotspot mutations in H3F3A and IDH1 define distinct epigenetic and biological subgroups of glioblastoma. Cancer Cell 2012;22(4):425–37.

20. Wu G, Broniscer A, McEachron TA, et al. Somatic histone H3 alterations in pediatric diffuse intrinsic pontine gliomas and non-brainstem glioblastomas. Nat Genet 2012;44(3):251–3.

21. McGirt MJ, Chaichana KL, Gathinji M, et al. Independent association of extent of resection with survival in patients with malignant brain astrocytoma. J Neurosurg 2009;110(1):156–62.

22. Aziz-Bose R, Monje M. Diffuse intrinsic pontine glioma: molecular landscape and emerging therapeutic targets. Curr Opin Oncol 2019;31(6):522–30.

23. Rechberger JS, Lu VM, Zhang L, et al. Clinical trials for diffuse intrinsic pontine glioma: the current state of affairs. Childs Nerv Syst 2020;36(1):39–46.

24. Krug B, De Jay N, Harutyunyan AS, et al. Pervasive H3K27 Acetylation Leads to ERV Expression and a Therapeutic Vulnerability in H3K27M Gliomas. Cancer Cell 2019;35(5):782–97.e8.

25. Wiese M, Hamdan FH, Kubiak K, et al. Combined treatment with CBP and BET inhibitors reverses inadvertent activation of detrimental super enhancer programs in DIPG cells. Cell Death Dis 2020;11(8):673.

26. Ren M, van Nocker S. In silico analysis of histone H3 gene expression during human brain development. Int J Dev Biol 2016;60(4–6):167–73.

27. Castel D, Philippe C, Kergrohen T, et al. Transcriptomic and epigenetic profiling of "diffuse midline gliomas, H3 K27M-mutant" discriminate two subgroups based on the type of histone H3 mutated and not supratentorial or infratentorial location. Acta Neuropathol Commun 2018;6(1):117.

28. Hoffman M, Gillmor AH, Kunz DJ, et al. Intratumoral genetic and functional heterogeneity in pediatric glioblastoma. Cancer Res 2019;79(9):2111–23.

29. Martin KR, Zhou W, Bowman MJ, et al. The genomic landscape of tuberous sclerosis complex. Nat Commun 2017;8:15816.

30. Franz DN, Belousova E, Sparagana S, et al. Efficacy and safety of everolimus for subependymal giant cell astrocytomas associated with tuberous sclerosis complex (EXIST-1): a multicentre, randomised, placebo-controlled phase 3 trial. Lancet 2013; 381(9861):125–32.

31. French JA, Lawson JA, Yapici Z, et al. Adjunctive everolimus therapy for treatment-resistant focal-onset seizures associated with tuberous sclerosis (EXIST-3): a phase 3, randomised, double-blind, placebo-controlled study. Lancet 2016;388(10056): 2153–63.

32. Krueger DA, Care MM, Holland K, et al. Everolimus for subependymal giant-cell astrocytomas in tuberous sclerosis. N Engl J Med 2010;363(19):1801–11.

33. Sturm D, Pfister SM, Jones DTW. Pediatric Gliomas: Current Concepts on Diagnosis, Biology, and Clinical Management. J Clin Oncol 2017;35(21):2370–7.

34. Ricker CA, Pan Y, Gutmann DH, et al. Challenges in Drug Discovery for Neurofibromatosis Type 1-Associated Low-Grade Glioma. Front Oncol 2016;6:259.

35. Laithier V, Grill J, Le Deley M-C, et al. Progression-free survival in children with optic pathway tumors: dependence on age and the quality of the response to chemotherapy–results of the first French prospective study for the French Society of Pediatric Oncology. J Clin Oncol 2003;21(24):4572–8.

36. Banerjee A, Jakacki RI, Onar-Thomas A, et al. A phase I trial of the MEK inhibitor selumetinib (AZD6244) in pediatric patients with recurrent or refractory low-grade glioma: a Pediatric Brain Tumor Consortium (PBTC) study. Neuro Oncol 2017;19(8): 1135–44.

37. Fangusaro JR, Onar-Thomas A, Young-Poussaint T, et al. A phase II prospective study of selumetinib in children with recurrent or refractory low-grade glioma (LGG): A Pediatric Brain Tumor Consortium (PBTC) study. J Clin Oncol 2017;35(15_suppl):10504.

38. Kaul A, Toonen JA, Cimino PJ, et al. Akt- or MEK-mediated mTOR inhibition suppresses Nf1 optic glioma growth. Neuro Oncol 2015;17(6):843–53.

39. Jones DTW, Hutter B, Jäger N, et al. Recurrent somatic alterations of FGFR1 and NTRK2 in pilocytic astrocytoma. Nat Genet 2013;45(8):927–32.

40. Zhang J, Wu G, Miller CP, et al. Whole-genome sequencing identifies genetic alterations in pediatric low-grade gliomas. Nat Genet 2013;45(6):602–12.

41. Jones DTW, Kocialkowski S, Liu L, et al. Tandem duplication producing a novel oncogenic BRAF fusion gene defines the majority of pilocytic astrocytomas. Cancer Res 2008;68(21):8673–7.

42. Guerreiro Stucklin AS, Ramaswamy V, Daniels C, et al. Review of molecular classification and treatment implications of pediatric brain tumors. Curr Opin Pediatr 2018;30(1):3–9.

43. Lassaletta A, Zapotocky M, Mistry M, et al. Therapeutic and Prognostic Implications of BRAF V600E in Pediatric Low-Grade Gliomas. J Clin Oncol 2017;35(25):2934–41.

44. Schindler G, Capper D, Meyer J, et al. Analysis of BRAF V600E mutation in 1,320 nervous system tumors reveals high mutation frequencies in pleomorphic xanthoastrocytoma, ganglioglioma and extra-

cerebellar pilocytic astrocytoma. Acta Neuropathol 2011;121(3):397–405.

45. Prabowo AS, Iyer AM, Veersema TJ, et al. BRAF V600E mutation is associated with mTOR signaling activation in glioneuronal tumors. Brain Pathol 2014;24(1):52–66.

46. Koelsche C, Wöhrer A, Jeibmann A, et al. Mutant BRAF V600E protein in ganglioglioma is predominantly expressed by neuronal tumor cells. Acta Neuropathol 2013;125(6):891–900.

47. Wang AC, Jones DTW, Abecassis IJ, et al. Desmoplastic Infantile Ganglioglioma/Astrocytoma (DIG/DIA) Are Distinct Entities with Frequent BRAFV600 Mutations. Mol Cancer Res 2018;16(10):1491–8.

48. Mistry M, Zhukova N, Merico D, et al. BRAF mutation and CDKN2A deletion define a clinically distinct subgroup of childhood secondary high-grade glioma. J Clin Oncol 2015;33(9):1015–22.

49. Tateishi K, Nakamura T, Yamamoto T. Molecular genetics and therapeutic targets of pediatric low-grade gliomas. Brain Tumor Pathol 2019;36(2):74–83.

50. Hargrave DR, Bouffet E, Tabori U, et al. Efficacy and Safety of Dabrafenib in Pediatric Patients with BRAF V600 Mutation-Positive Relapsed or Refractory Low-Grade Glioma: Results from a Phase I/IIa Study. Clin Cancer Res 2019;25(24):7303–11.

51. Dabrafenib Effective in Pediatric Glioma. Cancer Discov 2017;7(1):OF5.

52. Karajannis MA, Legault G, Fisher MJ, et al. Phase II study of sorafenib in children with recurrent or progressive low-grade astrocytomas. Neuro Oncol 2014;16(10):1408–16.

53. Solit DB, Rosen N. Resistance to BRAF inhibition in melanomas. N Engl J Med 2011;364(8):772–4.

54. Suvà ML, Louis DN. Next-generation molecular genetics of brain tumours. Curr Opin Neurol 2013;26(6):681–7.

55. Chheda ZS, Kohanbash G, Okada K, et al. Novel and shared neoantigen derived from histone 3 variant H3.3K27M mutation for glioma T cell therapy. J Exp Med 2018;215(1):141–57.

56. Mueller S, Taitt JM, Villanueva-Meyer JE, et al. Mass cytometry detects H3.3K27M-specific vaccine responses in diffuse midline glioma. J Clin Invest 2020. https://doi.org/10.1172/JCI140378.

57. Stafford JM, Lee C-H, Voigt P, et al. Multiple modes of PRC2 inhibition elicit global chromatin alterations in H3K27M pediatric glioma. Sci Adv 2018;4(10):eaau5935.

58. Lewis PW, Müller MM, Koletsky MS, et al. Inhibition of PRC2 activity by a gain-of-function H3 mutation found in pediatric glioblastoma. Science 2013;340(6134):857–61.

59. Fang D, Gan H, Cheng L, et al. H3.3K27M mutant proteins reprogram epigenome by sequestering the PRC2 complex to poised enhancers. Elife 2018;7.

60. Piunti A, Hashizume R, Morgan MA, et al. Therapeutic targeting of polycomb and BET bromodomain proteins in diffuse intrinsic pontine gliomas. Nat Med 2017;23(4):493–500.

61. Grasso CS, Tang Y, Truffaux N, et al. Functionally defined therapeutic targets in diffuse intrinsic pontine glioma. Nat Med 2015;21(6):555–9.

62. Chen K-Y, Bush K, Klein RH, et al. Reciprocal H3.3 gene editing identifies K27M and G34R mechanisms in pediatric glioma including NOTCH signaling. Commun Biol 2020;3(1):1–15.

63. Yu PB, Deng DY, Lai CS, et al. BMP type I receptor inhibition reduces heterotopic [corrected] ossification. Nat Med 2008;14(12):1363–9.

64. Diaz AK, Baker SJ. The genetic signatures of pediatric high-grade glioma: no longer a one-act play. Semin Radiat Oncol 2014;24(4):240–7.

65. Buczkowicz P, Hoeman C, Rakopoulos P, et al. Genomic analysis of diffuse intrinsic pontine gliomas identifies three molecular subgroups and recurrent activating ACVR1 mutations. Nat Genet 2014;46(5):451–6.

66. Clarke M, Mackay A, Ismer B, et al. Infant High-Grade Gliomas Comprise Multiple Subgroups Characterized by Novel Targetable Gene Fusions and Favorable Outcomes. Cancer Discov 2020;10(7):942–63.

67. Guerreiro Stucklin AS, Ryall S, Fukuoka K, et al. Alterations in ALK/ROS1/NTRK/MET drive a group of infantile hemispheric gliomas. Nat Commun 2019;10(1):4343.

68. Ziegler DS, Wong M, Mayoh C, et al. Brief Report: Potent clinical and radiological response to larotrectinib in TRK fusion-driven high-grade glioma. Br J Cancer 2018;119(6):693–6.

69. Olsen TK, Panagopoulos I, Meling TR, et al. Fusion genes with ALK as recurrent partner in ependymoma-like gliomas: a new brain tumor entity? Neuro Oncol 2015;17(10):1365–73.

70. Ng A, Levy ML, Malicki DM, et al. Unusual high-grade and low-grade glioma in an infant with PPP1CB-ALK gene fusion. BMJ Case Rep 2019;12(2). https://doi.org/10.1136/bcr-2018-228248.

71. Nakano Y, Tomiyama A, Kohno T, et al. Identification of a novel KLC1-ROS1 fusion in a case of pediatric low-grade localized glioma. Brain Tumor Pathol 2019;36(1):14–9.

72. Maruggi M, Malicki DM, Levy ML, et al. A novel KIF5B-ALK fusion in a child with an atypical central nervous system inflammatory myofibroblastic tumour. BMJ Case Rep 2018;2018. https://doi.org/10.1136/bcr-2018-226431.

73. Kiehna EN, Arnush MR, Tamrazi B, et al. Novel GOPC(FIG)-ROS1 fusion in a pediatric high-grade glioma survivor. J Neurosurg Pediatr 2017;20(1):51–5.

74. Chmielecki J, Bailey M, He J, et al. Genomic Profiling of a Large Set of Diverse Pediatric Cancers

Identifies Known and Novel Mutations across Tumor Spectra. Cancer Res 2017;77(2):509–19.

75. Coccé MC, Mardin BR, Bens S, et al. Identification of ZCCHC8 as fusion partner of ROS1 in a case of congenital glioblastoma multiforme with a t(6;12)(q21;q24.3). Genes Chromosomes Cancer 2016;55(9):677–87.

76. Aghajan Y, Levy ML, Malicki DM, et al. Novel PPP1CB-ALK fusion protein in a high-grade glioma of infancy. BMJ Case Rep 2016;2016.

77. El Ayoubi R, Boisselier B, Rousseau A. Molecular landscape of pediatric diffuse intrinsic pontine gliomas: about 22 cases. J Neurooncol 2017;134(2):465–7.

78. Fons NR, Sundaram RK, Breuer GA, et al. PPM1D mutations silence NAPRT gene expression and confer NAMPT inhibitor sensitivity in glioma. Nat Commun 2019;10(1):3790.

79. Ensan D, Smil D, Zepeda-Velázquez CA, et al. Targeting ALK2: an open science approach to developing therapeutics for the treatment of diffuse intrinsic pontine glioma. J Med Chem 2020;63(9):4978–96.

80. Cordero FJ, Huang Z, Grenier C, et al. Histone H3.3K27M Represses p16 to Accelerate Gliomagenesis in a Murine Model of DIPG. Mol Cancer Res 2017;15(9):1243–54.

81. Miklja Z, Pasternak A, Stallard S, et al. Molecular profiling and targeted therapy in pediatric gliomas: review and consensus recommendations. Neuro Oncol 2019. https://doi.org/10.1093/neuonc/noz022.

Clinical Trials

Molecularly Targeted Clinical Trials

Matthew A. Smith-Cohn, DO[a,b], Orieta Celiku, PhD[c], Mark R. Gilbert, MD[d,*]

KEYWORDS

- Glioblastoma • Heterogenicity • Targeted therapy • Blood-brain barrier • Synthetic lethality

KEY POINTS

- Glioblastomas are incurable malignant central nervous system cancers with an unmet need for new therapies.
- Intratumoral heterogenicity and redundancy of growth pathways make targeting individual pathways ineffective for most patients.
- The blood-brain barrier presents a challenge for drug delivery.
- Molecularly targeted clinical trial design requires robust biomarkers.
- Molecularly targeted therapies and synthetic lethality may benefit a subset of glioblastoma patients.

INTRODUCTION

Glioblastoma (GBM) is the most common primary brain tumor in adults, with approximately 12,000 new cases diagnosed each year in the United States.[1] The prognosis for patients with GBM remains dismal, with a median survival with surgery, chemotherapy, and radiation in patients eligible for clinical trials of only 15 months to 22 months.[2,3] Data from population-based registries report a median survival of fewer than 12 months if all patients are included.[4] Despite extensive research, there have not been significant advances in the past 30 years except for temozolomide with radiation therapy.[5,6]

The 2016 World Health Organization guideline update of central nervous system tumors led to recognizing molecular profiling of brain tumors as best practice.[2] Aside from improved clarity of diagnosis, molecular profiling of tumors can identify gene or gene product alterations potentially amenable to targeted therapy. In contrast to traditional chemotherapies, which broadly affect cells in the body, targeted therapies interfere with specific molecular changes unique to the cancer cells. Targeted therapies have shown efficacy in various cancers, including lymphoma, breast, colon, and lung, but have demonstrated success in only a small subset of primary brain tumor patients.[7–10] Because targeting a single mutation does not work for most malignant gliomas, exploiting a larger genomic context may be more effective. Synthetic lethality, or cell death resulting from simultaneous disabling of 2 genes, may be exploited to expand the therapeutic options of glioma patients. First observed by Bridges[11] in the early twentieth century when crossing fruit flies with certain nonallelic genes,[12] this approach as anticancer therapy is exemplified by the use of poly (adenosine diphosphate–ribose) polymerase (PARP) inhibitors in breast cancer patients with germline mutations in BRCA1 and BRCA2.[13,14] Successful utilization of synthetic lethality in GBM will depend on the ability to predict robust synthetic lethal relationships. This article discusses the successes and challenges of targeted

[a] Neuro-Oncology Branch, National Cancer Institute, National Institutes of Health, 37 Convent Drive, Building 37, Room 1016, Bethesda, MD 20892, USA; [b] Department of Neurology, The Johns Hopkins University School of Medicine, Baltimore, MD 21287, USA; [c] Neuro-Oncology Branch, National Cancer Institute, National Institutes of Health, 37 Convent Drive, Building 37, Room 1142, Bethesda, MD 20892, USA; [d] Neuro-Oncology Branch, National Cancer Institute, National Institutes of Health, Bethesda, MD 20892, USA
* Corresponding author. National Cancer Institute, National Institutes of Health, 9030 Old Georgetown Road, Bloch Building 82, Bethesda, MD 20814.
E-mail address: Mark.Gilbert@nih.gov

Neurosurg Clin N Am 32 (2021) 191–210
https://doi.org/10.1016/j.nec.2020.12.002
1042-3680/21/Published by Elsevier Inc.

therapy in brain tumors and reviews synthetic lethality as an attractive new approach to treating brain tumors.

DISCUSSION

The Food and Drug Administration (FDA) approval of tamoxifen in the 1970s for estrogen receptor–positive breast cancer signaled the start of personalized, targeted cancer medicine. Subsequent decades of research led to the discoveries of a diverse arsenal of new therapies with clinical benefits in various cancers, notably imatinib for Philadelphia chromosome–positive chronic myeloid leukemia.[15,16] Despite the success of molecularly targeted therapies in other cancers, however, these approaches have not demonstrated much success in GBM. This failure has been attributed to a variety of factors, including intratumoral genetic and transcriptional heterogeneity, redundant activating pathways or escape mechanisms, and delivery of a drug to therapeutic levels within tumor tissue through the blood-brain barrier (BBB).[9,10] Recent advances in molecular testing and tumor profiling, however, have led to a resurgence of interest in targeted therapy with the increasing recognition of more robust and potentially actionable alterations.

Molecular Classification and Potentially Actionable Alterations in Glioblastoma

Genomic, transcriptomic, epigenomic, and proteomic analysis of GBM has revealed distinct molecular subtypes with different clinical behaviors and therapeutic implications.[17] Work by The Cancer Genome Atlas (TCGA) classified GBM into 3 subtypes: classical, associated with EGFR amplification and CDKN2A deletion; mesenchymal, distinguished by NF1 deletions, elevated endothelial markers (cluster of differentiation 31 (CD31), vascular endothelial growth factor receptor-2 (VEGFR-2)), increased mitogen-activated protein kinase (MAPK) pathway activations, and decreased levels of mechanistic target of rapamycin (mTOR); and proneural, associated with PDGFRA amplification, IDH1 mutation, and proneural development gene expression. A fourth, neural subtype, later was attributed to neural tissue at the margin of the tumor.[18,19]

Other significant genomic alterations identified by TCGA include mutations in PIK3CA, PTEN, RB1, and TP53; genomic gains and losses involving MET, CDK6, CDK4, MDM2, and CDKN2A/CDKN2B codeletion; and oncogenic gene fusions, including fibroblast growth factor receptor 1 (FGFR1)-transforming acidic coiled coil 1 (TACC1), FGFR3-TACC3, Epidermal growth factor receptor (EGFR)-Septin 14 (SEPT14), and neurotrophic tropomyosin receptor kinase (NTRK).[19–21] More recently, methylation profiling of an extensive series of GBMs has identified the Receptor tyrosine kinase (RTK1)-type corresponding to the proneural subgroup, RTK2-type, comprising classical and mesenchymal GBM and GBM with Histone Family 3A (H3F3A) alterations as a unique subset.[22] Proteomic investigations of GBM found 2 subclasses with exclusive mutations. Proteomic cluster 1 (GPC1) exclusively had mutations in EGFRvIII and PIK3CA, whereas the second group, GPC2, was characterized by mutations in TP53, NF1, PTEN, RB1, and EGFR without the vIII gene fusion variant.[17] More recently, grade 4 gliomas are segregated by their Isocitrate dehydrogenase (IDH) (IDH1/IDH2) mutation status: tumors with wild-type IDH retain the designation of GBM, whereas tumors with IDH mutation now are labeled as grade 4 IDH-mutated astrocytoma.

Drawing from the molecular insights and successes of targeted therapies of other cancers, attempts have been made to extrapolate these successes to GBM, albeit with limited success for most patients.

Signals of Efficacy in Biomarker-Driven Therapy in Glioblastoma

Biomarkers are biological molecules indicative of a physiologic state and may include DNA, RNA, protein, or extracellular vesicles.[23] Biomarkers in oncology fall in a spectrum of prognostic (or indicative of a patient's overall outcome) versus predictive (or informative of the expected response to therapeutic intervention).[24] Some biomarkers have both attributes; for example, in breast cancer, HER2 amplification is both prognostic of a poor prognosis due to a more aggressive course without targeted therapy and predictive of therapeutic efficacy with HER2 targeting treatments, such as trastuzumab.[25] Similarly, IDH mutations are a prognostic marker of better survival for glioma patients and may be predictive of response to IDH and PARP inhibitors.[2,10,26,27] Some biomarkers are predictive of a lack of targeted therapy, as exemplified by a lack of efficacy of EGFR inhibitors targeting non–small cell lung cancers with concurrent mutation of EGFR and K-ras mutations, and lack of efficacy of BRAF inhibitors in mutant colon cancers and GBM with concurrent EGFR and BRAF mutations.[24,28] An established and regularly utilized molecular biomarker in GBM is methylguanine methyltransferase (MGMT) promotor methylation status. When this DNA repair gene is inactive through methylation of the gene promoter (which occurs in approximately 30% of GBMs), it is predictive of therapeutic efficacy of alkylating chemotherapy in IDH wild-type gliomas and possibly is prognostic of better survival or at least predictive of the benefit of radiation therapy without chemotherapy.[3,29,30] As discussed previously, robust complementary biomarkers are a necessity for successful targeted treatment and design of clinic trials.[23]

Relative to other cancers, biomarker-driven therapies in GBM are less established and have been mainly unsuccessful. Despite recent setbacks, targeted treatment of driver mutations and gene fusions in GBM has produced clinical benefit in rare subsets of patients exemplified in case reports and basket trials. Many clinical trials with active targeted therapy are under way for GBM patients (**Table 1**).

Most reports of the benefit of targeted therapy in GBM patients have been in driver mutations. BRAF mutations have been demonstrated to be a viable therapeutic target in a variety of cancers, including primary brain tumors through inhibition of BRAF and MEK, which is downstream in this kinase pathway.[31] A basket trial using trametinib, a MEK inhibitor, included 5 patients with anaplastic astrocytoma and 6 with GBM. One patient had a partial response, and 5 patients had stable disease, with 2 of the patients having disease stabilization that lasted more than 1 year.[4] Currently, a majority of reported cases of adult brain tumor patients with BRAF alterations are heavily pretreated, may have other current tumor-directed treatments, and had mixed use of different combinations of MEK and BRAF inhibitors making the results difficult to interpret.[28] A trial is under way evaluating the use of the MEK inhibitor binimetinib and BRAF inhibitor encorafenib in adults with recurrent BRAFV600E mutant GBM (NCT03973918). The IDH inhibitor ivosidenib has shown prolonged disease control in grade 2 and grade 3 IDH-mutant astrocytomas, but it is unknown if there is a benefit with grade 4 IDH-mutant astrocytomas.[27,32] Neurofibromatosis type 1–associated GBMs are uncommon and typically arise from lower-grade gliomas. A clinical benefit with MEK inhibitors was observed based on case report experiences.[33,34] Targeting of TSC2 mutation with the MTOR inhibitor everolimus in a GBM patient with Li-Fraumeni syndrome also showed a therapeutic response.[35] Gliosarcoma, a subtype of mesenchymal GBM with platelet-derived growth factor receptor (PDGFR) and KIT/SCF autocrine activation loops, has an ongoing phase II trial using sunitinib that targets these pathways (NCT03641326).

Although gene fusions occur in 30% to 50% of GBMs, only a select few have been associated with oncogenic biologic function.[36] Neurotrophic-tropomyosin receptor kinase (NTRK) fusions in adults with GBM are rare, but, similarly to other cancers with this alteration, have demonstrated a treatment response in case reports, including 45% volume reduction using entrectinib in a pontine astrocytoma patient harboring BCAN-NTRK1 fusion, and a partial response of subclonal periventricular lesion from 67 mm × 52 mm to 8 mm × 4 mm using larotrectinib in an adult with recurrent multifocal GBM with an EML4-NTRK3 fusion for 1 month.[37,38] Several basket trials are exploring NTRK inhibitors.[39] A pediatric patient with GBM harboring a Receptor-type tyrosine-protein phosphatase zeta-MET proto-oncogene (PTPRZ1-MET) fusion and treated with crizotinib had a partial response. An ongoing trial (NCT02978261) is evaluating the c-Met Inhibitor PLB1001 in patients with PTPRZ1-MET fusion recurrent high-grade gliomas. The targeting of FGFR-TACC fusions also has been explored. A phase 1 trial using the pan-fibroblast growth factor receptor (FGFR) tyrosine kinase inhibitor JNJ-42756493 reported a partial response in 2 GBM patients with FGFR3-TACC3 fusion.[40] There are currently are ongoing trials in recurrent glioma with FGFR3-TACC3 fusions (NCT01975701, NCT02824133).

A majority of targeted therapy studies in GBM have been derived from successes in systemic cancer. Even among systemic cancers, however, there is heterogenicity of responses of the same drug to the same mutation, which is not surprising given the heterogeneity in the genetic and epigenetic background in which these mutations occur.[10,41] Concomitant mutations can prevent therapeutic efficacy through the activation of alternative proliferation pathways. For example, EGFR mutations with concurrent EML4-ALK fusions or NRAS alterations lead to EGFR tyrosine kinase inhibitor resistance in non–small lung cancer. Similarly, targeted inhibition of BRAFV600E yields a response rate in 80% of melanoma versus 5% of colon cancers. It is hypothesized that this results from much higher expression in of EGFR in colon cancers, which results in adaptive feedback reactivation of MAPK signaling, leading to activation of other RAF kinases and subsequent resistance.[28]

Challenges to Success of Molecularly Targeted Therapy in Glioblastoma

Throughout the spectrum of cancer, the number of patients eligible for targeted therapy is relatively low, with the number of patients who benefit from targeted therapy even lower. A cross-

Table 1
Active glioblastoma trials using molecularly targeting agents

NCT Number	Drugs	Targets	Title	Phases
NCT02761070	Temozolomide, bevacizumab	VEGFA	Bevacizumab Alone vs Dose-dense Temozolomide Followed by Bevacizumab for Recurrent Glioblastoma, phase III	Phase 3
NCT02678975	Disulfiram, alkylating agents	ALDH2, DBH	Disulfiram in Recurrent Glioblastoma	Phase 2, Phase 3
NCT02573324	Temozolomide, ABT-414, placebo for ABT-414	EGFR	A Study of ABT-414 in Subjects with newly diagnosed Glioblastoma GBM With Epidermal Growth Factor Receptor (EGFR) Amplification	Phase 2, Phase 3
NCT02152982	Temozolomide, veliparib	PARP1, PARP2	Temozolomide With or Without Veliparib in Treating Patients With Newly Diagnosed Glioblastoma Multiforme	Phase 2, Phase 3
NCT03025893	Sunitinib, lomustine	PDGFRB, FLT4, KDR, FLT3, KIT, FLT1, CSF1R, PDGFRA, STMN4	A Phase II/III Study of High-Dose, Intermittent Sunitinib in Patients With Recurrent Glioblastoma Multiforme	Phase 2, Phase 3
NCT03970447	Temozolomide, lomustine, regorafenib	STMN4, FGFR2, PDGFRB, ABL1, BRAF, RAF1, FLT4, KDR, KIT, FGFR1, RET, FLT1, NTRK1, PDGFRA, EPHA2, TEK, DDR2, MAPK11, FRK	A Trial to Evaluate Multiple Regimens in Newly Diagnosed and Recurrent Glioblastoma	Phase 2, Phase 3
NCT02525692	ONC201	DRD2, AKT1, MAPK1	Oral ONC201 in Recurrent GBM, H3 K27M glioma, and Midline Glioma	Phase 2
NCT03363659	Disulfiram, temozolomide	ALDH2, DBH	Disulfiram and Copper Gluconate With Temozolomide in Unmethylated Glioblastoma Multiforme	Phase 2
NCT03973918	Encorafenib, binimetinib	BRAF V600, MAP2K1, MAP2K2	Study of Binimetinib With Encorafenib in Adults With Recurrent BRAF V600-Mutated HGG	Phase 2

NCT Number	Intervention	Targets	Title	Phase
NCT03919071	Dabrafenib mesylate, trametinib dimethyl sulfoxide	BRAF, MAP2K1, MAP2K2, MAPK1	Dabrafenib Combined With Trametinib After Radiation Therapy in Treating Patients With Newly-Diagnosed High-Grade Glioma	Phase 2
NCT02981940	Abemaciclib	CDK4, CDK6	A Study of Abemaciclib in Recurrent Glioblastoma	Phase 2
NCT03746080	Plerixafor, temozolomide	CXCR4	Whole Brain Radiation Therapy With Standard Temozolomide Chemo-Radiotherapy and Plerixafor in Treating Patients With Glioblastoma	Phase 2
NCT03600467	SEVI-D (seviteronel in combination with dexamethasone)	CYP17A1	Activity of Seviteronel in Patients With Androgen Receptor (AR)-Positive Glioblastoma	Phase 2
NCT03618667	GC1118	EGFR	GC1118 in Recurrent Glioblastoma Patients With High EGFR Amplification	Phase 2
NCT02844439	Tesevatinib	EGFR, ERBB1, HER2, ERBB2, VEGFR, EPHB4	Study of Tesevatinib Monotherapy in Patients With Recurrent Glioblastoma	Phase 2
NCT03216499	HIF-2α inhibitor PT2385	EPAS1	HIF-2 Alpha Inhibitor PT2385 in Treating Patients With Recurrent Glioblastoma	Phase 2
NCT04051606	Regorafenib	FGFR2, PDGFRB, ABL1, BRAF, RAF1, FLT4, KDR, KIT, FGFR1, RET, FLT1, NTRK1, PDGFRA, EPHA2, TEK, DDR2, MAPK11, FRK	Regorafenib in Bevacizumab Refractory Recurrent Glioblastoma	Phase 2
NCT02926222	Regorafenib, lomustine	FGFR2, PDGFRB, ABL1, BRAF, RAF1, FLT4, KDR, KIT, FGFR1, RET, FLT1, NTRK1, PDGFRA, EPHA2, TEK, DDR2, MAPK11, FRK, STMN4	Regorafenib in Relapsed Glioblastoma	Phase 2
NCT02137759	Standard temozolomide, belinostat	HDAC1, HDAC2, HDAC3, HDAC6	MRSI to Predict Response to RT/TMZ + Belinostat in GBM	Phase 2
NCT02977780	Temozolomide, neratinib, CC-115, anemaciclib	HER2, ERBB2, EGFR, MTOR, CKD4, CDK6	INdividualized Screening Trial of Innovative Glioblastoma Therapy (INSIGhT)	Phase 2

(continued on next page)

Table 1
(continued)

NCT Number	Drugs	Targets	Title	Phases
NCT02885324	Cabozantinib	KDR, RET, MET	Pilot Study of Cabozantinib for Recurrent or Progressive High-Grade Glioma in Children	Phase 2
NCT03581292	Temozolomide, veliparib	PARP1, PARP2	Veliparib, Radiation Therapy, and Temozolomide in Treating Patients With Newly Diagnosed Malignant Glioma Without H3 K27 M or BRAFV600 Mutations	Phase 2
NCT03212274	Olaparib	PARP1, PARP2, PARP3	Olaparib in Treating Patients With Advanced Glioma, Cholangiocarcinoma, or Solid Tumors With IDH1 or IDH2 Mutations	Phase 2
NCT03661723	Pembrolizumab, bevacizumab	PDCD1, VEGFA	Pembrolizumab and Reirradiation in Bevacizumab Naive and Bevacizumab Resistant Recurrent Glioblastoma	Phase 2
NCT02626364	Crenolanib	PDGFRA, PDGFRB, FLT3	Study of Crenolanib in Recurrent/Refractory Glioblastoma With PDGFRA Gene Amplification	Phase 2
NCT01817751	Sorafenib tosylate, valproic acid, sildenafil citrate	PDGFRB, BRAF, RAF1, FLT4, KDR, FLT3, KIT, FGFR1, RET, FLT1	Sorafenib Tosylate, Valproic Acid, and Sildenafil Citrate in Treating Patients With Recurrent High-Grade Glioma	Phase 2
NCT03522298	Paxalisib (GDC-0084)	PIK3CA	Safety, Pharmacokinetics and Efficacy of Paxalisib (GDC-0084) in Newly-diagnosed Glioblastoma	Phase 2
NCT03027388	LB-100	PP2A	Protein Phosphatase 2A Inhibitor, in Recurrent Glioblastoma	Phase 2
NCT01582269	LY2157299 monohydrate, lomustine, placebo	STMN4	A Study in Recurrent Glioblastoma (GBM)	Phase 2

NCT number	Interventions	Targets	Phase	Title
NCT03149003	DSP-7888 dosing emulsion, bevacizumab	VEGFA	Phase 2	A Study of DSP-7888 Dosing Emulsion in Combination With Bevacizumab in Patients With Recurrent or Progressive Glioblastoma Following Initial Therapy
NCT01903330	ERC1671, granulocyte macrophageecolony stimulating factor (GM-CSF), cyclophosphamide, oral control (sucrose pill) Injectable control (sodium chloride injection United States Pharmacopeia [0.9%]), bevacizumab	VEGFA	Phase 2	ERC1671/GM-CSF/Cyclophosphamide for the Treatment of Glioblastoma Multiforme
NCT03532295	Epacadostat, bevacizumab	VEGFA	Phase 2	INCMGA00012 and Epacadostat in Combination With Radiation and Bevacizumab in Patients With Recurrent Gliomas
NCT03743662	Bevacizumab, nivolumab	VEGFA, PDCD1	Phase 2	Nivolumab With Radiation Therapy and Bevacizumab for Recurrent MGMT Methylated Glioblastoma
NCT03463265	ABI-009, bevacizumab, temozolomide, lomustine, marizomib	VEGFA, STMN4	Phase 2	ABI-009 (Nab-Rapamycin) in Recurrent High Grade Glioma and Newly Diagnosed Glioblastoma
NCT01004874	Bevacizumab, temozolomide, topotecan	VEGFA, TOP1, TOP1MT	Phase 2	Avastin/Radiation (XRT)/Temozolomide (Temodar) Followed by Avastin/Temodar/Topotecan for Glioblastoma
NCT01062425	Cediranib maleate, temozolomide	VEGFR1, VEGFR2, VEGFR3	Phase 2	Temozolomide and Radiation Therapy With or Without Cediranib Maleate in Treating Patients With Newly Diagnosed Glioblastoma
NCT02974621	Cediranib, cediranib maleate, olaparib	VEGFR1, VEGFR2, VEGFR3, PARP1, PARP2, PARP3	Phase 2	Cediranib Maleate and Olaparib Compared to Bevacizumab in

(continued on next page)

Table 1
(continued)

NCT Number	Drugs	Targets	Title	Phases
			Treating Patients With Recurrent Glioblastoma	
NCT03856099	TTAC-0001	VEGFR2	TTAC-0001 Phase II Trial With Recurrent Glioblastoma Progressed on Bevacizumab	Phase 2
NCT03673787	Ipatasertib, atezolizumab	AKT1, PDCD1	A Trial of Ipatasertib in Combination With Atezolizumab	Phase 1, Phase 2
NCT02715609	Disulfiram, copper gluconate, temozolomide	ALDH2, DBH	Disulfiram/Copper With Concurrent Radiation Therapy and Temozolomide in Patients With Newly Diagnosed Glioblastoma	Phase 1, Phase 2
NCT03158389	APG101, alectinib, idasanutlin, atezolizumab, vismodegib, temsirolimus, palbociclib	ALK, SMO, MTOR, CDK4, CDK6	NCT Neuro Master Match (NOA-20)	Phase 1, Phase 2
NCT02586857	ACP-196	BTK	A Phase 1 b/2, Multicenter, Open-label Study of ACP-196 in Subjects With Recurrent Glioblastoma Multiforme (GBM)	Phase 1, Phase 2
NCT02942264	Zotiraciclib (TG02), temozolomide	CDK1, CDK2, CDK7, JAK2, CDK9, FLT3, FLK2, STK1	Zotiraciclib (TG02) Plus Dose-Dense or Metronomic Temozolomide Followed by Randomized Phase II Trial of Zotiraciclib (TG02) Plus Temozolomide vs Temozolomide Alone in Adults With Recurrent Anaplastic Astrocytoma and Glioblastoma	Phase 1, Phase 2
NCT01790503	PLX3397, temozolomide	CSF1R	A Phase 1 b/2 Study of PLX3397 + Radiation Therapy + Temozolomide in Patients With Newly Diagnosed Glioblastoma	Phase 1, Phase 2
NCT04121455	Olaptesed pegol	CXCL12		Phase 1, Phase 2

NCT Number	Agents	Molecular Targets	Title	Phase
NCT00669669	Carmustine, O6-benzylguanine, plerixafor, temozolomide	GSR, CXCR4	Glioblastoma Treatment With Irradiation and Olaptesed Pegol (NOX-A12) in MGMT Unmethylated Patients O6-Benzylguanine-Mediated Tumor Sensitization With Chemoprotected Autologous Stem Cell in Treating Patients With Malignant Gliomas	Phase 1, Phase 2
NCT00555399	Vorinostat, isotretinoin, temozolomide	HDAC1, HDAC2, HDAC3, HDAC6	Vorinostat, Isotretinoin and Temozolomide in Adults With Recurrent Glioblastoma Multiforme (GBM)	Phase 1, Phase 2
NCT00731731	Temozolomide, vorinostat	HDAC1, HDAC2, HDAC3, HDAC6	Vorinostat, Temozolomide, and Radiation Therapy in Treating Patients With Newly Diagnosed Glioblastoma Multiforme	Phase 1, Phase 2
NCT03684811	FT-2102, azacitidine, gemcitabine and cisplatin	IDH1, DNMT1	A Study of FT 2102 in Participants With Advanced Solid Tumors and Gliomas With an IDH1 Mutation	Phase 1, Phase 2
NCT01434602	Everolimus, sorafenib	MTOR, PDGFRB, BRAF, RAF1, FLT4, KDR, FLT3, KIT, FGFR1, RET, FLT1	Phase I-II Everolimus and Sorafenib in Recurrent High-Grade Gliomas	Phase 1, Phase 2
NCT03150862	BGB-290, temozolomide	PARP1, PARP2	A Study Assessing Pamiparib With Radiation and/or Temozolomide (TMZ) in Subjects With Newly Diagnosed or Recurrent Glioblastoma	Phase 1, Phase 2
NCT03914742	PARP inhibitor BGB-290, temozolomide	PARP1, PARP2	BGB-290 and Temozolomide in Treating Patients With Recurrent Gliomas With IDH1/2 Mutations	Phase 1, Phase 2
NCT03782415	MN-166, temozolomide	PDE3, PDE4, PD10, PDE11	Study to Evaluate Ibudilast and TMZ Combo Treatment in Newly Diagnosed and Recurrent Glioblastoma	Phase 1, Phase 2

(continued on next page)

Table 1
(continued)

NCT Number	Drugs	Targets	Title	Phases
NCT02331498	Pazopanib	PDGFRB, FLT4, KDR, KIT, FLT1, PDGFRA, FGF1, FGFR3, ITK, SH2B3	Phase I/II Study of Pazopanib + Temozolomide in Patients With Newly Diagnosed Glioblastoma Multiforme	Phase 1, Phase 2
NCT03466450	PF-04449913, temozolomide oral capsule	SMO	Glasdegib (PF-04449913) With Temozolomide Newly Diagnosed Glioblastoma	Phase 1, Phase 2
NCT02765165	USL311, lomustine	STMN4	Phase 1/2 Study of USL311 Alone and in Combination With Lomustine in Subjects With Advanced Solid Tumors and Relapsed/Recurrent Glioblastoma Multiforme (GBM)	Phase 1, Phase 2
NCT02770378	Temozolomide, aprepitant, minocycline, disulfiram, celecoxib, sertraline, captopril, itraconazole, ritonavir, auranofin	TACR1, VEGFA, ALOX5, rpsl, rpsD, MMP9, CASP1, CASP3, CYCS, ALDH2, DBH, PTGS2, PDPK1, SLC6A4, SLC6A3, ACE, MMP2, MMP9, ERG11, CYP51A1, pol, IKBKB, PRDX5	A Proof-of-concept Clinical Trial Assessing the Safety of the Coordinated Undermining of Survival Paths by 9 Repurposed Drugs Combined With Metronomic Temozolomide (CUSP9v3 Treatment Protocol) for Recurrent Glioblastoma	Phase 1, Phase 2
NCT03119064	Nanoliposomal irinotecan, temozolomide	TOP1, TOP1MT	BrUOG 329 GBM Onyvide With TMZ	Phase 1, Phase 2
NCT02611024	Lurbinectedin (PM01183), irinotecan	TOP1, TOP1MT	Pharmacokinetic Study of PM01183 in Combination With Irinotecan in Patients With Selected Solid Tumors	Phase 1, Phase 2
NCT03678883	9-ING-41, gemcitabine—21-d cycle, doxorubicin, lomustine, carboplatin, nab-paclitaxel, paclitaxel, gemcitabine—28 d cycle, irinotecan	TOP2A, STMN4, TUBB1, MAP2, BCL2, MAP4, MAPT, TOP1, TOP1MT	9-ING-41 in Patients With Advanced Cancers	Phase 1, Phase 2
NCT03213002	Capecitabine, temozolomide	TYMS	Oral Capecitabine and Temozolomide (CAPTEM) for Newly Diagnosed GBM	Phase 1, Phase 2

NCT01349660	Bevacizumab, BKM120	VEGFA	Combination of BKM120 and Bevacizumab in Refractory Solid Tumors and Relapsed/Refractory Glioblastoma Multiforme	Phase 1, Phase 2
NCT02330562	MRZ, bevacizumab	VEGFA	Stage 1: Marizomib + Bevacizumab in WHO Gr IV GBM; Stage 2: Marizomib Alone; Stage 3: Combination of Marizomib and Bevacizumab	Phase 1, Phase 2
NCT04004975	Anlotinib	VEGFR2, VEGFR3	Clinical Study on the Treatment of Recurrent Glioblastoma With Anlotinib	Phase 1, Phase 2
NCT04421378	Selinexor, temozolomide (temozolomide), lomustine (CCNU)	XPO1, STMN4	A Study of Selinexor in Combination With Standard of Care Therapy for Newly Diagnosed or Recurrent Glioblastoma	Phase 1, Phase 2
NCT01430351	Mefloquine, memantine hydrochloride, metformin hydrochloride, temozolomide	ADORA2A, HBA1	Temozolomide, Memantine Hydrochloride, Mefloquine, and Metformin Hydrochloride in Treating Patients With Glioblastoma Multiforme After Radiation Therapy	Phase 1
NCT02270034	Crizotinib	ALK, MET	Study to Evaluate Safety and Activity of Crizotinib With Temozolomide and Radiotherapy in Newly Diagnosed Glioblastoma	Phase 1
NCT03535350	Ibrutinib, temozolomide (temozolomide)	BTK	Ibrutinib With Radiation and Temozolomide in Patients With Newly Diagnosed Glioblastoma	Phase 1
NCT03224104	TG02, temozolomide	CDK1, CDK2, CDK7, JAK2, CDK9, FLT3, FLK2, STK1	Study of TG02 in Elderly Newly Diagnosed or Adult Relapsed Patients With Anaplastic Astrocytoma or Glioblastoma	Phase 1
NCT03231501	Epitinib succinate	EGFR	HMPL-813 in Treating Patients With Glioblastoma	Phase 1
NCT02101905	Lapatinib, lapatinib ditosylate	EGFR, ERBB2	Lapatinib Ditosylate Before Surgery in Treating Patients With Recurrent High-Grade Glioma	Phase 1

(continued on next page)

Table 1
(continued)

NCT Number	Drugs	Targets	Title	Phases
NCT02423525	Afatinib	EGFR, ERBB2, ERBB4	Safety Study of Afatinib for Brain Cancer	Phase 1
NCT02974738	PT2977	EPAS1	A Trial of PT2977 Tablets In Patients With Advanced Solid Tumors	Phase 1
NCT03374943	KB004	EPHA3	A Trial of KB004 in Patients With Glioblastoma	Phase 1
NCT00102648	Lonafarnib, temozolomide	Ftase	Lonafarnib and Temozolomide in Treating Patients With Glioblastoma Multiforme That Is Recurrent or Did Not Respond to Previous Treatment With Temozolomide	Phase 1
NCT03452930	Tinostamustine	HDAC1, HDAC2, HDAC3, HDAC6	Tinostamustine With or Without Radiation Therapy in Treating Patients With Newly Diagnosed MGMT-Unmethylated Glioblastoma	Phase 1
NCT00268385	Temozolomide, vorinostat	HDAC1, HDAC2, HDAC3, HDAC6	Vorinostat and Temozolomide in Treating Patients With Malignant Gliomas	Phase 1
NCT02381886	IDH305	IDH1	A Study of IDH305 in Patients With Advanced Malignancies That Harbor IDH1R132 Mutations	Phase 1
NCT03514069	Ruxolitinib, temozolomide	JAK1, JAK2	Ruxolitinib With Radiation and Temozolomide for Grade III Gliomas and Glioblastoma	Phase 1
NCT02133183	Sapanisertib	MTOR	Sapanisertib Before and After Surgery in Treating Patients With Recurrent Glioblastoma	Phase 1
NCT02142803	Sapanisertib	MTOR	TORC1/2 Inhibitor MLN0128 and Bevacizumab in Treating Patients	Phase 1

NCT ID	Drug	Target	Title	Phase
NCT02238496	Perifosine, temsirolimus	MTOR	Perifosine and Torisel (Temsirolimus) for Recurrent/Progressive Malignant Gliomas	Phase 1
NCT03749187	PARP inhibitor BGB-290, temozolomide	PARP1, PARP2	BGB-290 and Temozolomide in Treating Isocitrate Dehydrogenase (IDH)1/2-Mutant Grade I-IV Gliomas	Phase 1
NCT03426891	Pembrolizumab, vorinostat, temozolomide	PDCD1, HDAC1, HDAC2, HDAC3, HDAC6	Pembrolizumab and Vorinostat Combined With Temozolomide for Newly Diagnosed Glioblastoma	Phase 1
NCT04205357	Sulfasalazine	PTGS1, PTGS2, ALOX5, CHUK, IKBKB, SLC7A11, ACAT1, TBXAS1, PLA2G1B	Sulfasalazine and Stereotactic Radiosurgery for Recurrent Glioblastoma	Phase 1
NCT03463733	Hydroxyurea, temozolomide	RRM1	Hydroxy-urea and Temozolomide in Patients With a Recurrent Malignant Brain Tumor (Glioblastoma)	Phase 1
NCT03587038	OKN 007, temozolomide	SULF2	OKN-007 in Combination With Adjuvant Temozolomide Chemoradiotherapy for Newly Diagnosed Glioblastoma	Phase 1
NCT02192359	Irinotecan, irinotecan hydrochloride	TOP1, TOP1MT	Carboxylesterase-Expressing Allogeneic Neural Stem Cells and Irinotecan Hydrochloride in Treating Patients With Recurrent High-Grade Gliomas	Phase 1
NCT02644291	Mebendazole	TUBA1A, TUBB4B	Phase I Study of Mebendazole Therapy for Recurrent/Progressive Pediatric Brain Tumors	Phase 1
NCT01729260	Mebendazole	TUBA1A, TUBB4B	Mebendazole in Newly Diagnosed High-Grade Glioma Patients Receiving Temozolomide	Phase 1
NCT02669173	Capecitabine, bevacizumab	TYMS, VEGFA	Capecitabine + Bevacizumab in Patients With Recurrent Glioblastoma	Phase 1

(continued on next page)

Table 1
(continued)

NCT Number	Drugs	Targets	Title	Phases
NCT03722342	TTAC-0001 and pembrolizumab combination	VEGFR2	TTAC-0001 and Pembrolizumab Combination phase1b Trial in Recurrent Glioblastoma	Phase 1
NCT01849146	Adavosertib, temozolomide	WEE1	Adavosertib, Radiation Therapy, and Temozolomide in Treating Patients With Newly Diagnosed or Recurrent Glioblastoma	Phase 1
NCT04216329	Selinexor, temozolomide	XPO1	Selinexor (KPT-330) in Combination With Temozolomide and Radiation Therapy in Patients With Newly Diagnosed Glioblastoma	Phase 1

sectional study reported that 8.33% of 609,640 patients in 2018 were eligible for targeted treatment, but only 4.9% of all patients had a clinical benefit.[42] These numbers likely are even lower in GBM due to a multitude of issues, discussed previously, including impaired drug delivery because of the BBB, intratumoral genetic and transcriptional heterogeneity, redundant activating pathways or escape mechanisms, and inherent therapeutic resistance.[10,43]

The BBB presents a unique challenge in that it restricts the entry of more than 95% of FDA-approved drugs into the central nervous system, thereby preventing the delivery of therapeutic drug concentrations to brain cancer. Accordingly, targeted molecular therapies considered for clinical trials should demonstrate therapeutic levels within the brain and the entire tumor volume (both enhancing and nonenhancing).[9]

The genetic and transcriptional heterogenicity of GBM presents a challenge to targeting therapy in that subpopulations can respond to selective evolutionary pressures of targeted therapy, thereby resulting in treatment resistance.[10] Single-cell analysis studies found that frequently there are multiple subtypes (mesenchymal, classical, and so forth) within 1 GBM, including a population harboring stem cell properties.[43] Perceived potentially actionable alterations could be passenger mutations, instead of driver mutations amenable to therapy.[44] A notable example is that EGFR is overexpressed in 50% to 60% of GBM patients making it historically an attractive target. EGFR tyrosine kinase inhibitors and monoclonal antibody targeting EGFR, however, have failed to show clinical activity.[10] A later attempt to address intertumoral heterogenicity with a combination of EGFR tyrosine kinase inhibitor and mTOR inhibitors lead to dose-limiting toxicity and no therapeutic response.[20] Additionally, initial responses to the targeting of driver mutations often lack a durable treatment effect that has been reported in many cases.[28,38,45]

Further complicating the picture and targeted therapy for cancer, in general, are recent investigations showing that off-target toxicity rather than the on-target effects are responsible for the antitumor efficacy. A study using clustered regularly interspaced short palindromic repeats (CRISPR)-Cas9 mutagenesis evaluated a set of cancer drugs and drug targets and found that the effectiveness of drugs was unaffected by the loss of its putative target, indicating that these compounds kill cells via off-target effects. Therefore, providing experimental validation of the mechanism of action of cancer drugs in the preclinical setting would be critical before embarking on a clinical trial. Such verification may help decrease the number of therapies tested on humans that fail to provide any clinical benefit.[46] These challenges underscore the need to develop complementary approaches to direct targeting.

Synthetic Lethality and Future Approaches to Biomarker-Driven Strategies in Glioblastoma

A large number of currently active clinical trials (see **Table 1**) include a molecular targeting component and can be broadly divided into 2 classes: (1) trials whose eligibility criteria are based on the specific genetic alterations being targeted (for example, BRAFV600E, EGFRvIII, and IDH1 R132H), and (2) trials that target pathways frequently amplified over the disease course or as a response to treatment (for example, angiogenesis pathways or DNA repair pathways). The number of patients who can benefit from targeting specific genetic alterations in GBM is small. Many alterations in GBM are loss of function mutations or deletions, which makes their direct targeting difficult. The situation can be partially alleviated by expanding molecular testing to include gene expression profiling. The WINTHER trial (NCT01856296), which enrolled primarily patients with colon, head, and neck, and lung cancer, demonstrated that transcriptomic profiling can expand personalized cancer treatment.[47,48] The success of targeting amplified pathways requires elucidation of the biological mechanisms that are being affected by targeting, identification of predictive biomarkers of response, and inclusion of such biomarkers' status in the eligibility criteria to identify the patients most likely to benefit from the therapy. As illustrated by the failure of many antiangiogenesis therapies to elicit a sustained response in GBM, targeting biological pathways essential for survival is likely to activate compensatory mechanisms that ensure cell survival.[49] In this situation, treatment can be effective only when such compensation is disabled either by the disease (inactivating mutation or gene deletion) or by targeted therapy.

Molecular targeting often works best where the requirement for the target is increased in cancer cells compared with normal cells, due to either intrinsic genetic or epigenetic changes in the cancer cells or extrinsic microenvironmental changes.[50,51] One such dependency that can be exploited for therapeutic benefit is the dependency between 2 synthetic lethal partner genes: the loss of each gene individually can be tolerated by the cell, but their simultaneous loss leads to cell death (**Fig. 1**). For cancer cells in which 1 of the synthetic lethal partners is lost (via mutation or

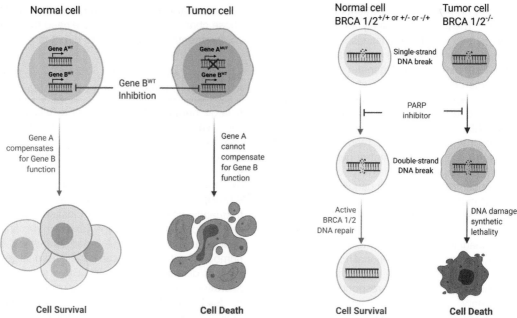

Fig. 1. Synthetic lethality. (*A*) Synthetic lethality arises when simultaneous loss of 2 genes results in cell death. (*B*) PARP inhibition is a selective anticancer therapy for BRCA1/2 mutant cancer cells. Created with BioRender.com. MUT, mutant; WT, wild-type.

deletion), targeting the second partner provides an effective and selective anticancer strategy: the cancer cells cannot tolerate the loss of the second partner, whereas normal cells largely are unaffected.[50] The first-discovered and most effective to-date anticancer therapy that exploits synthetic lethal interactions is inhibition of PARP (PARP1/PARP2) in breast cancer patients with germline mutations in BRCA1 and BRCA2.[13,14] PARP senses single-strand breaks in DNA and induce DNA damage response; its inhibition leads to accumulation of single and double-strand breaks in DNA. Loss-of-function mutations of BRCA1/2, which are required for homologous recombination and DNA break repair, renders cells unable to repair the accumulated DNA damage, and induces apoptosis (see **Fig. 1**). PARP inhibition has been considered a therapeutic approach in the context of non-BRCA1/2 mutations in situations where cells have increased reliance on homologous recombination for survival (either due to cytotoxic stress induced by treatment or reactive oxygen species, or other DNA repair enzyme mutations). This concept is being tested in brain tumors. For example, NCT03212274 is trialing PARP inhibition in advanced IDH1/2 mutated gliomas (because 2-hydroxygluterate produced by neomorphic IDH has been reported to suppress homologous

recombination), and NCT02152982 is trialing PARP inhibition in combination with temozolomide in newly diagnosed GBM.[26]

Several preclinical studies have demonstrated the potential of targeting other synthetic lethal interactions as anticancer therapies.[51–53] Barbie and colleagues,[51] for example, discovered that *TBK1* (encoding the tank binding kinase) is essential in *KRAS* mutation–driven cell lines. Chan and colleagues[52] showed that cancers with microsatellite instability depend on *WRN* helicase. The depletion of WRN-induced double-stranded DNA breaks and promoted apoptosis and cell-cycle arrest selectively in these models.[52] To date, however, few clinical studies have managed to exploit such interactions beyond PARP inhibition.[54] Some of the challenges associated with successfully translating these principles include the difficulty in experimentally determining synthetic lethal interactions, which theoretically entails knocking down all possible pairs of genes; the inability of preclinical models to fully recapitulate the patient disease; and the existence of multiple compensatory mechanisms, which lowers the magnitude of response (leading to synthetic sickness rather than death when a pair of genes is downregulated). In particular, the magnitude of the response may itself be dependent on a larger molecular context rather than be uniform across tumor subtypes.[55] Similarly, subclonal heterogeneity affects the likelihood of response.[56]

Given the limitations of preclinical testing and the extensive tumor heterogeneity, predicting robust synthetic lethal relationships is imperative for successfully translating the promise of synthetic lethal targeting. The advent of high-throughput screening and gene editing technologies facilitates large-scale screening and identification of synthetic pairs in vitro models.[57–60] The limitations of the experimental approaches are being overcome through computational and machine learning approaches that leverage knowledge from yeast screens, protein-protein information networks, metabolic and functional pathways, and biological principles.[61–63] The accumulation of large multiomics patient-tumor derived data sets from projects like TCGA enables novel integrative computational approaches that strengthen predictions through evidence from orthogonal data sources.[64–66] For example, Lee and colleagues'[65] approach of identification of clinically relevant synthetic lethality (ISLE) sequentially filters putative synthetic lethal pairs by taking into consideration evidence from cell line screens, evidence of negative pressure for selection of disabled putative pairs as gauged by lower than expected frequency of encountering such pairs in patient tumors, evidence of lower viability of tumors that exhibit disabled putative pairs and that can be assessed through the association of such disabled pairs with longer overall survival of the patients harboring such tumors, and evolutionary relatedness of the genes in a pair, which can indicate similarity of function.[65] Crucially, approaches like ISLE enable predicting targeted drug response for individual samples based on the genomic or transcriptomic status of the target's predicted synthetic lethal partners in the sample, effectively stipulating and improving the eligibility criteria for patient enrollment in clinical trials.

SUMMARY

Despite the advances and successes of molecularly targeted therapies in other malignancies, GBM remains among the most difficult to treat cancers, due to its robust heterogenicity and presence of the BBB preventing adequate delivery of most systemically administered agents. Traditional molecular targeted therapies work only in rare subsets of patients harboring a tumor with a true driver genomic alteration that continues to be required for tumor cell survival. Such driver targets, however, are unlikely to be identified for most brain tumors. Therefore, complementary

approaches that incorporate a larger genomic context in the decision process may overcome the limitations of direct targeting and deserve further investigation. The maturation of a master protocol incorporating multicenter clinical trial designs as exemplified by National Cancer Institute Molecular Analysis for Therapy Choice (NCI-MATCH) (encompassing 40 treatment arms and spanning more than 1100 clinical centers) combined with advances in next-generation sequencing technologies that are enabling extensive molecular profiling of tumors are providing unprecedented opportunities to make the next-generation brain cancer trials transformative.

CLINICS CARE POINTS

- Molecular evaluation of GBM is the standard of care for diagnostic clarity and identification of potential druggable alterations
- Targeted therapy benefits few GBM patients due to immense molecular heterogeneity
- Delivery of targeted drugs at therapeutic concentrations often is impeded by the BBB, making it essential to demonstrate therapeutic levels of drug within the brain and entire tumor volume in preclinical studies
- The therapeutic benefit seen with a small subset of GBM patients indicate that robust molecular markers and patient selection are critical
- Novel complementary treatment approaches based on synthetic lethal interactions may expand the promise of precision oncology

DISCLOSURE

The authors have nothing to disclose.

REFERENCES

1. Ostrom QT, Cioffi G, Gittleman H, et al. CBTRUS statistical report: primary brain and other central nervous system tumors diagnosed in the United States in 2012–2016. Neuro-Oncology 2019; 21(Supplement_5):v1–100.
2. Louis DN, Perry A, Reifenberger G, et al. The 2016 World Health Organization Classification of Tumors of the Central Nervous System: a summary. Acta Neuropathol 2016;131(6):803–20.
3. Hegi ME, Diserens A-C, Gorlia T, et al. MGMT gene silencing and benefit from temozolomide in glioblastoma. N Engl J Med 2005;352(10):997–1003.

4. Asklund T, Malmström A, Bergqvist M, et al. Brain tumors in Sweden: Data from a population-based registry 1999–2012. Acta Oncol 2015;54(3):377–84.

5. Stupp R, Mason WP, van den Bent MJ, et al. Radiotherapy plus Concomitant and Adjuvant Temozolomide for Glioblastoma. N Engl J Med 2005; 352(10):987–96.

6. Hegi ME, Stupp R. Withholding temozolomide in glioblastoma patients with unmethylated MGMT promoter—still a dilemma?: Table 1. Neuro Oncol 2015; 17(11):1425–7.

7. Touat M, Idbaih A, Sanson M, et al. Glioblastoma targeted therapy: updated approaches from recent biological insights. Ann Oncol 2017;28(7):1457–72.

8. Baudino T. Targeted cancer therapy: the next generation of cancer treatment. Curr Drug Discov Technol 2015;12(1):3–20.

9. Grossman SA, Romo CG, Rudek MA, et al. Baseline requirements for novel agents being considered for phase ii/iii brain cancer efficacy trials:conclusions from the adult brain tumor consortium's first workshop on cns drug delivery. Neuro-Oncology 2020; noaa142. https://doi.org/10.1093/neuonc/noaa142.

10. Chen R, Smith-Cohn M, Cohen AL, et al. Glioma Subclassifications and Their Clinical Significance. Neurotherapeutics 2017;14(2):284–97.

11. Bridges CB. The origin of variation. Amer Nat 1922; 56:51–63. Available at. https://www.journals.uchicago.edu/doi/pdfplus/10.1086/279847.

12. Nijman SMB. Synthetic lethality: General principles, utility and detection using genetic screens in human cells. FEBS Lett 2011;585(1):1–6.

13. Bryant HE, Schultz N, Thomas HD, et al. Specific killing of BRCA2-deficient tumours with inhibitors of poly(ADP-ribose) polymerase. Nature 2005; 434(7035):913–7.

14. Farmer H, McCabe N, Lord CJ, et al. Targeting the DNA repair defect in BRCA mutant cells as a therapeutic strategy. Nature 2005;434(7035):917–21.

15. Yan L, Rosen N, Arteaga C. Targeted cancer therapies. Chin J Cancer 2011;30(1):1–4.

16. Kantarjian HM, Talpaz M, O'Brien S, et al. Imatinib mesylate for Philadelphia chromosome-positive, chronic-phase myeloid leukemia after failure of interferon-alpha: follow-up results. Clin Cancer Res 2002;8(7):2177–87.

17. Oh S, Yeom J, Cho HJ, et al. Integrated pharmacoproteogenomics defines two subgroups in isocitrate dehydrogenase wildtype glioblastoma with prognostic and therapeutic opportunities. Nat Commun 2020;11(1):3288.

18. Wang Q, Hu B, Hu X, et al. Tumor Evolution of Glioma-Intrinsic Gene Expression Subtypes Associates with Immunological Changes in the Microenvironment. Cancer Cell 2017;32(1):42–56.e6.

19. Brennan CW, Verhaak RGW, McKenna A, et al. The somatic genomic landscape of glioblastoma. Cell 2013;155(2):462–77.

20. Prados MD, Byron SA, Tran NL, et al. Toward precision medicine in glioblastoma: the promise and the challenges. Neuro Oncol 2015;17(8):1051–63.

21. Okamura R, Boichard A, Kato S, et al. Analysis of NTRK Alterations in Pan-Cancer Adult and Pediatric Malignancies: Implications for NTRK-Targeted Therapeutics. JCO Precision Oncol 2018;(2):1–20.

22. Sturm D, Witt H, Hovestadt V, et al. Hotspot Mutations in H3F3A and IDH1 Define Distinct Epigenetic and Biological Subgroups of Glioblastoma. Cancer Cell 2012;22(4):425–37.

23. Henry NL, Hayes DF. Cancer biomarkers. Mol Oncol 2012;6(2):140–6.

24. Oldenhuis CNAM, Oosting SF, Gietema JA, et al. Prognostic versus predictive value of biomarkers in oncology. Eur J Cancer 2008;44(7):946–53.

25. Perez EA, Romond EH, Suman VJ, et al. Trastuzumab Plus Adjuvant Chemotherapy for Human Epidermal Growth Factor Receptor 2–Positive Breast Cancer: Planned Joint Analysis of Overall Survival From NSABP B-31 and NCCTG N9831. JCO 2014;32(33): 3744–52.

26. Sulkowski PL, Corso CD, Robinson ND, et al. 2-Hydroxyglutarate produced by neomorphic IDH mutations suppresses homologous recombination and induces PARP inhibitor sensitivity. Sci Transl Med 2017;9(375):eaal2463.

27. Mellinghoff IK, Ellingson BM, Touat M, et al. Ivosidenib in Isocitrate Dehydrogenase 1 – Mutated Advanced Glioma. JCO 2020. https://doi.org/10.1200/JCO.19. 03327.

28. Smith-Cohn M, Davidson C, Colman H, et al. Challenges of targeting BRAF V600E mutations in adult primary brain tumor patients: a report of two cases. CNS Oncol 2019;8(4):CNS48. https://doi.org/10. 2217/cns-2019-0018.

29. Wick W, Meisner C, Hentschel B, et al. Prognostic or predictive value of MGMT promoter methylation in gliomas depends on IDH1 mutation. Neurology 2013;81(17):1515–22.

30. Rivera AL, Pelloski CE, Gilbert MR, et al. MGMT promoter methylation is predictive of response to radiotherapy and prognostic in the absence of adjuvant alkylating chemotherapy for glioblastoma. Neuro-Oncology 2010;12(2):116–21.

31. Maraka S, Janku F. BRAF alterations in primary brain tumors. Discov Med 2018;26(141):51–60.

32. Louis DN, Wesseling P, Aldape K, et al. cIMPACT-NOW update 6: new entity and diagnostic principle recommendations of the cIMPACT-Utrecht meeting on future CNS tumor classification and grading. Brain Pathol 2020;bpa.12832. https://doi.org/10.1111/bpa.12832.

33. Lobbous, Bernstock, Coffee, et al. An update on neurofibromatosis type 1-associated gliomas. Cancers 2020;12(1):114.

34. Ameratunga M, McArthur G, Gan H, et al. Prolonged disease control with MEK inhibitor in neurofibromatosis type I-associated glioblastoma. J Clin Pharm Ther 2016;41(3):357–9.

35. Zureick AH, McFadden KA, Mody R, et al. Successful treatment of a *TSC2*-mutant glioblastoma with everolimus. BMJ Case Rep 2019;12(5):e227734.

36. Xu T, Wang H, Huang X, et al. Gene fusion in malignant glioma: an emerging target for next-generation personalized treatment. Translational Oncol 2018; 11(3):609–18.

37. Drilon A, Siena S, Ou S-HI, et al. Safety and antitumor activity of the multitargeted pan-TRK, ROS1, and ALK inhibitor entrectinib: combined results from two phase i trials (ALKA-372-001 and STARTRK-1). Cancer Discov 2017;7(4):400–9.

38. Schram AM, Taylor BS, Hechtman JF, et al. Abstract LB-302: potential role of larotrectinib (LOXO-101), a selective pan-TRK inhibitor, in NTRK fusion-positive recurrent glioblastoma. In: Dang CV, editor. Experimental and molecular therapeutics, Volume 77, Issue 13. American Association for Cancer Research; 2017. https://doi.org/10.1158/1538-7445. AM2017-LB-302. pp. LB-302. Available at: https://cancerres.aacrjournals.org/content/77/13_Supplement/LB-302. LB-302-LB-302.

39. Gambella A, Senetta R, Collemi G, et al. NTRK fusions in central nervous system tumors: a rare, but worthy target. IJMS 2020;21(3):753.

40. Tabernero J, Bahleda R, Dienstmann R, et al. Phase I dose-escalation study of JNJ-42756493, an oral pan-fibroblast growth factor receptor inhibitor, in patients with advanced solid tumors. J Clin Oncol 2015;33(30):3401–8.

41. Mroz EA, Rocco JW. The challenges of tumor genetic diversity: Tumor Diversity. Cancer 2017; 123(6):917–27.

42. Marquart J, Chen EY, Prasad V. Estimation of the Percentage of US Patients With Cancer Who Benefit From Genome-Driven Oncology. JAMA Oncol 2018; 4(8):1093.

43. Couturier CP, Ayyadhury S, Le PU, et al. Single-cell RNA-seq reveals that glioblastoma recapitulates a normal neurodevelopmental hierarchy. Nat Commun 2020;11(1):3406.

44. Gatenby RA, Cunningham JJ, Brown JS. Evolutionary triage governs fitness in driver and passenger mutations and suggests targeting never mutations. Nat Commun 2014;5:5499.

45. International Cancer Genome Consortium PedBrain Tumor Project. Recurrent MET fusion genes represent a drug target in pediatric glioblastoma. Nat Med 2016;22(11):1314–20.

46. Lin A, Giuliano CJ, Palladino A, et al. Off-target toxicity is a common mechanism of action of cancer drugs undergoing clinical trials. Sci Transl Med 2019;11(509):eaaw8412.

47. Rodon J, Soria J-C, Berger R, et al. Genomic and transcriptomic profiling expands precision cancer medicine: the WINTHER trial. Nat Med 2019;25(5): 751–8.

48. Batchelor TT, Reardon DA, de Groot JF, et al. Antiangiogenic Therapy for Glioblastoma: Current Status and Future Prospects. Clin Cancer Res 2014; 20(22):5612–9.

49. Gilbert MR, Dignam JJ, Armstrong TS, et al. A Randomized Trial of Bevacizumab for Newly Diagnosed Glioblastoma. N Engl J Med 2014;370(8): 699–708.

50. Hartwell LH. Integrating Genetic Approaches into the Discovery of Anticancer Drugs. Science 1997; 278(5340):1064–8.

51. Barbie DA, Tamayo P, Boehm JS, et al. Systematic RNA interference reveals that oncogenic KRAS-driven cancers require TBK1. Nature 2009; 462(7269):108–12.

52. Chan EM, Shibue T, McFarland JM, et al. WRN helicase is a synthetic lethal target in microsatellite unstable cancers. Nature 2019;568(7753):551–6.

53. Karpel-Massler G, Ishida CT, Bianchetti E, et al. Induction of synthetic lethality in IDH1-mutated gliomas through inhibition of Bcl-xL. Nat Commun 2017;8(1):1067.

54. Ashworth A, Lord CJ. Synthetic lethal therapies for cancer: what's next after PARP inhibitors? Nat Rev Clin Oncol 2018;15(9):564–76.

55. Ku AA, Hu H-M, Zhao X, et al. Integration of multiple biological contexts reveals principles of synthetic lethality that affect reproducibility. Nat Commun 2020;11(1):2375.

56. Hyman DM, Taylor BS, Baselga J. Implementing Genome-Driven Oncology. Cell 2017;168(4):584–99.

57. Whitehurst AW, Bodemann BO, Cardenas J, et al. Synthetic lethal screen identification of chemosensitizer loci in cancer cells. Nature 2007;446(7137): 815–9.

58. Williams SP, Barthorpe AS, Lightfoot H, et al. High-throughput RNAi screen for essential genes and drug synergistic combinations in colorectal cancer. Sci Data 2017;4(1):170139.

59. Shen JP, Zhao D, Sasik R, et al. Combinatorial CRISPR–Cas9 screens for de novo mapping of genetic interactions. Nat Methods 2017;14(6):573–6.

60. Han K, Jeng EE, Hess GT, et al. Synergistic drug combinations for cancer identified in a CRISPR screen for pairwise genetic interactions. Nat Biotechnol 2017;35(5):463–74.

61. Kranthi T, Rao SB, Manimaran P. Identification of synthetic lethal pairs in biological systems through

network information centrality. Mol Biosyst 2013; 9(8):2163.

62. Folger O, Jerby L, Frezza C, et al. Predicting selective drug targets in cancer through metabolic networks. Mol Syst Biol 2011;7(1):501.

63. Srivas R, Shen JP, Yang CC, et al. A Network of Conserved Synthetic Lethal Interactions for Exploration of Precision Cancer Therapy. Mol Cell 2016; 63(3):514–25.

64. Liany H, Jeyasekharan A, Rajan V. Predicting synthetic lethal interactions using heterogeneous data sources. Bioinformatics 2020;36(7):2209–16.

65. Lee JS, Das A, Jerby-Arnon L, et al. Harnessing synthetic lethality to predict the response to cancer treatment. Nat Commun 2018;9(1):2546.

66. Jerby-Arnon L, Pfetzer N, Waldman YY, et al. Predicting Cancer-Specific Vulnerability via Data-Driven Detection of Synthetic Lethality. Cell 2014;158(5):1199–209.

Novel Radiation Approaches

Rupesh Kotecha, MD[a,b,*], Martin C. Tom, MD[a,b], Minesh P. Mehta, MD[a,b]

KEYWORDS

• Radiation therapy • Radiotherapy • Glioblastoma • GBM • Trials • Protons • Carbon ions

KEY POINTS

• The standard dose/fractionation schedule for newly diagnosed glioblastoma is 60 Gy/30 fractions; alternative hypofractionated schedules (5–15 fractions) can be considered in select patients.
• The addition of multiparametric MRI, metabolic, and functional imaging to target volume delineation in radiotherapy is an active area of current investigation.
• Advances in particle therapy (protons, carbon ions, and boron neutron capture therapy) are currently being evaluated for patients with newly diagnosed and recurrent glioblastoma.
• Several re-irradiation strategies exist for recurrent patients, including stereotactic radiosurgery, fractionated stereotactic radiation therapy, hypofractionated radiotherapy, pulsed-reduced dose-rate radiotherapy, and particle therapy.

INTRODUCTION

The aggressive nature of glioblastoma necessitates a multimodal treatment regimen consisting of maximum safe resection and adjuvant chemoradiotherapy. Despite improvements in surgical techniques, advances in molecular diagnostics, and introduction of novel chemotherapeutic agents, biologically targeted treatments, and immunotherapy innovations, the locally progressive pattern of disease spread has only solidified the role of radiation therapy (RT) in the management of this disease. This article systematically addresses the key elements of RT, with an assessment of the key studies regarding dose and fractionation schedules, principles of target volume delineation, and role of particle therapy techniques to improve the therapeutic ratio of treatment. Finally, the role of RT at the time of relapse remains an evolving area, and emerging evidence of its value is reviewed in brief.

DOSE AND FRACTIONATION

The optimal dose, volume, and fractionation schedule was the subject of several legacy randomized clinical trials (**Table 1**).[1] Walker and colleagues[2] published a pooled analysis of 3 Brain Tumor Study Group trials that demonstrated that 60 Gy was associated with improved overall survival (OS) compared with 55 Gy, 50 Gy, or ≤45 Gy. Multiple studies subsequently assessed different RT dose-escalation strategies. One such approach is hyperfractionation, whereby RT is delivered using multiple smaller fractions delivered each day to a higher total dose. However, hyperfractionated RT delivered at 1.2 to 1.6 Gy per fraction twice daily up to 70.4 to 72 Gy

Conflicts of Interest: R. Kotecha: Honoraria from Elsevier, Elekta AB, Accuray Inc, Novocure Inc, and Viewray Inc. M.C. Tom: None. M.P. Mehta: Consulting for Zap, Mevion, Karyopharm, Tocagen, Astra-Zeneca. Board of Directors: Oncoceutics.
Cite Sources of Support (if applicable): This research received no specific grant from any funding agency in the public, commercial, or not-for-profit sectors.
[a] Department of Radiation Oncology, Miami Cancer Institute, Baptist Health South Florida, Miami, FL, USA;
[b] Herbert Wertheim College of Medicine, Florida International University, Miami, FL, USA
* Corresponding author. Department of Radiation Oncology, Miami Cancer Institute, Baptist Health South Florida, Office 1R203, Miami, FL 33176.
E-mail address: rupeshk@baptisthealth.net

Table 1
Clinical trials assessing different dose and fractionation schedules for newly diagnosed glioblastoma

Study	Key Population Criteria	Total Dose (Gy)	Number of Fractions	Dose per Fraction (Gy)	Interfraction Interval	Results
Ali et al,[3] 2018	694 patients with grade III (29%) or IV (71%) glioma	72 (with BCNU) 60 (with BCNU)	60 30	1.2 2	4–8 1 d	Hyperfractionated RT did not improve median OS (11.3 vs 13.1 mo, P = .20).
Andersen et al,[74] 1978	108 adults with grade IV astrocytoma (glioblastoma)	No RT 45	N/A 25 (5–6 fractions/wk)	N/A 1.8	N/A 1 d	RT improved OS at 6 mo (P<.005).
Bleehen et al,[75] 1991	474 patients with grade III (33%), III/IV (6%), or IV (61%) glioma	45 60	20 30	2.25 2	1 d 1 d	60 Gy improved median OS (12 vs 9 mo, P = .007).
Glinkski et al,[76] 1993	108 patients with grade III (59%) or IV (41%) astrocytoma	50 (WBRT) → 10 (tumor boost) 20 (WBRT) → 20 (WBRT) → 10 (tumor boost)	30 5 → 5 → 5	2 4 → 4 → 2	1 d 1 d; each course separated by 1 mo interval	Among grade IV, hypofractionated RT regimen improved 2 y OS (23% vs 10%, P<.05).
Keime-Guibert et al,[77] 2007	81 patients with glioblastoma, age ≥70, KPS ≥70	No RT (supportive care) 50	N/A 25	N/A 1.8	N/A 1 d	RT improved median OS (29.1 vs 16.9 wk, P = .002).
Kristiansen et al,[78] 1981	118 patients with grade III or IV astrocytoma	No RT (no CHT) 45 Gy (WBRT) 45 Gy (WBRT with bleomycin)	N/A 25 25	N/A 1.8 1.8	N/A 1 d 1 d	RT (but not bleomycin) improved median OS (10.8 vs 5.2 mo).
Malmström et al,[11] 2012	291 patients with glioblastoma, age ≥60	No RT (TMZ alone) 34 60	N/A 10 30	N/A 3.4 2	N/A 1 d 1 d	60 Gy worsened median OS (6 vs 8.3 [TMZ, P = .01] vs 7.5 [34 Gy, P = .24] mo).
Phillips et al,[79] 2003	68 patients with grade III (10%) or IV (90%) astrocytoma	35 60	10 30	3.5 2	1 d 1 d	Short course RT had similar median OS (8.7 vs 10.3 mo, P = .37).
Prados et al,[4] 2001	231 patients with glioblastoma	70.4 70.4 (with DMFO) 59.4 59.4 (with DMFO)	44 44 33 33	1.6 1.6 1.8 1.8	6–8 h (BID) 6–8 h (BID) 1 d 1 d	Hyperfractionated RT did not improve median OS (42 vs 41 wk, P = .75). No difference in OS with DMFO.

Study	Population	Dose (Gy)	Fractions	Dose/fraction	Frequency	Results
Roa et al,[10] 2004	100 patients with glioblastoma, age ≥60	40 60	15 30	2.67 2	1 d 1 d	Hypofractionated RT had similar median OS (5.6 vs 5.1 mo, $P = .57$).
Roa et al,[12] 2015	98 patients with glioblastoma, all elderly and/or frail	25 40	5 15	5 2.67	1 d 1 d	Short course RT (25 Gy) had noninferior median OS (7.9 vs 6.4 mo, $P = .988$).
Shin et al,[80] 1987	124 patients with grade III (71%) or IV (29%) astrocytoma	61.41 61.41 (with misonidazole) 58	69 (TID) 69 (TID) 30	0.89 0.89 1.93	3–4 h (TID) 3–4 h (TID) 1 d	Hyperfractionated RT improved median OS (39–49 vs 27 wk, $P<.001$). No difference in OS with misonidazole.
Walker et al,[16] 1978	303 patients with grade III (10%) or IV (90%) astrocytoma	Supportive care alone BCNU alone 50–60 (WBRT) 50–60 (WBRT with BCNU)	N/A N/A 25–35 25–35	N/A N/A 1.71–2 1.71–2	N/A N/A 1 d 1 d	RT improved median OS (34.5–37.5 vs 18.5 [BCNU] vs 14 [supportive care] weeks], $P = .001$).
Walker et al,[2] 1979	Pooled analysis of 621 patients with malignant gliomas enrolled on BTSG studies	≤45 50 55 60	25–35 25–35 25–35 25–35	1.71–2 1.71–2 1.71–2 1.71–2	1 d 1 d 1 d 1 d	60 Gy associated with improved survival over 55 Gy, 50 Gy, and ≤45 wk (42 vs 36 vs 28 vs 13.5 wk, respectively).

Abbreviations: BCNU, carmustine; BID, twice daily; BTSG, brain tumor study group; CHT, chemotherapy; DMFO, difluoromethylornithine; Gy, Gray; KPS, Karnofsky performance status; N/A, not applicable; OS, overall survival; RT, radiotherapy; TID, 3 times daily; TMZ, temozolomide; WBRT, whole brain RT.

provided no survival benefit compared with conventional RT.[3,4] The Radiation Therapy Oncology Group (RTOG) also evaluated a stereotactic radiosurgery (SRS) boost of 15 to 24 Gy before conventionally fractionated 60 Gy with BCNU (carmustine), but there was similarly no survival benefit.[5] Furthermore, trials assessing the addition of a brachytherapy boost using radioactive implants have also been negative.[6] As such, a conventionally fractionated dose of 60 Gy remains the standard of care for nonelderly patients with good performance status.[7] Recent studies have demonstrated the feasibility of doses of more than 60 Gy,[8,9] which provided the basis for the ongoing NRG BN001 phase II study (NCT02179086) assessing dose escalation using photons or protons with a simultaneous integrated boost technique to 75 Gy in 30 fractions.

Because glioblastoma is associated with an exceptionally poor prognosis in elderly and frail patients (5- to 9-month OS), several hypofractionated RT courses have been evaluated. Dose/fractionation schedules using 40 Gy/15 fractions,[10] 34 Gy/10 fractions,[11] and 25 Gy/5 fractions[12] have yielded similar survival outcomes in select patients. More recent data also established the safety and benefit of concurrent temozolomide with 40 Gy in 15 fractions among patients ≥65 years of age.[13]

PRINCIPLES OF TARGET VOLUME DELINEATION

RT target volumes for glioblastoma have evolved, but significant heterogeneity still exists across cooperative group guidelines.[7,14,15] Although early studies treated the whole brain to full dose, 3-dimensional imaging allowed treatment volumes to include only the partial brain at highest risk of recurrence, typically consisting of the resection cavity and contrast-enhancing (CE) residual tumor plus a 5-mm to 30-mm margin to account for microscopic disease.[7,14–16] Whereas the Adult Brain Tumor Consortium (ABTC), North Central Cancer Treatment Group (NCCTG)/Alliance, and Radiation Therapy Oncology Group (RTOG)/NRG include an initial T2/fluid-attenuated inversion recovery (FLAIR) target with a subsequent cone-down to the cavity and CE residual tumor, the European Organisation for Research and Treatment of Cancer (EORTC) uses a 1-phase approach based on the CE residual tumor and resection cavity alone, without intentionally targeting T2/FLAIR hyperintensity.[7,14] A detailed description of target volume variations is presented in **Table 2**, with corresponding examples of each in **Fig. 1**. Other

key principles of target volume delineation include limiting target expansions to anatomic barriers of tumor spread (eg, falx cerebri, tentorium cerebelli), while ensuring coverage of areas at risk of contiguous tumor spread despite crossing midline (eg, anterior and posterior commissures).[15]

Currently, there are at least 3 different advanced imaging strategies seeking to redefine target delineation for glioblastoma: multiparametric magnetic resonance (MR), MR spectroscopy, and functional imaging. Dynamic CE MRI analyzes relative cerebral blood volume,[17,18] cerebral blood flow, and vascular permeability.[19] Together with diffusion-weighted MRI, a surrogate for tumor cellularity,[20] these images can be integrated into a multiparametric imaging signature that has been associated with patterns-of-failure outcomes in glioblastoma.[21] A multi-institutional phase II trial (NCT02805179) is currently under way using this multiparametric advanced imaging approach to guide dose-intensified radiotherapy (75 Gy/30 fractions) and aims to evaluate the OS of patients treated with this paradigm. An initial report from the first 12 patients in this study demonstrated that the advanced imaging target volumes were approximately 2 times smaller than the T1 enhancement volumes and 10 times smaller than the FLAIR volumes, yet identified disparate high-risk areas, with only a 57% overlap with the enhancement region on MRI alone.[22] A different approach uses spectroscopic MRI (sMRI) to evaluate the regions of the brain with elevated choline-to-N-acetylaspartate ratios[23] and guide dose escalation to these areas of elevated tumor-related metabolic activity, which also correspond to the areas at risk for disease relapse.[24] Integration of a dose-escalation (75 Gy/30 fractions) approach to sMRI-defined high-risk regions has been successfully tested across multiple institutions using a cloud platform.[25] A phase II multi-institutional pilot study using sMRI-defined target volumes (NCT03137888) is also under way with co-primary endpoints of feasibility and incidence of adverse events; data from the first 18 patients have been promising.[25] Finally, functional imaging with novel amino acid PET radiotracers, in particular, [11C]-Methionine (MET) PET has been correlated with areas at risk of disease progression to guide treatment planning[26] and studies have even developed radiobiological models to determine the dose needed to these areas to reduce the risk of relapse.[27] Similarly, [18F]-Fluoroethyltyrosine (FET)-based target volume delineation has been used in clinical studies to augment volumes defined with anatomic MRI alone, with no documented marginal or distant failures.[28] Dose-

Table 2
Glioblastoma radiotherapy target volume delineation among cooperative groups

	ABTC	EORTC	NCCTG/Alliance	RTOG/NRG
One or 2 phase	Two-phase: 46 Gy → 14 Gy	One-phase 60 Gy	Two-phase: 50 Gy → 10 Gy	Two-phase: 46 Gy → 14 Gy
Initial CTV	T2, T1-CE, cavity + 5 mm	T1-CE, cavity + 2–3 cm	T2, T1-CE, cavity + 2 cm to block edge	T2, T1-CE, cavity + 2 cm
Boost CTV	T1-CE, cavity + 5 mm	N/A	T1-CE, cavity + 2 cm to block edge	T1-CE, cavity + 2 cm
PTV	Generally 3–5 mm	Generally 5–7 mm	N/A	3–5 mm

Abbreviations: ABTC, adult brain tumor consortium; CE, contrast enhancement; CTV, clinical target volume; EORTC, European Organisation for Research and Treatment of Cancer; Gy, Gray; NCCTG, North Central Cancer Treatment Group; PTV, planning target volume; RTOG, Radiation Therapy Oncology Group.

escalation studies (72 Gy/30 fractions) to FET-PET–based regions demonstrated that all local relapses occurred within the 60-Gy isodose volume[29]; therefore, trials are currently under way to compare FET-PET with MRI alone in randomized settings (NCT01252459).[30] Each of the aforementioned approaches has merits and limitations; however, the future is clearly transitioning from anatomically delineated to biologically defined target volumes.

PARTICLE THERAPY ADVANCES

The radiobiological properties of particle therapy (such as protons, carbon ions, and boron neutron capture therapy [BNCT]) hold the promise to overcome the radioresistant nature of glioblastoma via activation of several unique molecular pathways.[31] The dosimetric profile of particle therapy allows for most of the dose to be accumulated into the tumor with little dose deposition beyond the distal edge

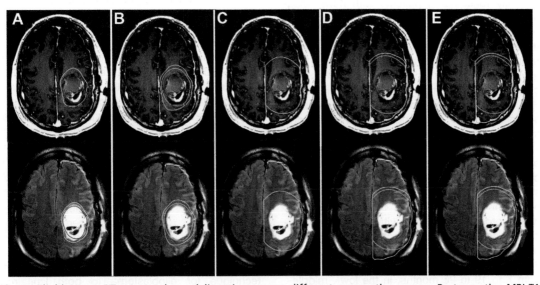

Fig. 1. Glioblastoma RT target volume delineation among different cooperative groups. Postoperative MRI T1 contrast-enhanced (*above*) and FLAIR (*below*) sequences. The gross tumor volume (GTV) initial is in yellow (97.73 cc) and GTV boost is in red (44.12 cc) (*A*). The ABTC volumes for clinical target volume (CTV) initial in cyan (46 Gy, 166.26 cc) and CTV boost in green (60 Gy, 81.83 cc) (*B*). The EORTC volume for the single phase CTV in green (60 Gy, 237.07 cc) (*C*). The NCCTG/Alliance volumes for CTV initial in cyan (50 Gy, 367.87 cc) and CTV boost in green (60 Gy, 237.07 cc) (*D*). The RTOG/NRG volumes for CTV initial in cyan (46 Gy, 367.87 cc) and CTV boost in green (60 Gy, 237.07 cc) (*E*).

of the treatment volume, resulting in superior dose conformality and reduced total integral dose to the brain.[32,33] As many of the central nervous system (CNS) organs-at-risk (OARs) have known dose-volume toxicity thresholds, particle therapy may allow for safer high-risk zone dose escalation, for example, in the hypoxic core.[34] Even reduction in integral dose to the brain alone with particle therapy (without any other benefits), and therefore the circulating blood pool, may reduce the treatment-induced lymphopenia observed with concurrent chemoradiotherapy, potentially translating into cost-effectiveness and improved survival.[35–37] Although limited data are currently available, several clinical trials have been recently completed or are under way, which may shed light on the use of particle therapy (**Table 3**).

Retrospective studies of proton therapy demonstrated the favorable safety, neurocognitive, and quality-of-life outcomes, and progression-free (PFS) and OS compared with photon series.[38–40] A phase II trial of 23 patients treated to a 90 Gy (with 57.6 Gy delivered with protons) resulted in a promising median OS of 20 months; most recurrences remained in-field and 30% developed symptomatic radiation necrosis.[41] Alternative approaches, such as hyper-fractionated concomitant boost techniques (50.4 Gy with photon therapy and 23.4 Gy cone-down) have resulted in reduced toxicities with similar OS (22 months).[38,42] The aforementioned NRG BN001 trial (NCT02179086) is currently randomizing patients with newly diagnosed glioblastoma to hypofractionated dose-escalated RT (75 Gy/30 fractions with photon therapy or proton therapy) or conventionally fractionated RT (60 Gy in 30 fractions with photon therapy) and will provide prospective assessment and comparable data with valuable information on OS, PFS, and treatment-related toxicities (including adverse events, neurocognitive function, and treatment-induced lymphopenia) (**Fig. 2**).

Carbon ion therapy has been evaluated in multiple phase I/II trials as a primary treatment modality or as a boost following photon therapy. In one study, 48 patients with high-grade gliomas (32 with glioblastoma) received 50 Gy/25 fractions with photon therapy along with nimustine hydrochloride followed by an 8 fraction boost with carbon ions in dose increments from 16.8 to 24.8 Gy. There was a stepwise increase in OS from 7 to 19 to 26 months, in the low-, middle-, and high-dose cohorts, respectively.[43] These promising results were evaluated in the recently completed CLEOPATRA trial (NCT01165671) in which patients were treated with photon therapy (50 Gy) and randomized to a proton therapy boost (10 Gy/5 fractions) or a carbon ion boost (dose-

escalation paradigm to 18 Gy/6 fractions)[44]; results are pending.

BNCT is a type of particle therapy that uses a 2-step approach to selectively target malignant cells. A boron-10 (^{10}B)-labeled compound is first delivered and selectively localizes in tumor cells in high concentrations that are subsequently irradiated with low-energy thermal neutrons.[45] The resulting reaction yields high linear-energy-transfer α-particles and ^{7}Li-particles traveling within a single cell's diameter, thus selectively damaging tumor cells while preserving normal cells. Historically, the availability of these epithermal neutrons has been restricted to reactor-based facilities, but novel accelerator-based approaches have led to a resurgence of this approach in hospital-based facilities. To date, only small trials using BNCT for newly diagnosed glioblastoma have been published, each using the ^{10}B compounds sodium borocaptate (BSH) and/or boronophenylalanine (BPA) with heterogeneous treatment delivery techniques, such as intraoperative BNCT or with the addition of conventional photon therapy.[46–51] A recently completed phase II multicenter study of BNCT using BSH and BPA with concurrent TMZ has preliminarily reported a promising median OS of 21.2 months (NCT00974987).[45,52]

RE-IRRADIATION STRATEGIES

Several re-irradiation strategies have been evaluated in patients with progressive or recurrent disease, including SRS, fractionated stereotactic RT (FSRT), intraoperative RT, hypofractionated RT, conventionally fractionated re-irradiation with pulsed-reduced dose-rate techniques (PRDR), and particle therapy. Given the heterogeneous disease cohorts included in each of these series, comparative analysis across studies cannot be performed and instead a re-treatment paradigm with consideration of patient-related, disease-related, and treatment-related factors with comprehensive evaluation in a multidisciplinary setting is recommended to tailor recommendations for each patient (**Fig. 3**).

Stereotactic Radiosurgery/Fractionated Stereotactic Radiotherapy

SRS/FSRT represents an attractive re-irradiation technique for glioblastoma to both limit re-irradiation volume and expedite treatment among a group of patients with short survival. Several phase I-II studies have reported various dosing strategies with or without systemic therapy, resulting in median survival of 6 to 12.5 months and crude radiation necrosis rates of 0% to 13%. An

Table 3
Current and ongoing clinical trials of particle therapy for newly diagnosed and recurrent glioblastoma

NCT Number	Study Name	Study Type	Phase	Initial vs Recurrent Disease	N	Particle Therapy Technique	Total Dose (Gy/fx)	Study Start Date	Estimated Completion Date	Primary Outcome
NCT02179086	NRG BN001	Randomized	II	Initial	606	Proton	75 Gy/30 fx	10/2021	05/2021	OS
NCT02824731	ProtoChoice-Hirn	Nonrandomized	II	Initial (supratentorial) Recurrent (>40 Gy in treatment area)	346	Proton	Initial: 54–60 Gy/30 fx Recurrent: 30 Gy/6 fx or 36 Gy/13 fx	07/2016	07/2026	Late toxicity (AE, QOL, or decreased brain function)
NCT01854554	NA	Randomized	II	Initial	90	Proton	60 Gy/30 fx	05/2013	05/2020	Time to cognitive failure
NCT04536649	NA	Randomized	III	Initial	369	Proton, Carbon ion	60 Gy/30 fx (proton) ± 15 Gy/3 fx carbon ion boost	10/2020	09/2025	OS
NCT01165671	CLEOPATRA	Randomized	II	Initial	100	Proton boost, Carbon ion boost	10 Gy/5 fx (protons) 18 Gy/6 fx (carbon ion)	07/2010	01/2015	OS
NCT00974987	NA	Nonrandomized	II	Initial	32	Boron neutron capture therapy	24 Gy/2 fx	09/2009	02/2016	OS
NCT01166308	CINDERELLA	Nonrandomized and randomized	I/II	Recurrent	56	Carbon ion	30–42 Gy/ 10–16 fx	12/2010	04/2016	1-y OS

Abbreviations: AE, adverse events; fx, fraction; N, number; NA, not available; OS, overall survival; PFS, progression-free survival; QOL, quality of life.

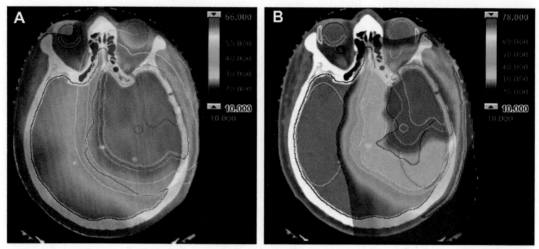

Fig. 2. Axial CT scans and corresponding isodose distributions for a patient enrolled onto the ongoing NRG BN001 clinical trial randomizing between (*A*) conventionally fractionated photon therapy (46 Gy in 23 fractions with a sequential boost to 60 Gy in 30 fractions) and (*B*) a dose-intensified schedule (75 Gy in 30 fractions with a simultaneous integrated boost of 51 Gy in 30 fractions, here depicted with proton therapy).

early dose-escalation study identified a maximum tolerated dose of 36 Gy/3 fractions.[53] The role of bevacizumab with SRS/FSRT re-irradiation (16 Gy in 1 fraction) was evaluated in a case control study that demonstrated a substantial reduction in the rate of radiation necrosis (43% vs 9%).[54] A 25-patient phase II study administered 30 Gy in 5 fractions with bevacizumab resulting in a median OS of 12.5 months and no radiation necrosis,[55] whereas another phase I study identified 33 Gy in 3 fractions as the maximum tolerated dose with bevacizumab.[56] Furthermore, a retrospective analysis of 297 patients with recurrent or residual glioblastoma treated with SRS found that bevacizumab was associated with improved OS, PFS, and reduced radiation necrosis.[57] Although the ideal dose/fractionation regimen has yet to be established, this approach should generally be limited to select patients with smaller target volumes (<5 cm).

Age
Prognosis
Performance status
Co-morbidities
Neurologic deficits
Patient preference

Local vs. marginal vs. out-of-field recurrence
Proximity to OAR's
Size of disease

Number and extent of prior surgeries
Number of prior therapies
Interval from initial RT

Favors SRS/SRT	**Favors Hypofractionation**	**Favors PRDR**
Example: 75 year old, KPS 70, distant recurrence, distant from OAR's, small size, 9 months from initial RT	Example: 62 year old, KPS 80, marginal recurrence, adjacent to OAR's, moderate size, 1 year from initial RT	Example: 48 year old, KPS 100, local recurrence, overlapping OAR's, large size, 5 years from initial RT

Fig. 3. Factors to consider for re-irradiation. KPS, Karnofsky performance status; SRT, stereotactic radiotherapy.

Hypofractionated Radiotherapy

Hypofractionated RT for re-irradiation may allow for expedited treatment compared with conventionally fractionated RT, while overcoming the toxicity associated with higher dose per fraction SRS/FSRT. However, early studies using hypofractionated RT doses of 20 to 50 Gy in 4 to 10 fractions (5 Gy per fraction) demonstrated high rates of radiation necrosis (23%–36%).[58,59] Subsequently, a lower dose per fraction regimen of 30 to 35 Gy in 10 fractions was found to have no grade 3 toxicity, but improved response rates compared with 24 Gy in 8 fractions.[60] Additional retrospective data from 147 patients supported a 35 Gy in 10 fractions regimen,[61] and led to the development of RTOG 1205, a multi-institutional phase II study of bevacizumab with or without hypofractionated RT (NCT01730950). Results were presented at the 2019 American Society of Radiation Oncology conference, demonstrating no difference in OS, but improved 6-month PFS with the addition of RT (54% vs 29%, $P = .001$).[62]

Pulsed-Reduced Dose-Rate

PRDR is a specialized technique that involves dividing the standard treatment delivery rate (4–6 Gy/min) into subfractions of approximately 0.2 Gy each, delivered at an effective dose-rate of 0.07 Gy/min.[63] Multiple series have demonstrated the safety of this approach with full-dose re-irradiation to large CNS target volumes, even with overlap of serial OARs.[64] Recently, the outcomes of a retrospective study of 80 patients with recurrent high-grade glioma (47 of whom received bevacizumab monotherapy and 33 were treated with PRDR and bevacizumab) reported improved PFS (4 vs 12 months) and OS (9 vs 16 months)[65] supporting this approach; additional results from a multicohort prospective study are forthcoming (NCT01743950).

Particle Therapy

Use of particle therapy approaches in the re-irradiation setting are limited to case series at present. In one study, patients were re-treated with a median dose of 33 Gy with proton therapy (following an initial median dose of 55 Gy and a median re-treatment interval of 16 months), resulting in a reported OS of 19.4 months.[66] The Proton Collaborative Group also reported a multi-institutional experience of re-irradiation in 45 patients to a median dose of 46.2 Gy with proton therapy (following an initial median dose of 60 Gy and a median re-treatment interval of 20 months), resulting in a reported OS of 14.2 months.[67] Prospective trials are under way to further evaluate these techniques, including the ongoing CINDERELLA trial in which patients with recurrent gliomas are randomized to carbon ion re-irradiation (dose escalation to 48 Gy in 16 fractions) or stereotactic photon RT (36 Gy in 18 fractions).[68] Several small studies have evaluated BNCT re-irradiation for recurrent malignant gliomas. A phase 1 study of 22 patients reported a median OS of 7 months following BNCT re-irradiation, whereas a more recent pilot study using BNCT re-irradiation followed by bevacizumab in 7 patients reported a median OS of 15.1 months.[69,70]

FUTURE DIRECTIONS

Although the median survival for patients with glioblastoma has remained disappointingly stagnant over the past 5 years, a number of prospective studies and clinical trials in radiation oncology have better defined key aspects of dose and fractionation, target volume delineation, particle therapies, and role of re-irradiation at the time of relapse. In addition, several innovative concepts related to radiotherapy technique and technology are currently in development. The introduction of MR linear accelerators in radiotherapy practice has allowed for frequent intrafraction imaging during chemoradiotherapy with observation of interfraction dynamic tumor morphologic changes; this may provide an avenue for on-line adaptive radiotherapy, especially in patients receiving hypofractionated treatments.[71] FLASH RT (delivered >40 Gy/s) has recently been demonstrated to provide tumor control without cognitive deficits in learning or memory in a glioblastoma mouse model; clinical systems are being outfitted with the necessary components to initiate clinical trials.[72] An in-beam PET scanner has been installed at the Italian National Center of Oncologic Hadrontherapy, which will allow for near real-time tracking and imaging of charged particles with millimetric accuracy.[73] These represent just a few of the exciting areas of RT research and development to support our overall mission to improve glioblastoma outcomes.

CLINICS CARE POINTS

- Conventionally fractionated radiotherapy to 60 Gy in 30 fractions is the standard dose for younger patients with glioblastoma with good performance status.
- Hypofractionated radiotherapy regimens are appropriate for elderly or poor performing patients who have a worse prognosis.

- Radiotherapy target volumes guidelines vary by cooperative groups.
- Several re-irradiation strategies are available, which should be chosen based on the unique clinical scenario, and are often administered in conjunction with bevacizumab.
- Owing to the poor prognosis of glioblastoma, patients should be enrolled on clinical trials when eligible.
- Numerous clinical trials assessing novel radiotherapy approaches are ongoing.

ACKNOWLEDGMENTS

None.

REFERENCES

1. Stupp R, Mason WP, van den Bent MJ, et al. Radiotherapy plus concomitant and adjuvant temozolomide for glioblastoma. N Engl J Med 2005;352(10): 987–96.
2. Walker MD, Strike TA, Sheline GE. An analysis of dose-effect relationship in the radiotherapy of malignant gliomas. Int J Radiat Oncol Biol Phys 1979; 5(10):1725–31.
3. Ali AN, Zhang P, Yung WKA, et al. NRG oncology RTOG 9006: a phase III randomized trial of hyperfractionated radiotherapy (RT) and BCNU versus standard RT and BCNU for malignant glioma patients. J Neurooncol 2018;137(1):39–47.
4. Prados MD, Wara WM, Sneed PK, et al. Phase III trial of accelerated hyperfractionation with or without difluoromethylornithine (DFMO) versus standard fractionated radiotherapy with or without DFMO for newly diagnosed patients with glioblastoma multiforme. Int J Radiat Oncol Biol Phys 2001;49(1):71–7.
5. Souhami L, Seiferheld W, Brachman D, et al. Randomized comparison of stereotactic radiosurgery followed by conventional radiotherapy with carmustine to conventional radiotherapy with carmustine for patients with glioblastoma multiforme: report of Radiation Therapy Oncology Group 93-05 protocol. Int J Radiat Oncol Biol Phys 2004;60(3):853–60.
6. Laperriere NJ, Leung PM, McKenzie S, et al. Randomized study of brachytherapy in the initial management of patients with malignant astrocytoma. Int J Radiat Oncol Biol Phys 1998;41(5):1005–11.
7. Cabrera AR, Kirkpatrick JP, Fiveash JB, et al. Radiation therapy for glioblastoma: Executive summary of an American Society for Radiation Oncology Evidence-Based Clinical Practice Guideline. Pract Radiat Oncol 2016;6(4):217–25.
8. Tsien C, Moughan J, Michalski JM, et al. Phase I three-dimensional conformal radiation dose escalation study in newly diagnosed glioblastoma: Radiation Therapy Oncology Group Trial 98-03. Int J Radiat Oncol Biol Phys 2009;73(3):699–708.
9. Tsien CI, Brown D, Normolle D, et al. Concurrent temozolomide and dose-escalated intensity-modulated radiation therapy in newly diagnosed glioblastoma. Clin Cancer Res 2012;18(1):273–9.
10. Roa W, Brasher PM, Bauman G, et al. Abbreviated course of radiation therapy in older patients with glioblastoma multiforme: a prospective randomized clinical trial. J Clin Oncol 2004;22(9):1583–8.
11. Malmstrom A, Gronberg BH, Marosi C, et al. Temozolomide versus standard 6-week radiotherapy versus hypofractionated radiotherapy in patients older than 60 years with glioblastoma: the Nordic randomised, phase 3 trial. Lancet Oncol 2012; 13(9):916–26.
12. Roa W, Kepka L, Kumar N, et al. International atomic energy agency randomized phase iii study of radiation therapy in elderly and/or frail patients with newly diagnosed glioblastoma multiforme. J Clin Oncol 2015;33(35):4145–50.
13. Perry JR, Laperriere N, O'Callaghan CJ, et al. Short-course radiation plus temozolomide in elderly patients with glioblastoma. N Engl J Med 2017; 376(11):1027–37.
14. Niyazi M, Brada M, Chalmers AJ, et al. ESTRO-ACROP guideline "target delineation of glioblastomas. Radiother Oncol 2016;118(1):35–42.
15. Kruser TJ, Bosch WR, Badiyan SN, et al. NRG brain tumor specialists consensus guidelines for glioblastoma contouring. J Neurooncol 2019;143(1):157–66.
16. Walker MD, Alexander E Jr, Hunt WE, et al. Evaluation of BCNU and/or radiotherapy in the treatment of anaplastic gliomas. A cooperative clinical trial. J Neurosurg 1978;49(3):333–43.
17. Cao Y, Tsien CI, Nagesh V, et al. Survival prediction in high-grade gliomas by MRI perfusion before and during early stage of RT [corrected]. Int J Radiat Oncol Biol Phys 2006;64(3):876–85.
18. Law M, Young RJ, Babb JS, et al. Gliomas: predicting time to progression or survival with cerebral blood volume measurements at dynamic susceptibility-weighted contrast-enhanced perfusion MR imaging. Radiology 2008;247(2):490–8.
19. Cao Y, Nagesh V, Hamstra D, et al. The extent and severity of vascular leakage as evidence of tumor aggressiveness in high-grade gliomas. Cancer Res 2006;66(17):8912–7.
20. Sugahara T, Korogi Y, Kochi M, et al. Usefulness of diffusion-weighted MRI with echo-planar technique in the evaluation of cellularity in gliomas. J Magn Reson Imaging 1999;9(1):53–60.
21. Wahl DR, Kim MM, Aryal MP, et al. Combining perfusion and high B-value diffusion MRI to inform prognosis and predict failure patterns in glioblastoma. Int J Radiat Oncol Biol Phys 2018;102(4):757–64.

22. Kim MM, Parmar HA, Aryal MP, et al. Developing a pipeline for multiparametric MRI-guided radiation therapy: initial results from a phase II clinical trial in newly diagnosed glioblastoma. Tomography 2019;5(1):118–26.

23. Law M, Cha S, Knopp EA, et al. High-grade gliomas and solitary metastases: differentiation by using perfusion and proton spectroscopic MR imaging. Radiology 2002;222(3):715–21.

24. Cordova JS, Kandula S, Gurbani S, et al. Simulating the effect of spectroscopic MRI as a metric for radiation therapy planning in patients with glioblastoma. Tomography 2016;2(4):366–73.

25. Gurbani S, Weinberg B, Cooper L, et al. The Brain Imaging Collaboration Suite (BrICS): a cloud platform for integrating whole-brain spectroscopic mri into the radiation therapy planning workflow. Tomography 2019;5(1):184–91.

26. Lee IH, Piert M, Gomez-Hassan D, et al. Association of 11C-methionine PET uptake with site of failure after concurrent temozolomide and radiation for primary glioblastoma multiforme. Int J Radiat Oncol Biol Phys 2009;73(2):479–85.

27. Erratum to: Iuchi T, Hatano K, Uchino Y, et al. Methionine uptake and required radiation dose to control glioblastoma. Int J Radiat Oncol Biol Phys 2015;93: 133-140. Int J Radiat Oncol Biol Phys 2016;94(1): 215.

28. Sherriff J, Tamangani J, Senthil L, et al. Patterns of relapse in glioblastoma multiforme following concomitant chemoradiotherapy with temozolomide. Br J Radiol 2013;86(1022):20120414.

29. Piroth MD, Pinkawa M, Holy R, et al. Integrated boost IMRT with FET-PET-adapted local dose escalation in glioblastomas. Results of a prospective phase II study. Strahlenther Onkol 2012;188(4): 334–9.

30. Oehlke O, Mix M, Graf E, et al. Amino-acid PET versus MRI guided re irradiation in patients with recurrent glioblastoma multiforme (GLIAA) - protocol of a randomized phase II trial (NOA 10/ARO 2013-1). BMC Cancer 2016;16(1):769.

31. Li F, Zhou K, Gao L, et al. Radiation induces the generation of cancer stem cells: A novel mechanism for cancer radioresistance. Oncol Lett 2016;12(5): 3059–65.

32. Lomax AJ. Charged particle therapy: the physics of interaction. Cancer J 2009;15(4):285–91.

33. Lomax A. Intensity modulation methods for proton radiotherapy. Phys Med Biol 1999;44(1):185–205.

34. Seidel S, Garvalov BK, Wirta V, et al. A hypoxic niche regulates glioblastoma stem cells through hypoxia inducible factor 2 alpha. Brain 2010;133(Pt 4): 983–95.

35. Dennis ER, Bussiere MR, Niemierko A, et al. A comparison of critical structure dose and toxicity risks in patients with low grade gliomas treated with IMRT versus proton radiation therapy. Technol Cancer Res Treat 2013;12(1):1–9.

36. Harrabi SB, Bougatf N, Mohr A, et al. Dosimetric advantages of proton therapy over conventional radiotherapy with photons in young patients and adults with low-grade glioma. Strahlenther Onkol 2016; 192(11):759–69.

37. Weber DC, Lim PS, Tran S, et al. Proton therapy for brain tumours in the area of evidence-based medicine. Br J Radiol 2020;93(1107):20190237.

38. Mizumoto M, Tsuboi K, Igaki H, et al. Phase I/II trial of hyperfractionated concomitant boost proton radiotherapy for supratentorial glioblastoma multiforme. Int J Radiat Oncol Biol Phys 2010;77(1): 98–105.

39. Fitzek MM, Thornton AF, Rabinov JD, et al. Accelerated fractionated proton/photon irradiation to 90 cobalt gray equivalent for glioblastoma multiforme: results of a phase II prospective trial. J Neurosurg 1999;91(2):251–60.

40. Adeberg S, Bernhardt D, Harrabi SB, et al. Sequential proton boost after standard chemoradiation for high-grade glioma. Radiother Oncol 2017;125(2): 266–72.

41. Fitzek MM, Thornton AF, Harsh Gt, et al. Dose-escalation with proton/photon irradiation for Daumas-Duport lower-grade glioma: results of an institutional phase I/II trial. Int J Radiat Oncol Biol Phys 2001; 51(1):131–7.

42. Mizumoto M, Yamamoto T, Takano S, et al. Long-term survival after treatment of glioblastoma multiforme with hyperfractionated concomitant boost proton beam therapy. Pract Radiat Oncol 2015; 5(1):e9–16.

43. Mizoe JE, Tsujii H, Hasegawa A, et al. Phase I/II clinical trial of carbon ion radiotherapy for malignant gliomas: combined X-ray radiotherapy, chemotherapy, and carbon ion radiotherapy. Int J Radiat Oncol Biol Phys 2007,69(2).390–6.

44. Combs SE, Kieser M, Rieken S, et al. Randomized phase II study evaluating a carbon ion boost applied after combined radiochemotherapy with temozolomide versus a proton boost after radiochemotherapy with temozolomide in patients with primary glioblastoma: the CLEOPATRA trial. BMC Cancer 2010;10:478.

45. Miyatake SI, Wanibuchi M, Hu N, et al. Boron neutron capture therapy for malignant brain tumors. J Neurooncol 2020;149(1):1–11.

46. Chanana AD, Capala J, Chadha M, et al. Boron neutron capture therapy for glioblastoma multiforme: interim results from the phase I/II dose-escalation studies. Neurosurgery 1999;44(6):1182–92 [discussion: 1192–3].

47. Busse PM, Harling OK, Palmer MR, et al. A critical examination of the results from the Harvard-MIT NCT program phase I clinical trial of neutron capture

therapy for intracranial disease. J Neurooncol 2003; 62(1–2):111–21.

48. Vos MJ, Turowski B, Zanella FE, et al. Radiologic findings in patients treated with boron neutron capture therapy for glioblastoma multiforme within EORTC trial 11961. Int J Radiat Oncol Biol Phys 2005;61(2):392–9.

49. Joensuu H, Kankaanranta L, Seppala T, et al. Boron neutron capture therapy of brain tumors: clinical trials at the finnish facility using boronophenylalanine. J Neurooncol 2003;62(1–2):123–34.

50. Henriksson R, Capala J, Michanek A, et al. Boron neutron capture therapy (BNCT) for glioblastoma multiforme: a phase II study evaluating a prolonged high-dose of boronophenylalanine (BPA). Radiother Oncol 2008;88(2):183–91.

51. Kawabata S, Miyatake S, Kuroiwa T, et al. Boron neutron capture therapy for newly diagnosed glioblastoma. J Radiat Res 2009;50(1):51–60.

52. Kawabata S, Miyatake S, Hiramatsu R, et al. Phase II clinical study of boron neutron capture therapy combined with X-ray radiotherapy/temozolomide in patients with newly diagnosed glioblastoma multiforme–study design and current status report. Appl Radiat Isot 2011;69(12):1796–9.

53. Schwer AL, Damek DM, Kavanagh BD, et al. A phase I dose-escalation study of fractionated stereotactic radiosurgery in combination with gefitinib in patients with recurrent malignant gliomas. Int J Radiat Oncol Biol Phys 2008;70(4):993–1001.

54. Park KJ, Kano H, Iyer A, et al. Salvage gamma knife stereotactic radiosurgery followed by bevacizumab for recurrent glioblastoma multiforme: a case-control study. J Neurooncol 2012;107(2):323–33.

55. Gutin PH, Iwamoto FM, Beal K, et al. Safety and efficacy of bevacizumab with hypofractionated stereotactic irradiation for recurrent malignant gliomas. Int J Radiat Oncol Biol Phys 2009;75(1):156–63.

56. Clarke J, Neil E, Terziev R, et al. Multicenter, Phase 1, Dose escalation study of hypofractionated stereotactic radiation therapy with bevacizumab for recurrent glioblastoma and anaplastic astrocytoma. Int J Radiat Oncol Biol Phys 2017;99(4):797–804.

57. Niranjan A, Monaco EA III, Kano H, et al. Stereotactic radiosurgery in the multimodality management of residual or recurrent glioblastoma multiforme. Prog Neurol Surg 2018;31:48–61.

58. Shepherd SF, Laing RW, Cosgrove VP, et al. Hypofractionated stereotactic radiotherapy in the management of recurrent glioma. Int J Radiat Oncol Biol Phys 1997;37(2):393–8.

59. Laing RW, Warrington AP, Graham J, et al. Efficacy and toxicity of fractionated stereotactic radiotherapy in the treatment of recurrent gliomas (phase I/II study). Radiother Oncol 1993;27(1):22–9.

60. Hudes RS, Corn BW, Werner-Wasik M, et al. A phase I dose escalation study of hypofractionated stereotactic radiotherapy as salvage therapy for persistent or recurrent malignant glioma. Int J Radiat Oncol Biol Phys 1999;43(2):293–8.

61. Fogh SE, Andrews DW, Glass J, et al. Hypofractionated stereotactic radiation therapy: an effective therapy for recurrent high-grade gliomas. J Clin Oncol 2010;28(18):3048–53.

62. Tsien C, Pugh S, Dicker AP, et al. Randomized Phase II trial of re-irradiation and concurrent bevacizumab versus bevacizumab alone as treatment for recurrent glioblastoma (NRG Oncology/RTOG 1205): Initial Outcomes and RT Plan Quality Report. Int J Radiat Oncol Biol Phys 2019;105(1, Supplement):S78.

63. Cannon GM, Tome WA, Robins HI, et al. Pulsed reduced dose-rate radiotherapy: case report : a novel re-treatment strategy in the management of recurrent glioblastoma multiforme. J Neurooncol 2007;83(3):307–11.

64. Murphy ES, Rogacki K, Godley A, et al. Intensity modulated radiation therapy with pulsed reduced dose rate as a reirradiation strategy for recurrent central nervous system tumors: An institutional series and literature review. Pract Radiat Oncol 2017; 7(6):e391–9.

65. Bovi JA, Prah MA, Retzlaff AA, et al. Pulsed reduced dose rate radiotherapy in conjunction with bevacizumab or bevacizumab alone in recurrent high-grade glioma: survival outcomes. Int J Radiat Oncol Biol Phys 2020;108(4):979–86.

66. Mizumoto M, Okumura T, Ishikawa E, et al. Reirradiation for recurrent malignant brain tumor with radiotherapy or proton beam therapy. Technical considerations based on experience at a single institution. Strahlenther Onkol 2013;189(8):656–63.

67. Saeed AM, Khairnar R, Sharma AM, et al. Clinical outcomes in patients with recurrent glioblastoma treated with proton beam therapy reirradiation: analysis of the multi-institutional proton collaborative group registry. Adv Radiat Oncol 2020;5(5):978–83.

68. Combs SE, Burkholder I, Edler L, et al. Randomised phase I/II study to evaluate carbon ion radiotherapy versus fractionated stereotactic radiotherapy in patients with recurrent or progressive gliomas: the CINDERELLA trial. BMC Cancer 2010;10:533.

69. Kankaanranta L, Seppala T, Koivunoro H, et al. L-boronophenylalanine-mediated boron neutron capture therapy for malignant glioma progressing after external beam radiation therapy: a Phase I study. Int J Radiat Oncol Biol Phys 2011;80(2):369–76.

70. Shiba H, Takeuchi K, Hiramatsu R, et al. Boron neutron capture therapy combined with early successive bevacizumab treatments for recurrent malignant gliomas - a pilot study. Neurol Med Chir (Tokyo) 2018;58(12):487–94.

71. Stewart J, Sahgal A, Lee Y, et al. Quantitating interfraction target dynamics during concurrent

chemoradiation for glioblastoma: a prospective serial imaging study. Int J Radiat Oncol Biol Phys 2021; 109(3):736–46. https://doi.org/10.1016/j.ijrobp.2020.10.002.

72. Montay-Gruel P, Acharya MM, Goncalves Jorge P, et al. Hypo-fractionated FLASH-RT as an effective treatment against glioblastoma that reduces neurocognitive side effects in mice. Clin Cancer Res 2021;27(3):775–84. https://doi.org/10.1158/1078-0432.CCR-20-0894.

73. Bisogni MG, Attili A, Battistoni G, et al. INSIDE in-beam positron emission tomography system for particle range monitoring in hadrontherapy. J Med Imaging (Bellingham) 2017;4(1):011005.

74. Andersen AP. Postoperative irradiation of glioblas-tomas. Results in a randomized series. Acta Radiol Oncol Radiat Phys Biol 1978;17(6):475–84.

75. Bleehen NM, Stenning SP. A Medical Research Council trial of two radiotherapy doses in the treat-ment of grades 3 and 4 astrocytoma. the medical research council brain tumour working party. Br J Cancer 1991;64(4):769–74.

76. Glinski B. Postoperative hypofractionated radio-therapy versus conventionally fractionated radiotherapy in malignant gliomas. A preliminary report on a randomized trial. J Neurooncol 1993; 16(2):167–72.

77. Keime-Guibert F, Chinot O, Taillandier L, et al. Radio-therapy for glioblastoma in the elderly. N Engl J Med 2007;356(15):1527–35.

78. Kristiansen K, Hagen S, Kollevold T, et al. Combined modality therapy of operated astrocytomas grade III and IV. Confirmation of the value of postoperative irradiation and lack of potentiation of bleomycin on survival time: a prospective multicenter trial of the Scandinavian Glioblastoma Study Group. Cancer 1981;47(4):649–52.

79. Phillips C, Guiney M, Smith J, et al. A randomized trial comparing 35Gy in ten fractions with 60Gy in 30 fractions of cerebral irradiation for glioblastoma multiforme and older patients with anaplastic astro-cytoma. Radiother Oncol 2003;68(1):23–6.

80. Shin KH, Urtasun RC, Fulton D, et al. Multiple daily fractionated radiation therapy and misonidazole in the management of malignant astrocytoma. A pre-liminary report. Cancer 1985;56(4):758–60.

Brain Tumor Vaccines

Justin Lee, BA, Benjamin R. Uy, MD, PhD, Linda M. Liau, MD, PhD, MBA*

KEYWORDS

- Brain tumor vaccines • Brain tumor immunotherapy • Dendritic cell vaccines • Peptide vaccines

KEY POINTS

- Vaccines are capable of mounting a peripheral immune response that can penetrate the blood brain barrier for the treatment of brain tumors.
- Peptide vaccines against epithelial growth factor receptor variant III, survivin, various heat shock protein complexes, and personalized tumor antigens have been developed for the treatment of glioblastoma.
- Dendritic cell vaccines can be designed against a variety of targets including tumor lysate, known antigens, and messenger RNA to combat high-grade gliomas and have demonstrated robust immune responses.

INTRODUCTION

Vaccines are regarded as one of the most impactful medical advancements because they have had tremendous success reducing morbidity and mortality associated with many infectious diseases. Modern vaccination began with Dr Edward Jenner's experiments to inoculate patients with cowpox—a mild, noncontagious disease—to prevent the far deadlier smallpox. Widespread vaccination led to the complete eradication of smallpox while continued technological advancement has resulted in the development of licensed vaccines for more than 30 diseases, which are estimated to save 2 to 3 million lives each year.[1,2]

Adaptive or acquired immunity is achieved through exposure to a pathogen or vaccination. This arm of the immune system is specific to particular pathogens and can provide long-lasting protection. Fundamentally, vaccines exert their effects by activating a patients' adaptive immune system against a target that resembles a pathogen or toxin. To accomplish successful immune system stimulation, 2 broad categories of vaccines have been developed: live attenuated vaccines and subunit vaccines.[3] Upon interacting with the vaccine, antigen-presenting cells (ie, macrophages, dendritic cells [DC], B cells) recognize the foreign antigens and load them onto major histocompatibility complex (MHC class I or II) for presentation to the adaptive arm of the immune system. Direct MHC I presentation to CD8+ cytotoxic T cells results in a cell-mediated response and the destruction of target cells. MHC II presentation to CD4+ helper T cells can further facilitate a cytotoxic response or stimulate a humoral immunity by activating B cells to produce antibodies. These antibodies can bind pathogens, resulting in neutralization and increased phagocytosis of antibody-bound antigen. Importantly, memory cells are also created and remain dormant until re-exposure to the infectious agent or toxin, resulting in restimulation of the immune cascade and pathogen elimination.[4]

Interest in using the immune system to fight malignancies has exploded in recent years.[5] Immunotherapies such as chimeric antigen receptor T cells prime engineered T cells to kill cancer cells and immune checkpoint inhibitors work to activate the immune system by disinhibiting tumor immune suppression.[6,7] One challenge in using the immune system stems from immune cells' ability to precisely distinguish "self" from "foreign" tissues to prevent autoimmunity. Most antigens expressed by cancers are self-antigens present on normal tissue, which may be slightly immunogenic or nonreactive. Therapeutic cancer vaccines have the potential to increase the immune

UCLA Department of Neurosurgery, David Geffen School of Medicine at UCLA, University of California Los Angeles, 300 Stein Plaza Driveway Suite 420 Los Angeles, CA 90095, USA
* Corresponding author.
E-mail address: LLIAU@mednet.ucla.edu

Neurosurg Clin N Am 32 (2021) 225–234
https://doi.org/10.1016/j.nec.2021.01.003
1042-3680/21/© 2021 Elsevier Inc. All rights reserved.

system's antitumor activity by training immune cells to target antigens expressed on cancers. Although vaccination has had tremendous success in preventing infectious disease and virally initiated cancers, namely, liver and cervical cancers caused by hepatitis B virus and human papillomavirus, respectively, vaccination as therapy against established disease has proven much more challenging.[8–10] Immune system evasion is a hallmark of cancers that represents a major hurdle for vaccine development. Cancers actively disguise themselves from immune cells by creating an immunosuppressive tumor microenvironment to dampen the immune system's cancer-fighting potential.[6] However, recent clinical results have shown clinical benefit and established therapeutic cancer vaccination as an attractive platform for further development.

In 2010, the US Food and Drug Administration approved the first therapeutic cancer vaccine (sipuleucel-T) composed of peripheral blood mononuclear cells stimulated against a recombinant fusion protein for the treatment of castration-resistant prostate cancer.[7] Therapeutic vaccines have since been developed for breast cancer, lung cancer, melanoma, pancreatic cancer, colorectal cancer, and renal cancer. These vaccines stimulate the immune system against tumor-associated antigens (TAAs), tumor-specific antigens, or neoantigens on malignant tumor cells. TAAs such as HER2/NEU are often overexpressed in malignancy, but are also expressed at lower levels in some healthy tissues.[11] One example of exploiting this increased expression of these genes in cancer includes the antibody-based immunotoxins against mesothelin, an overexpressed TAA. The treatment of advanced mesothelioma, as well as lung, pancreatic, and ovarian cancers demonstrated cancer regression without appreciable toxicity.[12] Tumor-specific antigens and neoantigens also present attractive targets because they are mutated antigens resulting from genomic instability and represent a unique cancer-specific target. However, these targets are not globally expressed across all tumor cells and are restricted to the subclonal populations within the heterogenous cancer. Previous work demonstrated the safety and immunogenicity of a vaccine targeting 20 predicted personal tumor neoantigens in melanoma, warranting further study.[13]

Although improvements have been made in the design and production of therapeutic vaccines, further developments are required to induce robust CD4[+] and CD8[+] effector function against tumor cells while avoiding induction of autoimmunity, immune reaction–like cytokine storm, or on-target off-tumor toxicity. Additionally, the efficacy of cancer vaccines and immunotherapy in general correlates with tumor mutational burden and microsatellite instability; as mutations increase, antigenic targets for the immune system to activate against also expands.[14] Innovations in cellular engineering have enabled adoptive cell therapy, where patients' own immune cells are isolated and either engineered or stimulated ex vivo to enhance their cancer-fighting capabilities.[15] DC vaccines are one type of adoptive therapy in which isolated DCs are stimulated with tumor markers ex vivo and reintroduced to the patient to activate cytotoxic and humoral immunity and importantly have the ability to target multiple antigens in parallel to enhance antitumor effects.[16]

Gliomas represent approximately 81% of newly diagnosed malignant primary brain tumors and glioblastomas are the most aggressive type, with less than 3% of patients surviving 5 years and a mean survival of less than 15 months.[17] Despite an increasingly comprehensive understanding of the molecular drivers of glioblastoma, targeted therapies have remained largely ineffective in improving prognosis beyond standard therapy of surgical resection, radiation, and chemotherapy.[18] Because of this poor prognosis, novel innovative treatments are needed such as cancer vaccines, which have the potential to overcome the challenges faced by previous treatments. However, vaccine development must still address challenges resulting from rapid growth, tumor heterogeneity, low tumor mutational burden, and immunosuppression in brain cancers.[19] Under physiologic conditions, the brain parenchyma is tightly shielded from the systemic immune system via the blood–brain barrier and minimal lymphatic vessels for antigen presenting cells to traffic to lymph nodes.[20] Additionally, microglia, brain resident macrophages, establish the bulk of the immune cell population, but have lower antigen-presenting capacity than other cells of the macrophage lineage.[21] Another important consideration for brain tumors is the recruitment of myeloid and lymphoid cells that play an integral role in supporting malignant growth. Tumor-associated macrophages represent the most abundant stromal cell type in glioblastoma, constituting 30% of the tumor mass and skew toward the immunosuppressive M2 phenotype, which inhibits CD4[+] and CD8[+] T-cell functions while inducing T regulatory cell differentiation.[22] T regulatory cells secrete IL-10 to contribute to immunosuppression and tumor-infiltrating lymphocytes display high levels of programmed death 1, CTLA-4, LAG3, TIM3, TIGIT, and CD39, which all indicate T-cell exhaustion.[23,24] These factors contribute to an immunosuppressive environment, or immunologically cold tumors, which generally demonstrate a poor response to immunostimulatory therapies such as therapeutic cancer vaccines.[20]

Advancements in neuro-oncology, including the discovery of new therapeutic targets, the development of mechanisms to increase tumor sensitivity to current immunotherapies, and an improvement in the tumor-specific pathway targeting have opened the doors to developing therapeutic vaccines for brain tumors.

PEPTIDE VACCINES

After the cloning of the first human TAA gene in the early 1990s, peptide vaccines were developed to stimulate patient's immune system against both TAAs and neoantigens.[25] Peptide vaccines offer the potential to induce T-cell–based killing and antibody production against foreign tumor antigens. They are generally made of amino acid sequences of various lengths attached to an immunogenic adjuvant to increase immunogenicity.[26] The administration of a synthetic or naturally occurring polypeptide vaccine results in uptake, processing, and presentation via MHC I on APCs, or direct insertion into MHC II, which ultimately leads to the activation of the adaptive immune response against the administered antigen. Through antigen-presenting cells interaction with naïve lymphocytes, CD8+ T cells directly targeting cancer cells or CD4+ T cells boosting antitumor immunity are activated as cancer-fighting agents (Fig. 1).[27,28]

One of the first protein-based vaccines was against epithelial growth factor receptor variant III (EGFRvIII), a cell membrane receptor unique to cancer cells. The EGFRvIII tumor-specific antigen results from a frame deletion mutation of exons 2 to 7 in the extracellular domain of EGFR, which creates a unique glycine residue between exons 1 and 8 that can be exploited therapeutically.[29–32] It is an attractive target for a peptide vaccine because it is expressed in breast, ovarian, and lung malignancies in addition to approximately 24% to 67% of glioblastoma cases, and it is absent in normal tissue.[33] The EGFRvIII peptide vaccine aims to stimulate a patient's immune system against EGFRvIII-positive glioblastoma cells. Phase I/II trials of CDX-110 (rindopepimut), a 14-mer peptide conjugated to the keyhole limpet hemocyanin (an immunostimulatory carrier protein) peptide vaccine injected intradermally, demonstrated safety,

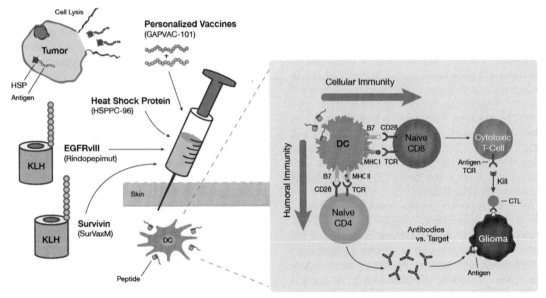

Fig. 1. Peptide and HSP vaccines. Peptides can be conjugated to immunogenic haptens (ie, keyhole limpet hemocyanin [KLH]) linked to EGFRvIII peptide (PEPvIII-KLH) rindopepimut or survivin peptide (Survivin-KLH, SurVaxM) for vaccine preparation and administered intradermally. Mixture of personalized peptide antigen vaccines (GAPVAC-101[APVAC1:unmutated + APVAC2:neoantigens]) based on patient tumor specific profile. Heat shock peptide-proteins complex-96 (HSPPC-96) is extracted from patient's tumor samples, purified, and injected in a similar manner as peptide vaccines. The antigen(s) recognized by antigen presentation cells (DCs) and presented to helper T-cells (CD4+) and cytotoxic T-cell lymphocytes (CTL, CD8+). Activated B-cells then produce antibodies to the peptide.

a tumor-specific immune response, and improved survival compared with matched control patients. However, the phase III double-blind randomized control trial (ACT IV) unfortunately showed no significant difference between the control and vaccine groups, and the trial was discontinued.[34–37] In the vaccine group, patients expressed increased EGFRvIII antibody production and the majority of resected recurrent tumors were negative for EGFRvIII. These data suggested that the EGFRvIII peptide vaccine successfully targeted EGFRvIII positive tumor cells but in the process selected for EGFRvIII negative or low expressing tumor cells. Therefore, in a heterogenous tumor such as glioblastoma, single antigen therapy may have very limited success rate despite measurable positive immune response.

Peptide vaccines have also been developed for additional glioma specific mutations including variants of the isocitrate dehydrogenase type 1 (IDH1) and histone-3 genes. IDH1 mutations most often occur at the Arg132 residue in the catalytic pocket, promoting malignant transformation and genomic hypermethylation.[38,39] More than 70% of diffuse grade II and III gliomas contain the IDH1(R132H) mutation, which is an immunogenic epitope that can be targeted via peptide vaccination.[40] Preclinical data demonstrated that IDH1(R132H) peptide vaccines are presented on MHC II and induce mutation-specific CD4$^+$ T-cell activation and antibody production.[41] Multiple phase I trials have been launched to determine vaccine safety (NCT02454634, NCT02193347).[42] Similarly, in aggressive midline gliomas, K27M mutations in the histone-3 gene result in methylation pattern alterations and subsequent changes in gene expression.[43] Preclinical work demonstrated that H3K27M peptide vaccines are presented via MHC I and elicit mutation-specific CD4$^+$ and CD8$^+$ immune responses in MHC-humanized mice.[44] A phase I clinical trial evaluating a synthetic peptide targeting the H3.3.K27 M protein is underway (NCT02960230).

Another target for peptide vaccination is survivin, a tumor-associated antigen that is a membrane inhibitor of apoptosis and regulator of the cell cycle. Its expression is absent in terminally differentiated tissues but present in various cancer types, including glioblastoma.[45] A peptide vaccine targeting survivin is currently under investigation. The vaccine uses a 15-mer survivin peptide linked to keyhole limpet hemocyanin (SurVaxM) to stimulate an immunogenic response. Early clinical trial data demonstrated antibody production and T-cell response to survivin vaccine. A phase I trial of recurrent malignant glioma patients with surviving-positive tumors

were given subcutaneous SurVaxM with sargramostim, a bone marrow stimulant, at 2-week intervals. SurVaxM administration was well tolerated. 6 of 8 immunologically evaluable patients demonstrated IgG production against the survivin peptide and increased survivin responsive CD4$^+$ and CD8$^+$ T cells. The median overall survival was 86.6 weeks from study entry with 7 of the 9 patients surviving more than 12 months.[46] An early phase II trial is underway for patients newly diagnosed with glioblastoma with restricted HLA types (HLA-A*02/03/11/24 haplotype) (https://clinicaltrials.gov/ct2/show/ NCT02455557). The data so far are optimistic with a 12-month overall survival of 94.2%.[47]

To overcome the challenges associated with single antigen therapies, peptide vaccines targeting multiple glioblastoma antigens have been developed as personalized therapeutic vaccines. This new strategy seeks to exploit multiple antigens to overcome the low mutational burden involving around 30 to 50 nonsynonymous mutations and the immunosuppressive environment of glioblastoma.[48] A recent study demonstrated that a multiepitope, personalized neoantigen-based vaccine based on patient's tumor transcriptomes and immunopeptidomes is feasible for patients with glioblastoma. This phase I/Ib study compared resected glioblastoma tissue with healthy tissue via whole-exome sequencing and RNA sequencing data to determine neoantigens. From these data and using patient-specific HLA allotype assessment, peptides with high predicted HLA binding affinity were designed and synthesized. The neoantigen peptide vaccine library was administered after radiotherapy and stimulated a neoantigen-specific T-cell response in patients with an increased concentration of circulating and tumor-infiltrating T cells in vaccine treated patients. While demonstrating that personalized neoantigens can favorably alter the immune landscape in a glioblastoma, tumor-infiltrating T cells after vaccination expressed multiple co-inhibitory receptors, consistent with an exhaustion phenotype.[49] An additional study, the phase I trial GAPVAC-101 of the Glioma Actively Personalized Vaccine Consortium, used both unmutated antigens and neoepitopes in an effort to increase immune cell activity against the limited glioblastoma target space. This study similarly demonstrated feasibility with an activation of CD8$^+$ T cells and the development of a sustained response via memory T cells using the unmutated APVAC1 antigen panel or a predominantly CD4$^+$ T-cell response using the APVAC2 neoantigen vaccine.[50]

Another type of peptide vaccine that has garnered interest for their immunogenic properties are heat shock proteins (HSPs). HSPs are produced by cells in response to stressful conditions and provide a physiologic link between the innate and adaptive immune systems through chaperoning antigens to APCs like DCs. During cell stress, HSPs are expressed intracellularly and bind misfolded proteins to prevent aggregation. HSPs loaded with protein may be released into circulation and bind to CD91 receptors on APCs to initiate both MCH I and II presentation.[51] In malignancy, HSPs bind to tumor specific neoantigens to activate both innate and adaptive immunity against patient-specific cancer mutations. To leverage this physiologic role of HSP, tumor cells are lysed and the HSPs of interest are isolated for intradermal vaccines. To date, HSP–antigen complexes have been used in a variety of cancer types including melanoma,[52,53] renal cell carcinoma,[54] colorectal cancer,[55] and gliobastoma,[55,56] and have been well-tolerated with a low toxicity. Despite optimistic findings in early phase clinical trials, a larger phase II randomized trial treating recurrent patients with glioblastoma with HSP peptide complex 96 (HSPPC-96) failed to show survival benefit when compared with

bevacizumab alone (overall survival 7.5 vs 10.7).[57] However, experiments measuring INF-γ release demonstrated increased tumor-specific peripheral blood mononuclear cells after exposure to autologous tumor lysate.[58] Because the data for patients with newly diagnosed glioma continue to demonstrate increased survival when programmed death ligand 1 is upregulated on myeloid cells, a phase II trial of HSPPC-96 with patients newly diagnosed with glioblastoma with and without programmed death 1 inhibitor pembrolizumab (NCT03018288) is underway.[59]

DENDRITIC CELL VACCINES

Different from peptide vaccines, which rely on a host's ability to direct pathogens to APCs, DC vaccines are directly primed against specific targets to mount a robust immune response against tumor cells. DCs are professional APCs capable of activating adaptive immunity through the presentation of epitopes that can be harnessed to combat tumor cells. Most autologous DC vaccines are made from DCs extracted from patients through leukapheresis and exposed ex vivo to tumor-associated antigens (peptides or messenger RNA) of choice. The cells are then

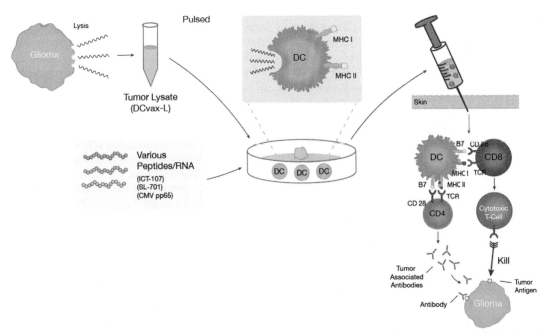

Fig. 2. DC vaccines. DCs isolated from peripheral blood leukapheresis are pulsed against tumor associated antigen, messenger RNA, or lysate, that is, *ICT107*: HER2, TRP-2, gp100, MAGE-1, IL13Ra2 and AIM-2, *SL701*: ILRa2, ephA2, surviving, *DCVax-L* (autologous tumor lysate), or *CMV pp65*. Primed DCs are then administered as a vaccine to patients peripherally. Following injection, DCs then recruit CTLs and stimulate antibody production against tumor epitopes. Activated cytotoxic T-cells and antibodies cross the blood brain barrier and target tumor cells with the surface receptor.

delivered either peripherally or intracranially to the patient to generate a cell-mediated and humoral immune response against various targets (**Fig. 2**). DC vaccines are capable of stimulating T cells to cross the blood–brain barrier. Additionally, they have a low toxicity profile. The ability of DCs to target multiple antigens provides an advantage compared with single antigen therapies when treating tumors with heterogeneous cell populations.

DCs pulsed with known antigens demonstrated an increased overall survival and immune response in preclinical models and clinical trials. In an early phase I study of multiple-peptide pulsed DC vaccine (ICT-107), in patients with newly diagnosed glioma with HLA-A1 or HLA-A2 and at least 1 TAA (HER2, TRP-2, gp100, MAGE-1, IL13-Rα2, or AIM-2) were given 3 intradermal doses of DCs pulsed with TAA along with standard chemotherapy and radiation. At an average follow-up of 40.1 months, 6 of 16 patients with newly diagnosed glioblastomas had no evidence of tumor recurrence. Overall, the phase I trial showed promise with an increased (median progression-free survival of 16.9 months and a median overall survival of 38.4 months).[60] In a randomized phase II multicenter trial (NCT01280552, n = 124), patients receiving the DCs pulsed with TAAs had greater progression-free survival without a significant improvement to overall survival (progression-free survival of 11.2 months vs 9.0 months [$P = .011$] and overall survival of 18.3 months vs 16.7 months [$P = .64$]).[61] Based on this trial, an HLA-A2 patient subpopulation was identified to have a significantly increased overall survival and increased responder rates for a phase III trial (STING, NCT02546102). Unfortunately, STING for HLA-A2 newly diagnosed glioma was terminated owing to an inability to secure funding. With the success of the multiple peptide vaccine, another autologous DC vaccine pulsed with known TAAs—IL13-Rα2, EphrinA2 and Survivin (trade name: SL701)—was developed. Currently, SL701 with or without Avastin (bevacizumab) is under phase II investigation (NCT02078648).[62]

Human cytomegalovirus (CMV) proteins are another interesting target being studied for DC vaccines. Some reports suggest that human CMV is frequently expressed in glioblastomas but absent in surrounding normal tissue.[63–65] CMV pp65 is a major CMV structural tegument protein found in a subset of glioblastoma cells. DCs pulsed with messenger RNA for pp65 generated T cells against CMV pp65. Early phase I trials for patients newly diagnosed with glioblastoma treated with DC pulsed with CMV pp65 messenger RNA demonstrated increased survival, safety, and significant immune response against pp65.[66,67] Larger phase II studies of DC-pp65 have since demonstrated reproducibility of previous clinical trial data with, an overall survival of 37.7 and 38.3 months in the ATTAC-GM and ATTAC-Td studies, respectively. The most recent study also demonstrated increased DC migration to the draining lymph nodes bilaterally.[68] Further trials will be conducted to examine CMV pp65 vaccine's efficacy alone or in combination with varlilumab for the activation of CD27+ lymphocytes (NCT03688178, NCT02465268).

Because DCs can mount an immune response to a series of known antigens, DCs exposed to unknown antigens through autologous tumor lysates could also generate systemic immune responses against a variety of tumor cells, with a possible benefit to overall survival. DCs pulsed with autologous human tumor lysate that is, either acid-eluted or freeze-thawed (DCVax-L) provide a patient-specific vaccine based on a patient's resected tumor and covers a wide array of epitopes. In a phase I trial, 12 patients (5 recurrent and 7 newly diagnosed patients) treated with DCVax-L showed an improved median progression-free survival (median progression-free survival of 19.9 months vs 8.2 months) and overall survival (median overall survival of 35.8 months vs 18.3 months) compared with historic controls with 50% survival at 2 years and 2 patients still alive at the time of publication (>58.0 and >48.4 months).[69] These patients are still alive today, over 16 years since the conclusion of this initial Phase I trial. Six of the 12 patients developed a systemic cytotoxic T-lymphocyte response on in vitro lysis assays, 4 of the 8 patients had tumor-infiltrating lymphocytes on reresection, and 1 patient showed objective MRI changes after injection. This phase I trial showed safety, bioactivity, and feasibility, and led to a randomized, multi-institute, double-blind, placebo-controlled phase III clinical trial (NCT00045968) of DCVax-L. The phase III trial compared chemoradiation (n = 99) with DCVax-L plus chemoradiation (n = 232) for patients newly diagnosed with glioblastoma in a 2:1 randomization, with crossover upon progression.[70] Because datalock was just recently completed at the time of this writing, the data remain blinded for this trial. However, a recent interim update showed that the overall survival seems to be favorable (intention-to-treat median overall survival of 23.1 months; 2-year survival rate of 46.2%; 3-year survival rate of 25.4%) and continues to be well-tolerated with low levels of adverse events. Also, as expected, the overall survival correlated with the extent of the resection.[51] In contrast, DC lysate In order to further enhance the efficacy of DCVax-L, a phase II randomized trial for recurrent glioma patients treated in combination with with DCVax-L in combination with with programmed death 1 blockade (NCT03014804) is underway.

SUMMARY

Glioblastoma treatments are in dire need of additional therapeutic options. Peptide and DC vaccines have demonstrated safety as potential treatments for brain tumors. A few treatments including SurVaxM and DCVax-L show early promising results with data from DCVax-L pending evaluation of phase III data. Cancer vaccines activate robust antitumor responses through immunostimulation against cancer antigens or transfusion of DCs stimulated ex vivo against tumor antigens to initiate adaptive immunity. Importantly, vaccines have shown the ability to induce antitumor T-cell trafficking and antibody production across the blood–brain barrier. GAPVAC-101 and DCVax-L also have the benefit of activating an immune response against multiple cancer antigens, and DCVax-L in particular can target unknown antigens by pulsing the cells with autologous tumor lysate, thereby potentially overcoming the problem of tumor heterogeneity. Recent results have demonstrated the potential for cancer vaccines to become an important therapeutic option in addition to surgery, radiation, and chemotherapy.

Although tumor vaccines have shown potential, there are still many opportunities to improve their cancer fighting capabilities. Activated T cells that migrate to the tumor face a harshly immunosuppressive environment and previous studies have demonstrated that vaccine-stimulated T cells exhibit many of the classic exhaustion markers once they engage with the cancer. To overcome these challenges, combination therapies incorporating both tumor vaccines and checkpoint inhibitors or immunostimulants are currently underway. Furthermore, vaccines targeting single antigens create selection pressure for tumor cells expressing the antigen at lower levels, which leads to therapeutic resistance. Vaccines targeting a broader cancer antigen landscape have been developed, but their efficacy must be validated and reproduced in larger studies. There have also been great strides made in using patient-specific tumor transcriptome or proteome data to develop personalize vaccines. This strategy can identify personalized neoantigens to combat the heterogenous glioblastoma tumor population, but the efficacy of targeting predicted neoantigens in glioblastoma is only theoretical and further research is needed to determine their effectiveness.

CLINICS CARE POINTS

- Brain tumor vaccines tested to date have generally been well-tolerated, with the most common side effects being moderate injection site reactions. However, severe adverse events, including toxic epidermal necrolysis, have been reported.

- Steroids diminish the general immune response to immunotherapy. In a small early phase clinical trial using neoantigen peptide vaccines, patients who received dexamethasone did not respond to therapy. Patients receiving brain tumor vaccines should be on minimal doses of steroids.

- Preliminary evidence on SurVaxM peptide has shown a median overall survival of 86.6 weeks and 2 phase I studies on multiepitope, personalized vaccines have shown potential in inducing T-cell responses in glioblastoma.

- An interim analysis of the intent-to-treat population in a phase III DCVax-L study demonstrated a median overall survival of 23.1 months from the surgery and a median overall survival of patients with methylated MGMT of 34.7 months from surgery; both represent a significant increase when compared with that of standard of care treatment.

- The benefits derived from therapeutic vaccines are often observed at later time points after treatment when compared with other therapy types. This factor is often demonstrated in the tail of survival curves.

ACKNOWLEDGMENTS

Supported by grants from the Eager Family Brain Tumor Research Fund, the Heart of the Brain Foundation, and the National Institutes of Health (UCLA Brain Tumor SPORE grant, P50 CA211015). The authors thank Gena Behnke for her assistance with figure creation.

REFERENCES

1. Riedel S. Edward Jenner and the history of smallpox and vaccination. Proc Bayl Univ Med Cent 2005; 18(1):21–5.

2. Delany I, Rappuoli R, De Gregorio E. Vaccines for the 21st century. EMBO Mol Med 2014;6(6):708–20.

3. Pulendran B, Ahmed R. Immunological mechanisms of vaccination. Nat Immunol 2011;12(6):509–17.

4. Clem AS. Fundamentals of Vaccine Immunology. J Glob Infect Dis 2011;3(1):73–8.

5. Farkona S, Diamandis EP, Blasutig IM. Cancer immunotherapy: the beginning of the end of cancer? BMC Med 2016;14:73.

6. Melief CJ M., Hall, T. van, Arens, R., et al. Therapeutic cancer vaccines. Available at: https://www.jci.org/articles/view/80009/pdf. 2015. https://doi.org/10.1172/JCI80009.

7. Kantoff PW, Higano CS, Shore ND, et al. Sipuleucel-T immunotherapy for castration-resistant prostate cancer. N Engl J Med 2010;363(5):411–22.

8. Meireles LC, Marinho RT, Van Damme P. Three decades of hepatitis B control with vaccination. World J Hepatol 2015;7(18):2127–32.

9. Schlom J. Therapeutic cancer vaccines: current status and moving forward. J Natl Cancer Inst 2012;104(8):599–613.

10. Lei J, Ploner A, Elfström KM, et al. HPV vaccination and the risk of invasive cervical cancer. N Engl J Med 2020;383(14):1340–8.

11. Ménard S, Tagliabue E, Campiglio M, et al. Role of HER2 gene overexpression in breast carcinoma. J Cell. Physiol. 2000;182(2):150–62.

12. Le DT, Brockstedt DG, Nir-Paz R, et al. A Live-Attenuated Listeria Vaccine (ANZ-100) and a live-attenuated listeria vaccine expressing mesothelin (CRS-207) for advanced cancers: phase I studies of safety and immune induction. Clin Cancer Res 2012;18(3):858–68.

13. Ott PA, Hodi FS, Robert C. CTLA-4 and PD-1/PD-L1 blockade: new immunotherapeutic modalities with durable clinical benefit in melanoma patients. Clin Cancer Res 2013;19(19):5300–9.

14. Snyder A, Makarov V, Merghoub T, et al. Genetic basis for clinical response to CTLA-4 blockade in melanoma. N Engl J Med 2014;371(23):2189–99.

15. June CH, O'Connor RS, Kawalekar OU, et al. CAR T cell immunotherapy for human cancer. Science 2018;359(6382):1361–5.

16. Perez CR, De Palma M. Engineering dendritic cell vaccines to improve cancer immunotherapy. Nat Commun 2019;10(1):5408.

17. Ostrom QT, Bauchet L, Davis FG, et al. The epidemiology of glioma in adults: a "state of the science" review. Neuro-oncology 2014;16(7):896–913.

18. Boussiotis VA, Charest A. Immunotherapies for malignant glioma. Oncogene 2018;37(9):1121–41.

19. Gool V, Willy S. Brain tumor immunotherapy: what have we learned so far? Front Oncol 2015;5:98.

20. Sampson JH, Gunn MD, Fecci PE, et al. Brain immunology and immunotherapy in brain tumours. Nat Rev Cancer 2020;20(1):12–25.

21. Carson MJ, Reilly CR, Sutcliffe JG, et al. Mature microglia resemble immature antigen-presenting cells. Glia 1998;22(1):72–85.

22. Kennedy BC, Showers CR, Anderson DE, et al. Tumor-associated macrophages in glioma: friend or foe? J Oncol 2013;2013:486912. Available at: https://www.hindawi.com/journals/jo/2013/486912/.

23. Nduom EK, Weller M, Heimberger AB. Immunosuppressive mechanisms in glioblastoma. Neuro-oncology 2015;17(Suppl 7):vii9–14.

24. Woroniecka K, Chongsathidkiet P, Rhodin K, et al. T-cell exhaustion signatures vary with tumor type and are severe in glioblastoma. Clin Cancer Res 2018;24(17):4175–86.

25. Li W, Joshi MD, Singhania S, et al. Peptide vaccine: progress and challenges. Vaccines (Basel) 2014;2(3):515–36.

26. Bijker MS, Melief CJ, Offringa R, et al. Design and development of synthetic peptide vaccines: past, present and future. Expert Rev Vaccin 2007;6(4):591–603.

27. Yamada A, Sasada T, Noguchi M, et al. Next-generation peptide vaccines for advanced cancer. Cancer Sci 2013;104(1):15–21.

28. Perez SA, von Hofe E, Kallinteris NL, et al. A new era in anticancer peptide vaccines. Cancer 2010;116(9):2071–80.

29. Humphrey PA, Gangarosa LM, Wong AJ, et al. Deletion-mutant epidermal growth factor receptor in human gliomas: effects of type II mutation on receptor function. Biochem Biophys Res Commun 1991;178(3):1413–20.

30. Sugawa N, Ekstrand AJ, James CD, et al. Identical splicing of aberrant epidermal growth factor receptor transcripts from amplified rearranged genes in human glioblastomas. Proc Natl Acad Sci U S A 1990;87(21):8602–6.

31. Wikstrand CJ, Reist CJ, Archer GE, et al. The class III variant of the epidermal growth factor receptor (EGFRvIII): characterization and utilization as an immunotherapeutic target. J Neurovirol 1998;4(2):148–58.

32. Wong AJ, Ruppert JM, Bigner SH, et al. Structural alterations of the epidermal growth factor receptor gene in human gliomas. Proc Natl Acad Sci U S A 1992;89(7):2965–9.

33. Heimberger AB, Hlatky R, Suki D, et al. Prognostic effect of epidermal growth factor receptor and EGFRvIII in glioblastoma multiforme patients. Clin Cancer Res 2005;11(4):1462–6.

34. Malkki H. Trial watch: glioblastoma vaccine therapy disappointment in Phase III trial. Nat Rev Neurol 2016;12(4):190.

35. Zussman BM, Engh JA. Outcomes of the ACT III study: rindopepimut (CDX-110) therapy for glioblastoma. Neurosurgery 2015;76(6):N17.

36. Schuster J, Lai RK, Recht LD, et al. A phase II, multicenter trial of rindopepimut (CDX-110) in newly

diagnosed glioblastoma: the ACT III study. Neuro-oncology 2015;17(6):854–61.

37. Sampson JH, Archer GE, Mitchell DA, et al. An epidermal growth factor receptor variant III-targeted vaccine is safe and immunogenic in patients with glioblastoma multiforme. Mol Cancer Ther 2009;8(10):2773–9.

38. Figueroa ME, Abdel-Wahab O, Lu C, et al. Leukemic IDH1 and IDH2 mutations result in a hypermethylation phenotype, disrupt TET2 function, and impair hematopoietic differentiation. Cancer Cell 2010; 18(6):553–67.

39. Cairns RA, Mak TW. Oncogenic isocitrate dehydrogenase mutations: mechanisms, models, and clinical opportunities. Cancer Discov 2013;3(7): 730–41.

40. Yan H, Parsons DW, Jin G, et al. IDH1 and IDH2 mutations in gliomas. N Engl J Med 2009;360(8): 765–73.

41. Schumacher T, Bunse L, Pusch S, et al. A vaccine targeting mutant IDH1 induces antitumour immunity. Nature 2014;512(7514):324–7.

42. Huang J, Yu J, Tu L, et al. Isocitrate dehydrogenase mutations in glioma: from basic discovery to therapeutics development. Front Oncol 2019;9:506.

43. Schwartzentruber J, Korshunov A, Liu XY, et al. Driver mutations in histone H3.3 and chromatin remodelling genes in paediatric glioblastoma. Nature 2012;482(7384):226–31.

44. Ochs K, Ott M, Bunse T, et al. K27M-mutant histone-3 as a novel target for glioma immunotherapy. OncoImmunology 2017;6(7):e1328340.

45. Das A, Tan WL, Teo J, et al. Expression of survivin in primary glioblastomas. J Cancer Res Clin Oncol 2002;128(6):302–6.

46. Fenstermaker RA, Ciesielski MJ, Qiu J, et al. Clinical study of a survivin long peptide vaccine (SurVaxM) in patients with recurrent malignant glioma. Cancer Immunol Immunother 2016;65(11):1339–52.

47. Ahluwalia M, Reardon D, Abad A, et al. ATIM-41. PHASE II TRIAL OF A SURVIVIN VACCINE (SurVaxM) For Newly Diagnosed Glioblastoma. Neuro Oncol. 2018;20(suppl_6):vi10.

48. Alexandrov LB, Nik-Zainal S, Wedge DC, et al. Signatures of mutational processes in human cancer. Nature 2013;500(7463):415–21.

49. Keskin DB, Anandappa AJ, Sun J, et al. Neoantigen vaccine generates intratumoral T cell responses in phase Ib glioblastoma trial. Nature 2019; 565(7738):234–9.

50. Hilf N, Kuttruff-Coqui S, Frenzel K, et al. Actively personalized vaccination trial for newly diagnosed glioblastoma. Nature 2019;565(7738):240–5.

51. McNulty S, Colaco CA, Blandford LE, et al. Heat-shock proteins as dendritic cell-targeting vaccines–getting warmer. Immunology 2013;139(4): 407–15.

52. Testori A, Richards J, Whitman E, et al. Phase III comparison of vitespen, an autologous tumor-derived heat shock protein gp96 peptide complex vaccine, with physician's choice of treatment for stage IV melanoma: the C-100-21 Study Group. J Clin Oncol 2008;26(6):955–62.

53. Eton O, Ross MI, East MJ, et al. Autologous tumor-derived heat-shock protein peptide complex-96 (HSPPC-96) in patients with metastatic melanoma. J Transl Med 2010;8:9.

54. Jonasch E, Wood C, Tamboli P, et al. Vaccination of metastatic renal cell carcinoma patients with autologous tumour-derived vitespen vaccine: clinical findings. Br J Cancer 2008;98(8):1336–41.

55. Mazzaferro V, Coppa J, Carrabba MG, et al. Vaccination with autologous tumor-derived heat-shock protein gp96 after liver resection for metastatic colorectal cancer. Clin Cancer Res 2003;9(9):3235–45.

56. Crane CA, Han SJ, Ahn B, et al. Individual patient-specific immunity against high-grade glioma after vaccination with autologous tumor derived peptides bound to the 96 KD chaperone protein. Clin Cancer Res 2013;19(1):205–14.

57. Bloch O, Shi Q, Anderson SK, et al. ATIM-14. alliance A071101: a phase II randomized trial comparing the efficacy of heat shock protein peptide complex-96 (hsppc-96) vaccine given with bevacizumab versus bevacizumab alone in the treatment of surgically resectable recurrent glioblastoma. Neuro Oncol 2017;19(suppl_6):vi29.

58. Ji N, Zhang Y, Liu Y, et al. Heat shock protein peptide complex-96 vaccination for newly diagnosed glioblastoma: a phase I, single-arm trial. JCI Insight 2018;3(10):e99145.

59. Bloch O, Lim M, Sughrue ME, et al. Autologous heat shock protein peptide vaccination for newly diagnosed glioblastoma: impact of peripheral PD-L1 expression on response to therapy. Clin Cancer Res 2017;23(14):3575–84.

60. Phuphanich S, Wheeler CJ, Rudnick JD, et al. Phase I trial of a multi-epitope-pulsed dendritic cell vaccine for patients with newly diagnosed glioblastoma. Cancer Immunol Immunother 2013;62(1):125–35.

61. Wen PY, Reardon DA, Armstrong TS, et al. A randomized double-blind placebo-controlled phase II trial of dendritic cell vaccine ICT-107 in newly diagnosed patients with glioblastoma. Clin Cancer Res 2019;25(19):5799–807.

62. Peereboom DM, Nabors LB, Kumthekar P, et al. Phase 2 trial of SL-701 in relapsed/refractory (r/r) glioblastoma (GBM): correlation of immune response with longer-term survival. J Clin Oncol 2018;36(15_suppl):2058.

63. Mitchell DA, Xie W, Schmittling R, et al. Sensitive detection of human cytomegalovirus in tumors and peripheral blood of patients diagnosed with glioblastoma. Neuro-oncology 2008;10(1):10–8.

64. Prins RM, Cloughesy TF, Liau LM. Cytomegalovirus immunity after vaccination with autologous glioblastoma lysate. N Engl J Med 2008;359(5):539–41.

65. Cobbs CS, Harkins L, Samanta M, et al. Human cytomegalovirus infection and expression in human malignant glioma. Cancer Res 2002;62(12):3347–50.

66. Batich KA, Reap EA, Archer GE, et al. Long-term survival in glioblastoma with cytomegalovirus pp65-targeted vaccination. Clin Cancer Res 2017; 23(8):1898–909.

67. Mitchell DA, Batich KA, Gunn MD, et al. Tetanus toxoid and CCL3 improve dendritic cell vaccines in mice and glioblastoma patients. Nature 2015; 519(7543):366–9.

68. Batich KA, Mitchell DA, Healy P, et al. Once, twice, three times a finding: reproducibility of dendritic cell vaccine trials targeting cytomegalovirus in glioblastoma. Clin Cancer Res 2020;26(20):5297–303.

69. Liau LM, Prins RM, Kiertscher SM, et al. Dendritic cell vaccination in glioblastoma patients induces systemic and intracranial T-cell responses modulated by the local central nervous system tumor microenvironment. Clin Cancer Res 2005;11(15): 5515–25.

70. Liau LM, Ashkan K, Tran DD, et al. First results on survival from a large Phase 3 clinical trial of an autologous dendritic cell vaccine in newly diagnosed glioblastoma. J Transl Med 2018;16(1):142.

The Current Landscape of Immune Checkpoint Blockade in Glioblastoma

Oluwatosin O. Akintola, MBBS, MS[a],*, David A. Reardon, MD[b]

KEYWORDS

- Glioblastoma (GBM) • Immunotherapy • Immune checkpoint inhibitor (ICI)
- Immune checkpoint blockade • Programmed cell death receptor 1 (PD-1)
- Programmed cell death ligand 1 (PD-L1) • Cytotoxic T- lymphocyte–associated protein 4 (CTLA-4)

KEY POINTS

- Immune checkpoint blockade has revolutionized the management of many solid malignancies.
- Similar positive results have not been duplicated in the treatment of glioblastoma with immune checkpoint blockade.
- There are ongoing studies to further evaluate the potential role of immune checkpoint blockade in the management of glioblastoma.
- Multimodal immunotherapy for glioblastoma is under active investigation, and results are expected to direct the future role of immunotherapy in glioblastoma.
- Identification of reliable biomarkers of response to immunotherapy treatment is essential to optimizing response in patients with glioblastoma.

BACKGROUND

Outcomes for patients with glioblastoma remains one of the poorest in oncology. Despite the emergence of multimodal therapies, prognosis is poor, with fewer than 50% of patients surviving for 1 year, and only 5% surviving beyond 5 years.[1] Immunotherapy focused on immune checkpoint blockade (ICB) has proven to be a successful approach in the management of patients with many different oncology indications. Despite tremendous interest in immunotherapies for high-grade gliomas, disease response has been low in clinical studies thus far. The theory of a largely immunosilent central nervous system (CNS) milieu as originally defined by Medawar's skin allograft transplantation studies[2] has been contested in more recent work documenting active lymphatics in the CNS[3,4] and is not consistent with known immune activation associated with CNS infections and neuroinflammatory conditions.

Multilayered immunosuppressive mechanisms deployed by glioblastoma cells complicate the quest to attack these tumors with immunotherapy. High-grade glioma cells express CD95 (Fas/apoptosis antigen 1) ligand, which induces apoptosis and T-cell suppression in the glioma microenvironment.[5,6] Similarly, the ligand for Programmed Death-1 (PD-L1) is upregulated in the glioblastoma microenvironment and has been shown to suppress T-cell recruitment and induces T-cell apoptosis.[7–9] Activation of the PD-1/PD-L1 pathway leads to a cascade of immunosuppressive mechanisms, including inhibition of tumor cell apoptosis, peripheral T effector cell exhaustion, and conversion of T effector cells to regulatory T cells (Tregs).[10] Multiple studies have shown that Treg cells also

[a] Center for Neuro-Oncology, Dana-Farber Cancer Institute, Massachusetts General Hospital Cancer Center, 450 Brookline Avenue, Boston, MA 02215-5450, USA; [b] Center for Neuro-Oncology, Dana-Farber Cancer Institute, Harvard Medical School, 450 Brookline Avenue, Boston, MA 02215-5450, USA
* Corresponding author.
E-mail address: oluwatosin_akintola@dfci.harvard.edu

Neurosurg Clin N Am 32 (2021) 235–248
https://doi.org/10.1016/j.nec.2020.12.003
1042-3680/21/© 2020 Elsevier Inc. All rights reserved.

accumulate in the glioblastoma microenvironment to prevent the antiglioma immune response.[11–13] In addition, high-grade glioma cells secrete immunosuppressive factors, such as interleukin-10 (IL-10) and transforming growth factor-β (TGF-β).[14,15] Furthermore, the microenvironment of GBM tumors is characterized by a dominant population of myeloid cells, which can account for up to 40% of GBM tumors, and are programmed to exhibit a highly immunosuppressive phenotype.[16–18] Combined, these protective strategies form sophisticated escape routes from immune surveillance, thereby contributing to the development and progression of glioblastoma tumors. These immune escape mechanisms are discussed extensively in later sections.

Despite the emerging challenges associated with the immunosuppressed glioblastoma microenvironment, the efficacy of ICB in other cancers continues to fuel interest to further investigate these agents in neurooncology. Numerous immunotherapy approaches to glioblastoma are under evaluation, including immunomodulation with immune checkpoint inhibitors (ICIs; cytotoxic T-lymphocyte–associated antigen [anti-CTLA-4], anti–PD-1, anti–PD-L1 monoclonal antibodies); tumor antigen-specific and tumor-associated vaccines; adoptive T-cell therapies (chimeric antigen receptor T cells and bispecific T-cell engagers); and oncolytic virus therapies.[19]

THE BIOLOGICAL BASIS FOR IMMUNE CHECKPOINT INHIBITION

Evasion of the immune system by tumor cells is a major determinant of the proliferation and growth of malignant cells. At tumorigenesis, the immune system attempts to eliminate malignant cells beginning with presentation of tumor antigens by antigen-presenting cells (APC) to T cells. Antigen presentation triggers multiple sequential steps, including T-cell priming, clonal selection of antigen-specific T cells, activation and proliferation in secondary lymphoid tissues, trafficking of T cells to tumor sites, initiation of effector functions at target sites, and recruitment of other effector immune cells via cytokines and membrane ligand signaling.[20] Each step is coordinated by a balance between costimulatory/agonistic and antagonistic/inhibitory signals known as immune checkpoint proteins (checkpoints such as CTLA-4, PD-1, BTLA, VISTA, TIM-3, LAG3, and CD47; costimulatory molecules such as CD 28, CD137, OX40, and GITR) (Fig. 1). Inhibitory checkpoint proteins normally function physiologically as reins that dampen the amplitude and potency of T-cell–mediated responses.[21] This balance is essential

for the prevention of autoimmunity. Nonetheless, tumor cells can exploit this normally protective mechanism by dysregulated expression of immune checkpoint proteins that can provide a mechanism of immune evasion.

The authors focus here on the classical inhibitory immune checkpoint molecules for which multiple therapeutic targets have been developed: CTLA-4 and the PD-1 pathway.

Cytotoxic T-Lymphocyte–Associated Antigen-4

CTLA-4 was identified as a major immune modulator after the discovery that CD28 costimulation plays a critical role in the activation of T cells.[22,23] Presentation of antigen proteins alone is insufficient to trigger T-cell activation because costimulatory signals in addition to T-cell receptor (TCR) engagement of foreign peptide antigen–major histocompatibility complexes (MHC) are needed to trigger T-cell activation, priming, and clonal expansion. The primary costimulatory signal is the interaction of CD28 expressed on T cells with B7-1 (CD80) and B7-2 (CD86) expressed on the surface of specialized APC.[24] B7-1 and B7-2 provide positive costimulatory signals through CD28 (Fig. 2). CTLA-4 is a homolog of CD28 that binds both B7-1 and B7-2 with greater affinity than CD28.[25,26] CTLA-4 is upregulated following TCR-tumor peptide bound MHC complex (pMHC) binding. Its expression by T cells is most active 2 to 3 days following TCR engagement.[27,28] CTLA-4

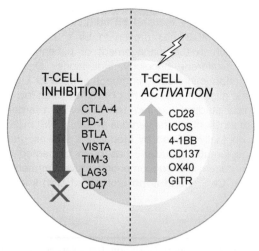

Fig. 1. Costimulatory immune modulatory proteins expressed by T cells to enhance T-cell activation (green). Coinhibitory immune modulatory proteins expressed following the interaction of the antigen pMHC complex with the TCR to produce attenuation of T-cell activity (red).

hinders TCR signaling by competing with the costimulatory CD28 molecule for the B7 ligands B7-1 and B7-2 (see **Fig. 2**). Because CTLA-4 has higher avidity and affinity for CD80 and CD86, it outcompetes CD28 in binding both ligands.[29,30] CTLA-4 binding limits CD28 downstream signaling (primarily mediated by PI3K and AKT), thereby dampening the stimulation of T cells.[31,32] In addition, CTLA-4 downregulates the expression of B7 ligands on APC through modulating cytokines, such as IL-10 or TGF-β, or via transendocytosis.[33] Thus, CTLA-4 primarily functions to attenuate T-cell activity at sites of T-cell priming in lymphatic tissues. Because of its central role in regulating T-cell activation, inhibition by CTLA4 is normally critical for self-tolerance and avoidance of autoimmunity.

Once the role of CTLA-4 as a negative regulator of T-cell responses was established, the possibility that blockade of immune inhibition engineered by CTLA-4 and B7-1/B7-2 interactions might augment T-cell responses to tumor cells and enhance antitumor immunity was explored. Leach and colleagues[34] provided early evidence that CTLA-4 blockade using antibodies enhanced antitumor immune responses in vivo. In mice transfected with colon carcinoma cells who were treated with anti-CTLA-4 or anti-CD28 injections, anti–CTLA-4–treated mice showed significant reduction in tumor growth.

Currently, ipilimumab is the only human CTLA-4-blocking antibody currently approved by the Food and Drug Administration (FDA).[35,36] Other CTLA-4 targeting agents, such as tremelimumab (a fully human monoclonal antibody against CTLA-4), are also under investigation in multiple cancer types.[37]

Programmed Death-1 and Programmed Death Ligand 1/2 Pathway

PD-1 or CD279 is another inhibitory molecule secreted during T-cell priming and activation. It is a cell surface receptor encoded by the *Pdcd1* gene. PD-1 is expressed by T lymphocytes, B cells, dendritic cells, macrophages, and natural killer cells. Its immunosuppressive activity is multifold. In chronic inflammatory states (eg, chronic infections and malignancies), persistent PD-1 expression causes T cells to enter into a state of metabolic exhaustion.[38,39] Like CTLA-4, PD-1 also counteracts the stimulatory signal induced by TCR engagement with CD28 via its ligands.[40] PD-L1 engages with PD-1 to provide inhibitory signals to suppress activated CD4$^+$, CD8$^+$ cells and to induce T-cell apoptosis.[41] When PD-1 engages with its ligands PD-L1 (B7-H1) and PD-L2 (B7-H2), dephosphorylation of protein tyrosine phosphatases (PTPs), such as SHP2, occurs.[42] PTP dephosphorylation leads to antagonism of positive signals typically mediated by TCR and CD28, and the inhibition of downstream signaling pathways (**Fig. 3**). The result is decreased T-cell activation, proliferation, survival, and cytokine production.[40] Although PD-L1 is expressed primarily by tumor cells and myeloid cells (such as macrophages), PD-L2 is nearly exclusively expressed some myeloid cells. This myeloid activity is essential to the inhibition of immunity, as myeloid cell expression of PD-L1/2 contributes to the inhibition of T cells in the tumor microenvironment.[43]

Altogether, the PD-1 and PD-L1/2 pathway triggers immunosuppressive mechanisms, including cytokines that lead to the inhibition of tumor cell apoptosis, peripheral T effector cell anergy, and conversion of T effector cells to Tregs.[44–46]

PD-L1 staining has been reported in glioblastoma tissues to varying extents and expression differs in molecular glioblastoma subtypes. Berghoff and colleagues[7] reported prominent expression of PD-L1 by glioma cells in most of their human glioblastoma samples. They reported low PD-L1 expression in proneural glioblastoma subtypes; meanwhile, high PD-L1 expression was observed in the mesenchymal glioblastoma

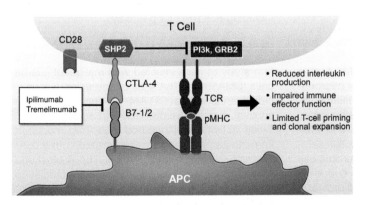

Fig. 2. CTLA-4 inhibits TCR signaling, thereby limiting interleukin production, T-cell priming, and survival. Anti-CTLA antibodies act to block this pathway.

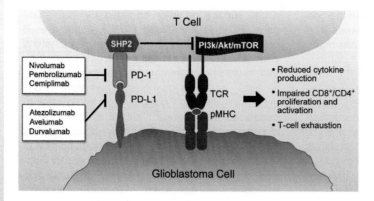

Fig. 3. PD-1/PD-L1 interaction inhibits TCR signaling to impair T-cell proliferation and to induce T-cell exhaustion. Anti–PD-1 and anti–PD-L1 antibodies act to block this pathway.

subtypes. Similarly, Heiland and colleagues[47] showed that PD-L1 expression was elevated in high-grade gliomas compared with lower-grade gliomas. They also reported increased PD-L1 expression in mesenchymal glioma types. PD-L1 presence in the glioblastoma microenvironment was associated with activation of the MAPK pathway. Finally, Nduom and colleagues[48] showed that most GBM tumors (61%) demonstrated PD-L1 expression as defined by detection among ≥1% of cells.

Therapeutic antibodies against PD-L1 (atezolizumab, avelumab, and durvalumab) and PD-1 (nivolumab, pembrolizumab, and cemiplimab) have been developed. These agents have demonstrated varying levels of efficacy in different cancer types (**Table 1**).

Beyond the Cytotoxic T-Lymphocyte–Associated Antigen-4, Programmed Death-1/Programmed Death Ligand-1 Pathways

T cells recruited into the glioblastoma tumor environment tend to overexpress PD-1, CTLA-4, and other inhibitory regulators (TIM-3, LAG-3, CD160, 2B4, TIGIT, CD39, and BTLA).[49,50] The immunosuppressive glioblastoma microenvironment is further enhanced by the expression of PD-L1 by microglia. PD-L1 expression by microglial cells is amplified when in close proximity to GBM cells, which in turn may promote apoptosis of cytotoxic T cells, thereby sparing glioma cells from T-cell–mediated killing.[51]

Tumor-infiltrating myeloid cells (TIM) further enhance immune resistance in the tumor microenvironment. Myeloid cells derived from healthy tissues typically express immunostimulatory cytokines to stimulate the proliferation and antitumor function of T cells and natural killer cells. In contrast, tumor-associated macrophages (TAMs) have poor antigen-presenting capability and produce factors that suppress T-cell proliferation and activity. Mantovani and Sica[52] showed

that exposure to IL-4 and IL-10 in tumors may induce TAMs to develop an immunosuppressive polarized type II phenotype, and these are referred to as M2 macrophages.

TAMs markedly infiltrate the tumor microenvironment. Macrophage differentiation, growth, and infiltration are regulated by several growth factors, including colony stimulating factor-1 (CSF-1). Treatments such as radiation, chemotherapy, and immunotherapies induce CSF-1 secretion from tumor cells, which promotes the influx of myeloid cells into the tumor microenvironment.[43] Overexpression of CSF-1 and chemokine (C-C motif) ligand 2 (CCL2), regulatory molecules for macrophages, has been associated with poor prognosis in multiple solid malignancies,[53] including glial tumors. Ding and colleagues[54] showed that M2-type macrophages were present in all glioma grades with higher expression levels associated with higher-grade gliomas. Flow cytometry studies demonstrate that tumor-infiltrating monocytes/macrophages from patients with GBM exhibit increased expression of PD-L1 (B7-H1).[55] Although PD-L1 was previously understood to be secreted by glioma cells, studies suggest that TIMs may in fact be the major source of PD-L1 in the glioma microenvironment.[43,56] Therefore, TIMs form a critical component of glioma immunosuppression that is influenced by many factors, including PD-1/PD-L1 pathway.

PRECLINICAL STUDIES

In a study of mice injected with malignant glioma cells (SMA560), CTLA-4 blockade using a monoclonal antibody to CTLA-4 produced long-term survival in some treated mice. In addition, CD4+ T-cell activity was restored and Treg-mediated immunosuppression was ameliorated.[57] In a subsequent study, combining anti–CTLA-4 blockade with granulocyte-macrophage colony-stimulating factor (GM-CSF) expressing whole glioma cell vaccination was shown to successfully increase

Table 1
Selected Food and Drug Administration–approved immune checkpoint blockade agents for solid malignancies[a]

Tumor Type	ICB Agent	Immune Checkpoint Target	Year of FDA Approval
Melanoma			
Melanoma (unresectable or metastatic)	Ipilimumab	CTLA-4	2011
Melanoma (progressed following treatment with ipilimumab)	Nivolumab	PD-1	2014
Melanoma (unresectable or metastatic)	Pembrolizumab	PD-1	2014
Melanoma (BRAF wild type)	Ipilimumab + nivolumab	CTLA-4 + PD-1	2015
Melanoma (adjuvant)	Ipilimumab	CTLA-4	2015
Melanoma (any BRAF status)	Ipilimumab + nivolumab	CTLA-4 + PD-1	2016
Lung/pleural malignancies			
Non–small cell lung cancer	Nivolumab	PD-1	2015
Non–small cell lung cancer	Pembrolizumab	PD-1	2015
Non–small cell lung cancer	Atezolizumab	PD-L1	2016
Non–small cell lung cancer	Durvalumab	PD-L1	2018
Small cell lung cancer (extensive)	Atezolizumab	PD-L1	2019
Mesothelioma	Nivolumab + ipilimumab	PD-1 + CTLA-4	2020
Genitourinary carcinomas			
Renal cell carcinoma	Nivolumab	PD-1	2015
Urothelial carcinoma	Atezolizumab	PD-L1	2016
Urothelial carcinoma	Avelumab	PD-L1	2017
Urothelial carcinoma	Durvalumab	PD-L1	2017
Urothelial carcinoma	Nivolumab	PD-1	2017
Urothelial carcinoma	Pembrolizumab	PD-1	2017
Renal cell carcinoma	Ipilimumab + nivolumab	CTLA-4 + PD-1	2018
Gastrointestinal tract/hepatobiliary tumors			
MSI-high, MMR-deficient metastatic colorectal cancer	Nivolumab	PD-1	2017
Microsatellite instability (MSI)-high or Mismatch repair (MMR)-deficient solid tumors of any histology	Pembrolizumab	PD-1	2017
Hepatocellular carcinoma	Nivolumab	PD-1	2017
Gastric and gastroesophageal carcinoma	Pembrolizumab	PD-1	2017
Other cutaneous cancers			
Merkel cell carcinoma	Avelumab	PD-L1	2017
Merkel cell carcinoma	Pembrolizumab	PD-1	2018
Advanced cutaneous squamous cell carcinoma	Cemiplimab	PD-1	2018

[a] Summary of FDA approval for selected immune checkpoint blockade therapies granted as of October 2020.

survival in glioma-injected mice.[58] Another murine experiment showed that mice harboring an intracranial GL-261 glial tumor had improved survival when treated with single-agent or combination monoclonal antibodies against PD-1, PD-L1, and CTLA with the greatest benefit reported in mice treated with the combination of PD-1 plus CTLA-4 blockade.[59]

Additional studies investigated combining ICB with standard therapies, such as radiation. Zeng and colleagues treated mice inoculated with GL-261 glioma tumors with anti–PD-1 antibody only or radiation plus anti–PD-1 antibody. They reported no significant survival benefit in the antibody-alone arm (27 days), but longer survival was noted in the radiation plus anti–PD-1 antibody arm (53 days).[60] They also reported increased glioma infiltration by $CD8^+$ effector cells and downregulation of Tregs.[60] These results suggested that immune checkpoint blockade could work synergistically with radiation to create a proinflammatory tumor environment against glioma cells.

Although these preclinical studies promised significant efficacy of immune checkpoint blockade in gliomas, this promise has not been achieved in clinical studies. One reason for the disconnect between preclinical and clinical experiences is that GL-261, the most widely used syngeneic mouse orthotopic glioma cell line used in murine ICI experiments,[57,59,61] exhibits robust immunogenicity and capacity to propagate an immune response. This murine tumor has been shown to possess a striking tumor mutational burden,[62] whereas human malignant glioma tumors typically exhibit a low tumor mutational burden (TMB).[63] The low mutational load in human GBM tumors has been demonstrated to be a prognosticator of poor response to ICB therapies.[64] Genoud and colleagues[65] introduced a murine glioma model (SB28) with a low mutational burden and poor immunogenic activity, which is more comparable to human glioma tumors. Murine GBM models that are less intrinsically immunogenic may be more informative to guide immunotherapy drug development for GBM patients.

CLINICAL STUDIES

Several anti–CTLA-4, anti–PD-1, and anti–PD-L1 antibodies have been tested in the context of brain tumors and in other solid tumors, including a number that have received approval by the FDA (see **Table 1**). Ipilimumab, a fully humanized monoclonal antibody that inactivates CTLA4, was first approved by the FDA for unresectable, advanced (stage III or IV) melanoma in 2011.[66] Multiple studies have also demonstrated activity of ipilimumab against brain metastases, including an open-label phase 2 trial, which reported a 24% response rate to ipilimumab among corticosteroid-naïve patients with brain metastases treated with ipilimumab.[67]

Clinical trials investigating blockade of the PD-1/PD-L1 pathway have shown efficacy in the treatment of many solid cancers. PD-1/PD-L1 pathway inhibition has also shown encouraging activity for some patients with brain metastases.[68]

Programmed Death-1/Programmed Death Ligand-1 Blockade in Glioblastoma

Nivolumab

Results of the first randomized phase 3 trial to evaluate immune checkpoint inhibition in patients with glioblastoma (CheckMate-143) were recently reported.[69] In this open-label trial, patients with first recurrence of glioblastoma after standard chemoradiation therapy were randomized 1:1 to 3 mg/kg of nivolumab (n = 184) or 10 mg/kg of bevacizumab (n = 185) every 2 weeks. Median overall survival (OS) was similar in both groups at 9.8 months (95% confidence interval [CI], 8.2–11.8 months) with nivolumab versus 10.0 months (95% CI, 9.0–11.8 months) with bevacizumab (hazard ratio [HR], 1.04; 95% CI, 0.83–1.30; $P = .76$). However, a planned subgroup analysis demonstrated that patients with MGMT methylated tumors and no baseline steroid use showed improved survival with nivolumab with a median OS of 17 months (n = 31) versus 10.1 months for bevacizumab (n = 25). Mean progression-free survival (PFS) disfavored nivolumab (1.5 months for nivolumab and 3.5 months for bevacizumab; $P < .001$). Similarly, the objective response rate (ORR) in evaluable patients in the nivolumab (n = 153) arm versus bevacizumab (n = 156) arm was 7.8% and 23%, respectively. Notably in those who achieved response, the effect was more durable for nivolumab (11.1 months) versus bevacizumab (5.3 months). Steroid use seemed to confound the clinical benefit picture, as patients in the nivolumab cohort who were on steroids at baseline had a median OS of 7 months compared with 12.6 months among patients without baseline steroid use. Similar rates of grade 3 or 4 treatment-related adverse effects (TRAEs) were observed in both arms: nivolumab (18.1%) and bevacizumab (15.2%).[69]

CheckMate-498[70] is an open-label, randomized phase 3 study that compares the OS of nivolumab or temozolomide (TMZ), each in combination with radiotherapy and then after radiotherapy, in patients with newly diagnosed MGMT-unmethylated GBM. Data from CheckMate-498 remain unpublished at this time. However, in May 2019, Bristol-Myers Squibb (BMS) announced that CheckMate-498 did not meet its primary endpoint of OS on final analysis.[71]

CheckMate-548 is a placebo-controlled, blinded, randomized phase 3 study evaluating nivolumab combined with concurrent standard chemoradiation versus standard of care in patients with newly diagnosed MGMT-methylated glioblastoma. BMS announced that the trial did not meet one of its primary endpoints, PFS, in September

2019.[72] Outcome for the primary endpoint of median OS has not been released.

Pembrolizumab

Keynote-028 is a basket study of pembrolizumab for various tumor types that included an arm for recurrent glioblastoma (n = 26). Patients received pembrolizumab 10 mg/kg every 2 weeks for up to 24 months. The primary end point was ORR per RECIST v. 1.1 guidelines. Among GBM patients, there was 1 partial response (n = 25; ORR, 4.0%, 95% CI, 0.1–20.4); 12 patients (48.0%) had stable disease. Median PFS was 2.8 months (95% CI, 1.9–9.1), and median OS was 14.4 months (95% CI, 10.3–not reached). TRAEs were reported in 19 (73.1%) patients, most commonly fatigue and rash (n = 6 each, 23.1%). Four (15.4%) patients experienced grade 3 or 4 TRAEs (lymphopenia, type 2 diabetes mellitus, arthritis, and syncope). None of the patients died or discontinued pembrolizumab because of a treatment-related adverse event.[73]

Another phase 2 study (NCT02337491) investigated the use of pembrolizumab (200 mg intravenously [IV] every 3 weeks) with bevacizumab (cohort A) or without (cohort B) bevacizumab (10 mg/kg IV every 2 weeks), in bevacizumab-naïve patients at first or second recurrence of glioblastoma.[74] The primary endpoint was PFS at 6 (PFS-6) months per RANO guidelines for each cohort. PFS-6 was 26% (95% CI, 16.3–41.5) in cohort A and 6.7% (95% CI, 1.6–25.4) in cohort B. Median OS was 8.8 months (95% CI, 7.7–14.2) in cohort A and 10.3 months (95% CI, 8.5–12.5) in cohort B. There were no grade 4 or 5 TRAEs reported. Grade 2 or 3 TRAEs occurred in ≥10% patients, including cohort A, hypertension (50%), fatigue (18%), headache (16%), infection (14%), and proteinuria (14%); cohort B, headache (30%) and fatigue (17%).

Atezolizumab

Atezolizumab is a humanized monoclonal antibody directed against PD-L1. It is approved in the treatment of patients with advanced metastatic urothelial carcinoma after the failure of platinum-based chemotherapy and the treatment of patients with metastatic non–small cell lung carcinoma.[75,76] There are multiple ongoing phase 1/2 studies evaluating atezolizumab for GBM, including combinations with (1) standard chemoradiation (NCT03174197); (2) D2C7-IT, a dual-specific EGFRwt/EGFRvIII monoclonal antibody (NCT04160494); and (3) ipatasertib, a selective inhibitor of AKT isoforms 1/2/3 (NCT03673787). The results of these trials have not been released.

Durvalumab

Durvalumab is a humanized monoclonal antibody directed against PD-L1 approved for the treatment of patients with advanced urothelial carcinoma.[77] Preliminary results of a phase 2 study of durvalumab (NCT02336165) that includes 1 arm of newly GBM diagnosed patients and 4 arms of recurrent GBM patients showed overall acceptable tolerability of the drug. The study is ongoing, and finalized data on efficacy are expected in the near future.[78]

Avelumab

Avelumab is a PD-L1 inhibitor approved for the treatment of metastatic Merkel-cell carcinoma, metastatic urothelial carcinoma, and advanced renal cell carcinoma.[79] NCT03341806 is an ongoing phase 1 study evaluating avelumab combined with laser interstitial thermal therapy (LITT) in patients with recurrent glioblastoma.

Cytotoxic T-Lymphocyte–Associated Antigen-4 Blockade in Glioblastoma

In an exploratory phase 1 cohort of CheckMate-143, the tolerability and efficacy of nivolumab and ipilimumab in recurrent glioblastoma were tested. In a small cohort, the addition of ipilimumab to nivolumab did not appear to improve OS, and nivolumab monotherapy was better tolerated when compared with combination therapy.[80] In a case series of 20 patients with recurrent glioblastoma treated with ipilimumab and bevacizumab, 31% of patients showed a partial response, 31% had stable disease, and 38% had disease progression.[81] There are limited studies testing ipilimumab or CTLA-4 blockade in glioblastoma. The Ipi-Glio trial testing adjuvant ipilimumab with temozolomide versus temozolomide alone was recently announced.[82] NCT02794883 is an active phase 2 trial designed to test tremelimumab (anti–CTLA-4 monoclonal antibody) and durvalumab (anti–PD-L1 antibody) as monotherapies and combination therapies among patients with recurrent malignant glioma.

MULTIMODAL IMMUNOTHERAPIES IN GLIOBLASTOMA

Given the heterogeneity of glioblastoma tumors and the multiple immune escape mechanisms deployed by these tumors, combinatorial treatment approaches will likely be required to achieve meaningful therapeutic benefit. Current strategies include combining immune checkpoint inhibitors, cytotoxic therapy, including radiation therapy, antiangiogenesis agents, targeted therapies, and other immunotherapy modalities (**Table 2**).

Combination with Oncolytic Viruses

There are multiple clinical trials underway that are currently evaluating oncolytic viruses combined

Table 2
Selected active, recruiting clinical trials of immune checkpoint blockade in high-grade gliomas[a]

Clinical Trial Number	Intervention	Combinational Strategy	Phase	Disease	Primary Outcome Measure
NCT03367715	Nivolumab + Ipilimumab + Short-course radiotherapy	Anti-PD-1 + Anti–CTLA-4 +Radiation therapy	2	Newly diagnosed, MGMT unmethylated glioblastoma	OS
NCT04396860	Ipilimumab + Nivolumab + radiation vs standard chemoradiation	Anti–CTLA-4 + Anti-PD-1 + Radiation therapy	2/3	Newly diagnosed, MGMT unmethylated glioblastoma	PFS OS
NCT04013672	Pembrolizumab + SurVaxM	Anti-PD-1 + Tumor-specific antigen vaccine	2	Recurrent glioblastoma	PFS
NCT03018288	Radiation + temozolomide + pembrolizumab ± Heat shock protein peptide-complex (HSPPC-96)	Anti-PD-1 + Chemoradiation + Tumor-derived peptide vaccine	2	Newly diagnosed glioblastoma	OS
NCT04479241	PVSRIPO and pembrolizumab	Anti-PD-1 + Oncolytic virus	1	Recurrent glioblastoma	Safety and tolerability
NCT03341806	Avelumab + LITT	Anti-PD-L1 + Laser interstitial thermotherapy	1	Recurrent glioblastoma	ORR Dose-limiting toxicity
NCT04160494	Atezolizumab + D2C7-IT	Anti-PD-L1 + EGFRwt/VIII immunotoxin	1	Recurrent (World Health Organization) grade IV malignant glioma	Tolerability
NCT02866747	Durvalumab + Hypofractionated stereotactic radiotherapy	Anti-PD-L1 + Radiation therapy	1/2	Recurrent glioblastoma	OS Dose-limiting toxicity

[a] Selected active, recruiting clinical trials as of October 2020.

with checkpoint inhibitors. Oncolytic viruses induce immunogenic cell death leading to increased tumor antigen release. Coadministration of anti–PD-1 or anti–CTLA 4 antibody will decrease compensatory enhanced expression of inhibitory immune checkpoints in this setting, thereby allowing the development of a robust immune response. The CAPTIVE trial (NCT02798406) is an ongoing phase 2 study investigating the oncolytic adenovirus DNX-2401 and pembrolizumab in patients with recurrent glioblastoma.[83]

Combination with Vaccines

Integrating tumor vaccines with immune checkpoint inhibitors has been shown to improve long-term survival in murine glioma studies.[58,84] NCT02287428 is an ongoing phase 1 study evaluating a personalized neoantigen cancer vaccine derived from glioma-specific protein-coding mutations in combination with pembrolizumab and radiation therapy. An autologous tumor lysate-loaded dendritic cell vaccine is being tested in combination with ICB in a phase 1 clinical trial among patients with recurrent glioblastoma (NCT04201873).

CHALLENGES OF IMMUNE CHECKPOINT INHIBITION THERAPY

Biomarkers that may predict response to ICB are emerging for many cancers, but their utility for GBM patients is not well understood. High-tumor mutational variance has been associated with an increased rate of immunogenic neoantigens that could trigger a robust immune response.[85] However, glioblastoma tumors exhibit a relatively small tumor mutational variance compared with other solid tumors.[86] Temozolomide, a cornerstone of glioblastoma treatment, is myelosuppressive and has been shown to increase the proportion of exhausted T cells in mice.[86] T-cell exhaustion can reduce the response to checkpoint blockade, suggesting that baseline T-cell exhaustion may be a negative biomarker of response. Immunophenotyping of the glioblastoma microenvironment has shown a paucity of immune-effector cells.[87] TAM and Tregs are immunosuppressive cells that are prevalent in glioblastoma tissues.[88,89]

Furthermore, molecular genetic abnormalities of GBM tumors may lead to immunomodulation of the GBM TME and may contribute to differentiating ICB responders from nonresponders. In their retrospective analysis of 66 patients with recurrent GBM who received anti–PD-1 therapy, Zhao and colleagues[90] identified distinct molecular genetic signatures in 17 patients who were responders

(14 months OS) versus 49 patients who were non-responders (10 months OS). Genomic and transcriptomic analysis of both cohorts revealed *PTEN* mutations to be associated with immunosuppressive gene signatures that were more enriched in nonresponders, whereas there was enrichment of MAPK pathway alterations (PTPN11, BRAF) in responders. Interestingly, studies in melanoma have shown that loss of PTEN function in tumor cells correlates with decreased T-cell recruitment, decreased T-cell–mediated cell death, and poorer outcomes with PD-1 inhibitor therapy.[91] Furthermore, Zhao and colleagues[90] also demonstrated that failure of immune checkpoint therapy may occur because of posttreatment genetic immune-editing. In their analysis of the clonal alterations of mutations after treatment, they found 3 missense mutations (MYPN R409H, UBQLN3 R159W, CYP27B1 G194E) that were present before anti–PD-1 therapy but were not detectable after immune checkpoint therapy. These results suggest that immune checkpoint therapy may lead to immune editing and loss of immunogenic mutations as a mechanism of treatment resistance.

In addition, questions about the optimal timing of ICB for patients with glioblastoma remain unanswered. Data suggest that cytoreductive surgery may increase efficacy by reducing residual tumor burden to be attacked by the mounted anticancer immune response. However, the best opportunity window (ie, before resection of recurrent tumor or after resection of recurrent tumor) remains unclear. Cloughesy and colleagues[92] conducted a randomized trial comparing 2 arms of pembrolizumab: before (neoadjuvant) and after (adjuvant) surgery versus adjuvant therapy only in 35 patients with recurrent, surgically resectable glioblastoma. Patients who received the neoadjuvant pembrolizumab arm (n = 16) had significantly improved OS (13.7 vs 7.5 months, $P = .04$) and PFS (3.3 vs 2.4 months, $P = .03$) compared with the adjuvant pembrolizumab (n = 19) only. The investigators also reported an increase in transcription of genes related to T-cell expansion and interferon-γ responsiveness in patients treated with neoadjuvant pembrolizumab. These findings support the hypothesis that neoadjuvant use of immune checkpoint inhibitors may enhance immune responses and improve efficacy of ICB.

Clinically, corticosteroids for the management of symptomatic cerebral edema among patients with glioblastoma present another potential challenge to immunotherapy. Corticosteroids, which are routinely used to decrease cerebral edema in patients with brain tumors, are immunosuppressive. Data on the impact of steroids on ICB in solid malignancies have been mixed, with some studies showing reduced efficacy[93,94] and other studies reporting no significant effect.[95,96]

Immune-related adverse events (irAEs) are the primary toxicities of ICIs. These side effects are generally more severe when combined CTLA-4 and PD-1/PD-L1 inhibition therapies are used and less prevalent with PD-1/PD-L1 monotherapy. They can affect multiple organs simultaneously and may become life-threatening if not addressed. Some of the most commonly reported irAEs include colitis, pneumonitis, hepatitis, myocarditis, hypophysitis, and encephalitis.[97] For these reasons, patients receiving ICIs are regularly monitored for treatment-related complications.

FUTURE DIRECTIONS

Identification of reliable biomarkers of response to immune checkpoint blockade and other immunotherapies is critical to the success of these approaches in patients with glioblastoma. The spectrum of possible predictive biomarkers is wide, and the expression of these biomarkers is highly variable with conflicting data on the strength of their association with survival.[98,99] Studies investigating other mechanisms of immune evasion, such as downregulated expression of MHC class I and II molecules[100,101] in the glioma environment, should also be considered. Given the number of molecules involved in the T-cell activation pathway (inhibitory molecules, such as BTLA, VISTA, TIM-3, LAG3, and CD47; co-stimulatory molecules, such as CD137, OX40, and GITR), the potential for combinatorial immunotherapy strategies in cancer and glioma treatment is promising.

SUMMARY

The management of hematologic and solid malignancies with immunotherapies, such as immune blockade, has yielded remarkably favorable results. In contrast, clinical studies investigating ICB in patients with glioblastoma have yielded disappointing results thus far. Nevertheless, several exciting immunotherapeutic approaches, including combinatorial regimens, are being investigated to overcome challenges associated with the dominantly immunosuppressive tumor microenvironment in order to generate effective antiglioma responses. Results of ongoing clinical trials are expected to clarify the future role of immune checkpoint blockade and other immunotherapies in the management of glioblastoma.

CLINICS CARE POINTS

- Immune checkpoint blockade in patients with glioblastoma has yielded disappointing results thus far.
- Results of ongoing clinical trials are expected to clarify the future role of immune checkpoint blockade and other immunotherapies in the management of glioblastoma.
- Corticosteroids are frequently prescribed to glioblastoma patients to treat symptomatic cerebral edema. However, these agents have immunosuppressive effects that may limit efficacy of immunotherapy approaches in patients with glioblastoma.
- Immune checkpoint inhibitors may cause immune-related adverse events, which range from mild to marked in severity that require proactive monitoring to mitigate as well as specialized care.

DISCLOSURE

O.O. Akintola has nothing to disclose. D.A. Reardon is an advisor to Abbvie; Advantagene; Agenus; Amgen; Bayer; Bristol-Myers Squibb; Celldex; DelMar; EMD Serono; Genentech/Roche; Imvax; Inovio; Medicenna Biopharma, Inc; Merck; Merck KGaA; Monteris; Novocure; Oncorus; Oxigene; Regeneron; Stemline; Sumitono Dainippon Pharma; Taiho Oncology, Inc.

REFERENCES

1. Ostrom Q, Gittleman H, Liao P. CBTRUS statistical report: primary brain and central nervous system tumors diagnosed in the United States in 2007–2011. Neuro Oncol 2014;16(Suppl 4):iv1–63.
2. Medawar PB. Immunity to homologous grafted skin; the fate of skin homografts transplanted to the brain, to subcutaneous tissue, and to the anterior chamber of the eye. Br J Exp Pathol 1948; 29(1):58–69.
3. Louveau A, Smirnov I, Keyes TJ, et al. Structural and functional features of central nervous system lymphatic vessels. Nature 2015;523(7560):337–41.
4. Di Lorenzo N, Palma L, Nicole S. Lymphocytic infiltration in long-survival glioblastomas: possible host's resistance. Acta Neurochir 1977;39(1–2): 27–33.
5. Weller M, Weinstock C, Will C, et al. CD95-dependent T-cell killing by glioma cells expressing CD95 ligand: more on tumor immune escape, the CD95 counterattack, and the immune privilege of the brain. Cell Physiol Biochem 1997;7(5):282–8.

6. Badie B, Schartner J, Prabakaran S, et al. Expression of Fas ligand by microglia: possible role in glioma immune evasion. J Neuroimmunol 2001; 120(1–2):19–24.

7. Berghoff AS, Kiesel B, Widhalm G, et al. Programmed death ligand 1 expression and tumor-infiltrating lymphocytes in glioblastoma. Neuro Oncol 2015;17(8):1064–75.

8. Butte MJ, Keir ME, Phamduy TB, et al. Programmed death-1 ligand 1 interacts specifically with the B7-1 costimulatory molecule to inhibit T cell responses. Immunity 2007;27(1):111–22.

9. Avril T, Saikali S, Vauléon E, et al. Distinct effects of human glioblastoma immunoregulatory molecules programmed cell death ligand-1 (PDL-1) and indoleamine 2,3-dioxygenase (IDO) on tumour-specific T cell functions. J Neuroimmunol 2010;225(1–2): 22–33.

10. Francisco LM, Sage PT, Sharpe AH. The PD-1 pathway in tolerance and autoimmunity. Immunol Rev 2010;236(1):219–42.

11. Grauer OM, Nierkens S, Bennink E, et al. CD4+ FoxP3+ regulatory T cells gradually accumulate in gliomas during tumor growth and efficiently suppress antiglioma immune responses in vivo. Int J Cancer 2007;121(1):95–105.

12. El Andaloussi A, Lesniak MS. CD4+ CD25+ FoxP3+ T-cell infiltration and heme oxygenase-1 expression correlate with tumor grade in human gliomas. J Neurooncol 2007;83(2):145–52.

13. Andaloussi AE, Lesniak MS. An increase in CD4+ CD25+ FOXP3+ regulatory T cells in tumor-infiltrating lymphocytes of human glioblastoma multiforme. Neuro Oncol 2006;8(3):234–43.

14. Hishii M, Nitta T, Ishida H, et al. Human glioma-derived interleukin-10 inhibits antitumor immune responses in vitro. Neurosurgery 1995;37(6): 1160–7.

15. Qiu B, Zhang D, Wang C, et al. IL-10 and TGΓ-β2 are overexpressed in tumor spheres cultured from human gliomas. Mol Biol Rep 2011;38(5): 3585–91.

16. Gabrusiewicz K, Ellert-Miklaszewska A, Lipko M, et al. Characteristics of the alternative phenotype of microglia/macrophages and its modulation in experimental gliomas. PLoS One 2011;6(8): e23902.

17. Chen Z, Feng X, Herting CJ, et al. Cellular and molecular identity of tumor-associated macrophages in glioblastoma. Cancer Res 2017;77(9):2266–78.

18. Wei J, Chen P, Gupta P, et al. Immune biology of glioma-associated macrophages and microglia: functional and therapeutic implications. Neuro Oncol 2020;22(2):180–94.

19. Medikonda R, Dunn G, Rahman M, et al. A review of glioblastoma immunotherapy. J Neurooncol 2020. https://doi.org/10.1007/s11060-020-03448-1.

20. Pardoll DM. The blockade of immune checkpoints in cancer immunotherapy. Nat Rev Cancer 2012; 12(4):252–64.

21. Zou W, Chen L. Inhibitory B7-family molecules in the tumour microenvironment. Nat Rev Immunol 2008;8(6):467–77.

22. June CH, Ledbetter JA, Gillespie MM, et al. T-cell proliferation involving the CD28 pathway is associated with cyclosporine-resistant interleukin 2 gene expression. Mol Cell Biol 1987;7(12):4472–81.

23. Thompson CB, Lindsten T, Ledbetter JA, et al. CD28 activation pathway regulates the production of multiple T-cell-derived lymphokines/cytokines. Proc Natl Acad Sci U S A 1989;86(4):1333–7.

24. Lanier LL, O'Fallon S, Somoza C, et al. CD80 (B7) and CD86 (B70) provide similar costimulatory signals for T cell proliferation, cytokine production, and generation of CTL. J Immunol 1995;154(1): 97–105.

25. Brunet J-F, Denizot F, Luciani M-F, et al. A new member of the immunoglobulin superfamily—CTLA-4. Nature 1987;328(6127):267–70.

26. Harper K, Balzano C, Rouvier E, et al. CTLA-4 and CD28 activated lymphocyte molecules are closely related in both mouse and human as to sequence, message expression, gene structure, and chromosomal location. J Immunol 1991;147(3):1037–44.

27. Walunas TL, Lenschow DJ, Bakker CY, et al. CTLA-4 can function as a negative regulator of T cell activation. Immunity 1994;1(5):405–13.

28. Brunner MC, Chambers CA, Chan FK-M, et al. CTLA-4-mediated inhibition of early events of T cell proliferation. J Immunol 1999;162(10):5813–20.

29. Schwartz J-CD, Zhang X, Fedorov AA, et al. Structural basis for co-stimulation by the human CTLA-4/B7-2 complex. Nature 2001;410(6828):604–8.

30. Stamper CC, Zhang Y, Tobin JF, et al. Crystal structure of the B7-1/CTLA-4 complex that inhibits human immune responses. Nature 2001;410(6828): 608–11.

31. Kane LP, Andres PG, Howland KC, et al. Akt provides the CD28 costimulatory signal for up-regulation of IL-2 and IFN-γ but not TH 2 cytokines. Nat Immunol 2001;2(1):37–44.

32. Pages F, Ragueneau M, Rottapel R, et al. Binding of phosphatidyl-inositol-3-OH kinase to CD28 is required for T-cell signalling. Nature 1994; 369(6478):327–9.

33. Qureshi OS, Zheng Y, Nakamura K, et al. Trans-endocytosis of CD80 and CD86: a molecular basis for the cell-extrinsic function of CTLA-4. Science 2011;332(6029):600–3.

34. Leach DR, Krummel MF, Allison JP. Enhancement of antitumor immunity by CTLA-4 blockade. Science 1996;271(5256):1734–6.

35. Larkin J, Chiarion-Sileni V, Gonzalez R, et al. Combined nivolumab and ipilimumab or monotherapy

in untreated melanoma. N Engl J Med 2015;373(1): 23–34.

36. Eggermont AM, Chiarion-Sileni V, Grob J-J, et al. Prolonged survival in stage III melanoma with ipilimumab adjuvant therapy. N Engl J Med 2016; 375(19):1845–55.

37. Comin-Anduix B, Escuin-Ordinas H, Ibarrondo FJ. Tremelimumab: research and clinical development. Onco Targets Ther 2016;9:1767.

38. Barber DL, Wherry EJ, Masopust D, et al. Restoring function in exhausted CD8 T cells during chronic viral infection. Nature 2006;439(7077):682–7.

39. Pauken KE, Wherry EJ. Overcoming T cell exhaustion in infection and cancer. Trends Immunol 2015; 36(4):265–76.

40. Sharpe AH, Pauken KE. The diverse functions of the PD1 inhibitory pathway. Nat Rev Immunol 2018;18(3):153.

41. Wintterle S, Schreiner B, Mitsdoerffer M, et al. Expression of the B7-related molecule B7-H1 by glioma cells: a potential mechanism of immune paralysis. Cancer Res 2003;63(21):7462–7.

42. Yokosuka T, Takamatsu M, Kobayashi-Imanishi W, et al. Programmed cell death 1 forms negative costimulatory microclusters that directly inhibit T cell receptor signaling by recruiting phosphatase SHP2. J Exp Med 2012;209(6):1201–17.

43. Antonios JP, Soto H, Everson RG, et al. Immunosuppressive tumor-infiltrating myeloid cells mediate adaptive immune resistance via a PD-1/PD-L1 mechanism in glioblastoma. Neuro Oncol 2017;19(6):796–807.

44. Terme M, Ullrich E, Aymeric L, et al. IL-18 induces PD-1–dependent immunosuppression in cancer. Cancer Res 2011;71(16):5393–9.

45. Freeman GJ, Long AJ, Iwai Y, et al. Engagement of the PD-1 immunoinhibitory receptor by a novel B7 family member leads to negative regulation of lymphocyte activation. J Exp Med 2000;192(7): 1027–34.

46. Cai J, Wang D, Zhang G, et al. The role of PD-1/PD-L1 axis in Treg development and function: implications for cancer immunotherapy. Onco Targets Ther 2019;12:8437.

47. Heiland DH, Haaker G, Delev D, et al. Comprehensive analysis of PD-L1 expression in glioblastoma multiforme. Oncotarget 2017;8(26):42214.

48. Nduom EK, Wei J, Yaghi NK, et al. PD-L1 expression and prognostic impact in glioblastoma. Neuro Oncol 2015;18(2):195–205.

49. Woroniecka K, Chongsathidkiet P, Rhodin K, et al. T-cell exhaustion signatures vary with tumor type and are severe in glioblastoma. Clin Cancer Res 2018;24(17):4175–86.

50. Mirzaei R, Sarkar S, Yong VW. T cell exhaustion in glioblastoma: intricacies of immune checkpoints. Trends Immunol 2017;38(2):104–15.

51. Parsa AT, Waldron JS, Panner A, et al. Loss of tumor suppressor PTEN function increases B7-H1 expression and immunoresistance in glioma. Nat Med 2007;13(1):84–8.

52. Mantovani A, Sica A. Macrophages, innate immunity and cancer: balance, tolerance, and diversity. Curr Opin Immunol 2010;22(2):231–7.

53. Qian B-Z, Pollard JW. Macrophage diversity enhances tumor progression and metastasis. Cell 2010;141(1):39–51.

54. Ding P, Wang W, Wang J, et al. Expression of tumor-associated macrophage in progression of human glioma. Cell Biochem Biophys 2014;70(3): 1625–31.

55. Bloch O, Crane CA, Kaur R, et al. Gliomas promote immunosuppression through induction of B7-H1 expression in tumor-associated macrophages. Clin Cancer Res 2013;19(12):3165–75.

56. Lamano JB, Lamano JB, Li YD, et al. Glioblastoma-derived IL6 induces immunosuppressive peripheral myeloid cell PD-L1 and promotes tumor growth. Clin Cancer Res 2019;25(12): 3643–57.

57. Fecci PE, Ochiai H, Mitchell DA, et al. Systemic CTLA-4 blockade ameliorates glioma-induced changes to the CD4+ T cell compartment without affecting regulatory T-cell function. Clin Cancer Res 2007;13(7):2158–67.

58. Agarwalla P, Barnard Z, Fecci P, et al. Sequential immunotherapy by vaccination with GM-CSF expressing glioma cells and CTLA-4 blockade effectively treats established murine intracranial tumors. J Immunother 2012;35(5):385.

59. Reardon DA, Gokhale PC, Klein SR, et al. Glioblastoma eradication following immune checkpoint blockade in an orthotopic, immunocompetent model. Cancer Immunol Res 2016;4(2):124–35.

60. Zeng J, See AP, Phallen J, et al. Anti-PD-1 blockade and stereotactic radiation produce long-term survival in mice with intracranial gliomas. Int J Radiat Oncol Biol Phys 2013;86(2):343–9.

61. Belmans J, Van Woensel M, Creyns B, et al. Immunotherapy with subcutaneous immunogenic autologous tumor lysate increases murine glioblastoma survival. Sci Rep 2017;7(1):1–11.

62. Johanns TM, Ward JP, Miller CA, et al. Endogenous neoantigen-specific CD8 T cells identified in two glioblastoma models using a cancer immunogenomics approach. Cancer Immunol Res 2016; 4(12):1007–15.

63. Lawrence MS, Stojanov P, Polak P, et al. Mutational heterogeneity in cancer and the search for new cancer-associated genes. Nature 2013;499(7457): 214–8.

64. Fridman WH, Zitvogel L, Sautès–Fridman C, et al. The immune contexture in cancer prognosis and treatment. Nat Rev Clin Oncol 2017;14(12):717.

65. Genoud V, Marinari E, Nikolaev SI, et al. Responsiveness to anti-PD-1 and anti-CTLA-4 immune checkpoint blockade in SB28 and GL261 mouse glioma models. Oncoimmunology 2018;7(12): e1501137.

66. Hodi FS, O'Day SJ, McDermott DF, et al. Improved survival with ipilimumab in patients with metastatic melanoma. N Engl J Med 2010; 363(8):711–23.

67. Margolin K, Ernstoff MS, Hamid O, et al. Ipilimumab in patients with melanoma and brain metastases: an open-label, phase 2 trial. Lancet Oncol 2012;13(5):459–65.

68. Gadgeel SM, Lukas RV, Goldschmidt J, et al. Atezolizumab in patients with advanced non-small cell lung cancer and history of asymptomatic, treated brain metastases: exploratory analyses of the phase III OAK study. Lung Cancer 2019;128: 105–12.

69. Reardon DA, Brandes AA, Omuro A, et al. Effect of nivolumab vs bevacizumab in patients with recurrent glioblastoma: the CheckMate 143 phase 3 randomized clinical trial. JAMA Oncol 2020;6(7): 1003–10.

70. Sampson JH, Omuro AMP, Preusser M, et al. A randomized, phase 3, open-label study of nivolumab versus temozolomide (TMZ) in combination with radiotherapy (RT) in adult patients (pts) with newly diagnosed, O-6-methylguanine DNA methyltransferase (MGMT)-unmethylated glioblastoma (GBM): CheckMate-498. J Clin Oncol 2016; 34(15_suppl):TPS2079.

71. Squibb B-M. Bristol-Myers Squibb announces Phase 3 CheckMate-498 study did not meet primary endpoint of overall survival with Opdivo (nivolumab) plus radiation in patients with newly diagnosed MGMT-unmethylated glioblastoma multiforme [press release]. In: May; 2019.

72. Squibb B-M. Bristol Myers Squibb provides update on Phase 3 Opdivo (nivolumab) CheckMate-548 trial in patients with newly diagnosed MGMT-methylated glioblastoma multiforme [press release]. In: September; 2019.

73. Reardon DA, Kim T-M, Frenel J-S, et al. ATIM-35. Results of the phase IB keynote-028 multi-cohort trial of pembrolizumab monotherapy in patients with recurrent PD-L1-positive glioblastoma multiforme (GBM). Neuro Oncol 2016;18(suppl_6): vi25–6.

74. Reardon DA, Nayak L, Peters KB, et al. Phase II study of pembrolizumab or pembrolizumab plus bevacizumab for recurrent glioblastoma (rGBM) patients. J Clin Oncol 2018;36(15_suppl):2006.

75. Powles T, Durán I, Van Der Heijden MS, et al. Atezolizumab versus chemotherapy in patients with platinum-treated locally advanced or metastatic urothelial carcinoma (IMvigor211): a multicentre,

76. open-label, phase 3 randomised controlled trial. Lancet 2018;391(10122):748–57.

77. Rittmeyer A, Barlesi F, Waterkamp D, et al. Atezolizumab versus docetaxel in patients with previously treated non-small-cell lung cancer (OAK): a phase 3, open-label, multicentre randomised controlled trial. Lancet 2017;389(10066):255–65.

78. Powles T, O'Donnell PH, Massard C, et al. Efficacy and safety of durvalumab in locally advanced or metastatic urothelial carcinoma: updated results from a phase 1/2 open-label study. JAMA Oncol 2017;3(9):e172411.

79. Reardon DA, Kaley TJ, Dietrich J, et al. Phase 2 study to evaluate safety and efficacy of MEDI4736 (durvalumab [DUR]) in glioblastoma (GBM) patients: An update. Journal of Clinical Oncology 2017;35(15_suppl):2042–2042.

80. Heery CR, O'Sullivan-Coyne G, Madan RA, et al. Avelumab for metastatic or locally advanced previously treated solid tumours (JAVELIN Solid Tumor): a phase 1a, multicohort, dose-escalation trial. Lancet Oncol 2017;18(5):587–98.

81. Omuro A, Vlahovic G, Lim M, et al. Nivolumab with or without ipilimumab in patients with recurrent glioblastoma: results from exploratory phase I cohorts of CheckMate 143. Neuro Oncol 2018;20(5): 674–86.

82. Carter T, Shaw H, Cohn-Brown D, et al. Ipilimumab and bevacizumab in glioblastoma. Clin Oncol 2016;28(10):622–6.

83. Brown NF, Ng SM, Brooks C, et al. A phase II open label, randomised study of ipilimumab with temozolomide versus temozolomide alone after surgery and chemoradiotherapy in patients with recently diagnosed glioblastoma: the Ipi-Glio trial protocol. BMC Cancer 2020;20(1):1–5.

84. Zadeh G, Lang F, Daras M, et al. ATIM-24. Interim results of a phase II multicenter study of the conditionally replicative oncolytic adenovirus DNX-2401 with pembrolizumab (Keytruda) for recurrent glioblastoma; captive study (Keynote-192). Neuro Oncol 2018;20(Suppl 6):vi6.

85. Duraiswamy J, Kaluza KM, Freeman GJ, et al. Dual blockade of PD-1 and CTLA-4 combined with tumor vaccine effectively restores T-cell rejection function in tumors. Cancer Res 2013;73(12): 3591–603.

86. Schumacher TN, Schreiber RD. Neoantigens in cancer immunotherapy. Science 2015;348(6230): 69–74.

87. Hodges TR, Ott M, Xiu J, et al. Mutational burden, immune checkpoint expression, and mismatch repair in glioma: implications for immune checkpoint immunotherapy. Neuro Oncol 2017;19(8): 1047–57.

88. Han S, Zhang C, Li Q, et al. Tumour-infiltrating CD4+ and CD8+ lymphocytes as predictors of

clinical outcome in glioma. Br J Cancer 2014;
110(10):2560–8.

88. Vidyarthi A, Agnihotri T, Khan N, et al. Predominance of M2 macrophages in gliomas leads to
the suppression of local and systemic immunity.
Cancer Immunol Immunother 2019;68(12):
1995–2004.

89. Fecci PE, Mitchell DA, Whitesides JF, et al.
Increased regulatory T-cell fraction amidst a diminished CD4 compartment explains cellular immune
defects in patients with malignant glioma. Cancer
Res 2006;66(6):3294–302.

90. Zhao J, Chen AX, Gartrell RD, et al. Immune and
genomic correlates of response to anti-PD-1 immunotherapy in glioblastoma. Nat Med 2019;25(3):
462–9.

91. Peng W, Chen JQ, Liu C, et al. Loss of PTEN promotes resistance to T cell–mediated immunotherapy. Cancer Discov 2016;6(2):202–16.

92. Cloughesy TF, Mochizuki AY, Orpilla JR, et al. Neoadjuvant anti-PD-1 immunotherapy promotes a survival benefit with intratumoral and systemic
immune responses in recurrent glioblastoma. Nat
Med 2019;25(3):477–86.

93. Parakh S, Park JJ, Mendis S, et al. Efficacy of anti-
PD-1 therapy in patients with melanoma brain metastases. Br J Cancer 2017;116(12):1558–63.

94. Queirolo P, Spagnolo F, Ascierto PA, et al. Efficacy
and safety of ipilimumab in patients with advanced
melanoma and brain metastases. J Neurooncol
2014;118(1):109–16.

95. Downey SG, Klapper JA, Smith FO, et al. Prognostic factors related to clinical response in patients with metastatic melanoma treated by CTL-
associated antigen-4 blockade. Clin Cancer Res
2007;13(22):6681–8.

96. Garant A, Guilbault C, Ekmekjian T, et al. Concomitant use of corticosteroids and immune checkpoint
inhibitors in patients with hematologic or solid neoplasms: a systematic review. Crit Rev Oncol Hem-
atol 2017;120:86–92.

97. Martins F, Sofiya L, Sykiotis GP, et al. Adverse effects of immune-checkpoint inhibitors: epidemiology, management and surveillance. Nat Rev
Clin Oncol 2019;16(9):563–80.

98. Heimberger AB, Sun W, Hussain SF, et al. Immunological responses in a patient with glioblastoma
multiforme treated with sequential courses of temozolomide and immunotherapy: case study. Neuro
Oncol 2008;10(1):98–103.

99. Crane CA, Han SJ, Ahn B, et al. Individual patient-
specific immunity against high-grade glioma after
vaccination with autologous tumor derived peptides bound to the 96 KD chaperone protein. Clin
Cancer Res 2013;19(1):205–14.

100. Qian J, Luo F, Yang J, et al. TLR2 promotes glioma
immune evasion by downregulating MHC class II
molecules in microglia. Cancer Immunol Res
2018;6(10):1220–33.

101. Zagzag D, Salnikow K, Chiriboga L, et al. Downregulation of major histocompatibility complex antigens in invading glioma cells: stealth invasion of
the brain. Lab Invest 2005;85(3):328–41.

CAR T Cells

Thilan Tudor, BA[a], Zev A. Binder, MD, PhD[a],*, Donald M. O'Rourke, MD[b]

KEYWORDS

- Chimeric antigen receptor • Chimeric antigen receptor T cell • Glioblastoma • Immunotherapy
- Trial • CAR-T

KEY POINTS

- Chimeric antigen receptor T cells (CAR-T) cells are reengineered T cells that express a fusion protein targeting a specific glioblastoma (GBM) tumor antigen.
- CAR construct design and manufacture process in the context of GBM leverages many of the same development principles that were used in the development and approval process of CAR-T cells for hematologic malignancies.
- The GBM tumor microenvironment presents numerous challenges to effective immunotherapy, including a stressful metabolic environment and a markedly immunosuppressive cytokine signature.
- In-human studies of CAR-T cell therapies demonstrate reasonable safety and tolerability and preliminary evidence of antitumor activity and appropriate trafficking to tumor sites, but limited persistence of these therapeutic agents and minimal durability of clinical response.
- Ongoing and emergent trials address novel frontiers in CAR-T therapeutic design for GBM, including multiantigen targeting, lymphodepletion preconditioning, and in vivo visualization of CAR-T trafficking, to improve therapeutic efficacy, reduce antigen escape and tumor recurrence, and advance clinical development.

INTRODUCTION

Glioblastoma (GBM), the most common primary malignant brain tumor in adults, is associated with extremely poor survival outcomes and is a universally fatal disease.[1] Standard of care therapy for newly diagnosed GBM involves maximal safe resection, subsequent radiotherapy and concurrent temozolomide (TMZ; 75 mg/m^2/d for 6 weeks), followed by maintenance TMZ (150–200 mg/m^2/d for first 5 consecutive days of a 28-day cycle for six cycles),[2,3] and is associated with poor survival outcomes, especially for patients with residual or multifocal disease.[3–5] The advancing therapeutic landscape for GBM is limited in scope, with only three novel therapies receiving Food and Drug Administration approval since 2005: (1) bevacizumab, a humanized anti–vascular endothelial growth factor (VEGF) monoclonal antibody treatment; (2) TMZ, an oral chemotherapeutic agent; and (3) a tumor-treating fields device that interferes with aberrant cell proliferation. A growing evidence base implicates the host adaptive immune response in the pathogenesis of GBM and overturns the prior characterization of the central nervous system (CNS) as an immune-privileged niche.[6]

Chimeric antigen receptor T cells (CAR-T) are an innovative immunotherapy approach to GBM, in which reengineered T cells express a fusion protein that targets a specific tumor antigen. When the CAR-T cell has associated with its targeted antigen, the reengineered T cell is activated and results in cytokine release, cytolytic degranulation,

[a] University of Pennsylvania, 3600 Hamilton Walk, Stemmler Hall, Room 176, Philadelphia, PA 19104; [b] John Templeton, Jr. M.D. Professor in Neurosurgery, Hospital of the University of Pennsylvania, 3400 Spruce St. Philadelphia, PA 19104, USA
* Corresponding author. Department of Neurosurgery, University of Pennsylvania, 3600 Hamilton Walk, Stemmler Hall, Room 176, Philadelphia, PA 19104.
E-mail address: Zev.Binder@pennmedicine.upenn.edu
Twitter: @ZevBinder (Z.A.B.); @DrORourke2 (D.M.O.)

Neurosurg Clin N Am 32 (2021) 249–263
https://doi.org/10.1016/j.nec.2020.12.005
1042-3680/21/

tumor cell killing, and T-cell proliferation.[7] CAR-T therapy development has been a watershed moment in cellular therapy for relapsed or refractory hematologic malignancies. CD19-directed CAR-T cells first received approval in 2017, with two products, tisagenlecleucel (Kymriah) and axicabtagene ciloleucel (Yescarta), delivering durable clinical outcomes for patients with advanced acute lymphoblastic leukemia and large B-cell lymphoma, respectively.[8,9] Investigators are currently working to recapitulate the success of CAR-T therapies for solid tumors including GBM[10]; however, there are unique challenges that are associated with therapeutic delivery in CNS malignancies, including bioavailability, immune cell trafficking, durability of response, and a hostile tumor microenvironment.[11,12]

CHIMERIC ANTIGEN RECEPTOR T CELLS
Chimeric Antigen Receptor T Cells Design Overview for Glioblastoma

CAR-T cells involve the ex vivo reengineering of a patient's or donor's peripheral T-cell population to express a CAR tailored to a specific antigen that is expressed on the surface of tumor cells.[10,13] The CAR construct itself includes multiple structural and functional intracellular domains that confer the reengineered T-cell population desirable therapeutic attributes. These fusion proteins contain an extracellular single chain variable fragment antigen recognition domain, a transmembrane domain, and an intracellular T-cell activation domain.[13]

The intracellular domain of the CAR construct contains the T-cell coreceptor CD3ζ and its immunoreceptor tyrosine-based activation motifs. Following antigen recognition and endodomain receptor clustering, the activation signal is transmitted to the T cell.[13] CAR-T cell design has evolved from its initial iterations to incorporate novel design elements that enable more potent costimulatory signaling. Second-generation CAR constructs include a single costimulatory molecule, such as 4-1BB or CD28 that is fused to CD3ζ to deliver a more potent immunotherapy.[12,14] Third-generation CARs contain two costimulatory domains linked to CD3ζ. These costimulatory domains improve CAR-T therapeutic efficacy and durability of response compared with first-generation constructs.[15]

T-Cell Harvesting

The autologous CAR-T manufacturing process for GBM generally reflects the same common steps that apply to CAR-T design for nonsolid malignancies.[16] The patient undergoes leukapheresis to harvest the peripheral blood mononuclear cells that contain the T-cell population that serves as the backbone of the reengineered immunotherapy. After cell washing, the apheresis product can then undergo enrichment or depletion of certain subpopulations.

Activation

To mimic T-cell activation in vivo, addition of OKT3, an anti-CD3 monoclonal antibody, or interleukin (IL)-2 is a common approach to stimulate T cells.[16] Coculture with lymphoblastoid cell lines, which are Epstein-Barr virus–infected peripheral blood mononuclear cells, can also stimulate T cells in what is termed the rapid expansion protocol.[16] CD3/CD28 antibody coated beads and artificial antigen-presenting cells represent emergent stimulation protocols that can be used to reduce GBM CAR-T manufacture time and are under current investigation.[17]

Chimeric Antigen Receptor T Cells Construct Delivery

Following stimulation, the T cells are transfected using plasmids or transduced with retroviral or lentiviral vectors containing the CAR construct. Lentiviral vectors are beneficial because they can transduce nondividing cells, excluding G-0 phase.[18] In contrast, retroviruses only transduce actively dividing cells and therefore rely on robust ex vivo T-cell proliferation.[16] A plasmid-based approach, in which naked DNA is electroporated into T cells, offers cost benefits compared with viral transduction methods,[19] yet is comparatively limited by its low efficiency of stable transfection into T cells.[20] Transduction efficiencies for the viral methods vary, with GBM CAR-T trials indicating a range between 5% and 26% in a lentiviral vector approach[5] and 18% and 67% for a retroviral vector approach.[21]

Expansion

CAR-T cells are expanded using an ex vivo culture medium that often contains cytokines and other stimulating factors that encourage T-cell proliferation. This critical step can take place either before or after the transfection or transduction of the CAR-T construct and may vary by investigator. Expansion can take place in a variety of settings, including T-flasks, culture plates or bags, and rocking bioreactors.[22] The culture media contains gamma-chain cytokines that support T-cell proliferation, with IL-2, IL-7, IL-15, and IL-21 as common additions.[12,23] The addition of support cytokines and expansion methodology used is trial-dependent and may influence the phenotypic distribution of the final infusion product.

Infusion

Following activation, transfection or transduction, and expansion, the CAR-T product is often phenotypically characterized and infused into the patient.[6] Lymphodepletion of GBM CAR-T patients before infusion is an avenue that is of particular interest. TMZ has been used as a lymphodepleting preconditioning agent in a trial setting for GBM patients.[12,24] Although it is hypothesized that lymphodepletion may yield benefits in terms of in vivo CAR-T expansion and persistence,[24] current GBM CAR-T trials demonstrate no benefit of chemotherapy preconditioning before infusion.[5,25]

CHIMERIC ANTIGEN RECEPTOR T CELLS DELIVERY IN THE CENTRAL NERVOUS SYSTEM

CAR-T delivery in the context of the CNS presents unique challenges with respect to engraftment, bioavailability, antitumor efficacy, and safety. The blood-brain barrier (BBB) is a highly selective physiologic boundary that connects brain capillary endothelial cells with the surrounding luminal and abluminal membranes[6,11] and is a critical structural and functional determinant of immune trafficking and immunotherapy delivery in the CNS.

The BBB, along with the glia limitans, formed by the fusion of astrocytes processes that line the basement membrane of the CNS, form a tightly controlled barrier.[26] The BBB specifically limits entry to activated T cells, but not to their naive counterparts. Therefore, only in settings of neuroinflammation or permissive signaling environment can T cells cross the BBB and enter the parenchymal tissue.[26–28] Given the challenges of trafficking CAR-T cells into parenchymal tissue, many GBM CAR-T trials have focused on local intracavitary and intraventricular delivery in favor of intravenous delivery.

Intravenous Delivery

Intravenous delivery of GBM CAR-T products is a viable approach even in the face of the unique challenges that the CNS poses for therapeutic delivery and bioavailability. Because the BBB and glia limitans are frequently dysregulated in the context of GBM,[29,30] systemic delivery may be a viable option. O'Rourke and colleagues[5] and Ahmed and colleagues[21] used intravenous delivery for their respective CAR-T trials. Both groups tracked engraftment of the CAR-T product in the tumor following intravenous delivery.

Intracavitary/Intratumoral Delivery

Multiple GBM CAR-T trials have successfully demonstrated intracavitary/intratumoral delivery as a means to overcome the structural and functional boundary imposed by the BBB and glia limitans. Brown and colleagues[17] and Keu and colleagues[31] provide preliminary evidence that intracavitary delivery appropriately localizes to GBM resection sites. The [^{18}F]FHBG PET-based imaging assay that was used to track CAR-T[+] cells indicated that the intracavitary delivery of the modified cytotoxic T lymphocytes trafficked to intracranial tumor sites.[31]

Intraventricular Delivery

Intraventricular delivery represents a potentially successful approach for a subset of GBM patients with spinal involvement of disease. Brown and colleagues[32] pursued intraventricular infusions following six cycles of intracavitary delivery of the IL13BBζ–CAR T CAR in a 50-year-old patient with recurrent GBM with leptomeningeal disease because of the appearance of spinal metastatic lesions during the course of the initial intracranial infusions. Subsequent intraventricular infusions completely eliminated all metastatic lesions.[32] Throughout the infusions delivered via a catheter in the lateral ventricle, CAR-T[+] cell numbers detected in the cerebrospinal fluid seemed to be directly associated with tumor burden and inflammatory cytokine levels.[32]

TUMOR MICROENVIRONMENT IN GLIOBLASTOMA

There are many unique considerations for CAR-T delivery, in addition to local delivery to the CNS, which are relevant to GBM patients. The GBM tumor microenvironment is an immunosuppressive and metabolically stressful niche that impairs immunotherapeutic efficacy. There are many soluble immunosuppressive factors, cytokines, and immune cells that attenuate the antitumor response.[11,33] GBM cells secrete IL-6, IL-10, transforming growth factor-β, and other anti-inflammatory cytokines that dampen cytotoxic antitumor immune responses.[33] Regulatory T cells, tumor-associated macrophages, immunosuppressive-type macrophages, microglia, and myeloid-derived suppressor cells also characterize the anti-inflammatory condition associated in GBM.[34–36]

Furthermore, the hypoxic and metabolically stressful microenvironment is a hallmark feature of GBM. Hypoxia has been shown to potentiate the immunosuppressive effects of other tumoral anti-inflammatory factors and contributes to the renewal of glioma-like stem cell population that may confer chemotherapy and irradiation.[37] Nutrient insufficiency is also characteristic of the dysregulated metabolic state in GBM. T cells encounter a glucose supply-demand mismatch in the GBM tumor microenvironment, because the glucose-poor niche does not provide sufficient glucose supply to meet the high glycolytic activity of T cells needed to maintain proliferation and effector capacity.[11,34] In addition to dysfunctional glucose metabolism, other metabolic substrates, including tryptophan, arginine, lactate, and lysine, can have deleterious effects on protein translation and T-cell function.[38]

SPATIAL AND TEMPORAL GLIOBLASTOMA HETEROGENEITY

There are many forms of heterogeneity in the GBM tumor microenvironment, including variation in cell type, mitotic activity, vascular pattern, and necrosis.[39] Common CAR-T targets for GBM, including epidermal growth factor receptor (EGFR) variant III (EGFRvIII), IL13Rα2, and human epidermal growth factor receptor 2 (HER2), demonstrate heterogeneity at the level of the patient in spatial and temporal dimensions.[21,40,41] This intratumoral variability presents a challenge to effective CAR-T delivery. In EGFRvIII- and IL13Rα2-directed CAR-T trials, investigators noted that target antigen quantitative expression varied regionally within the tumor[5] and that CAR-T cell trafficking to distant tumoral sites away from target intracranial lesions is possible.[31] Temporal heterogeneity is also evident, with next-generation sequencing of GBM patient lesions suggesting that there is selective expansion or regression of tumor subpopulations with unique molecular signatures when treated with radiation or chemotherapy.[42]

Antigen escape is a phenomenon in which tumor cells avoid CAR-T-directed killing by expressing alternate forms of the target antigen. Loss of target antigen has been documented in GBM CAR-T trials for EGFRvIII- and IL13Rα2-directed CAR-T constructs,[5,32] which may serve as a mechanism for decreased postinfusion expansion of the CAR-T product and attenuated efficacy from a monovalent CAR-T construct. Antigen escape poses many challenges for effective CAR-T design, because single-antigen targeting may be insufficient to stimulate a durable CAR-T response postinfusion.

TARGETS OF INTEREST IN GLIOBLASTOMA
IL13Rα2

IL13Rα2, a high-affinity IL-13 receptor, is an attractive target antigen for GBM CAR-T therapy given its upregulation in high-malignancy disease, specificity for GBM cells, and limited expression in normal brain parenchyma.[11,43] Approximately 58% of World Health Organization grade IV gliomas have upregulation of this receptor, and this overexpression has been linked with poor survival outcomes.[44]

HER2

HER2 is another attractive target antigen for the purposes of CAR design for GBM patients. HER2 encodes a transmembrane glycoprotein with intracellular tyrosine kinase activity[45] and is well-characterized with respect to the pathogenesis of breast cancer. Although HER2-positive GBM is not common, initial studies suggested that 15% to 17% of GBM expressed the transmembrane protein by immunohistochemistry and that expression is linked to poor survival outcomes.[46–48] A second-generation HER2-specific CAR construct demonstrated strong antitumor activity in an orthotopic xenogeneic mouse model.[49] The same research group subsequently initiated the first GBM CAR-T study that addressed HER2-positive GBM patients with progressive disease.[21]

EGFRvIII

EGFR is a receptor tyrosine kinase that is commonly amplified or mutated in human GBM.[50] EGFRvIII is the most common variant of EGFR in human tumors and results from the in-frame deletion of exons 2 to 7 that creates a novel glycine at the junction of exons 1 and 8.[51,52] The truncated variant leads to constitutive signaling in the Ras-mitogen-activated protein kinase pathway and is associated with more malignant GBM.[53] EGFRvIII is expressed in approximately 30% of newly diagnosed patients[51] and has been associated with mixed survival outcomes. Although earlier studies suggested that EGFRvIII was a poor prognostic indicator,[53–55] more recent and larger studies have not demonstrated any significant predictive power associated with the variant.[56]

CHIMERIC ANTIGEN RECEPTOR T CELLS CLINICAL TRIALS FOR GLIOBLASTOMA PATIENTS
IL13Rα2 Trials

The first human study of first-generation IL13Rα2-directed CAR-T cells with repeated intracavitary administration in three patients with recurrent GBM provided promising results regarding the safety and efficacy of the immunotherapy

(**Table 1**).[17] An IL-13-zetakine construct, an MHC-independent CAR, recognizes IL13Rα2 using a unique IL-13 ligand with a point mutation (E13Y) to reduce binding affinity and attenuate off-target reactivity to the more commonly expressed IL13Ra2/IL4Ra complex. The CAR-T infusions, delivered through a catheter/reservoir system, had a favorable safety profile, with no dose-limiting toxicities recorded. However, there were two grade 3 headaches attributable to one subject, and a grade 3 neurologic event associated with another patient that were possibly related to CAR-T administration. A rapid inflammatory response after T-cell infusion followed by necrosis favored antitumor activity over progressive disease or previous treatment effect.

The City of Hope research group that oversaw the first IL13Rα2 study followed up with a subsequent trial using a second-generation IL13Rα2-directed CAR that incorporated at 4-1BB costimulatory domain in a 50-year-old GBM patient.[32] The patient presented with recurrent multifocal GBM with leptomeningeal disease with unmethylated O6-methylguanine–DNA methyltransferase (MGMT) promoter, wild-type IDH1, and IL13Rα2 H-score of 100. The patient initially received six cycles of intracavitary infusions; however, because of progression at distal sites and the emergence of spinal metastases, a catheter was placed to enable intraventricular delivery. Following 10 cycles of intraventricular infusions, all spinal metastases were completely eliminated. In contrast with the earlier study, the research group observed a more favorable safety profile with the second-generation construct, with no grade 3 or higher adverse events observed and no dose-limiting toxicities. Of note, the data indicated that IL13Rα2-directed CARs may modulate the GBM tumor microenvironment. There were significant increases in proinflammatory cytokines throughout the 7-day infusion cycle, including interferon-γ, tumor necrosis factor-α, IL-2, IL-5, IL-6, IL-8, and host immune cell populations, such as CD19+ B cells and CD11b+CD15+ granulocytes in the cerebrospinal fluid. Similar to their previous trial, expansion and persistence of the second-generation IL13Rα2-directed CAR in this patient was limited in later infusions. After a substantial clinical response of 7.5 months following the initiation of the intracavitary and intraventricular infusions, GBM recurred at four novel sites. Immunohistochemistry analysis confirmed low IL13Rα2 expression, suggesting lower target antigen expression may be associated with disease recurrence at novel locations.

The localization of anti-IL13Rα2 CAR-T therapies to the appropriate compartment within the CNS is a critical therapeutic feature for antitumor activity. Keu and colleagues[31] developed a PET-based visualization methodology using [18F] FHBG, a fluorine-18 radiolabeled analogue of penciclovir, to monitor in vivo trafficking of HSV1-tk expressing IL13Rα2-directed CAR-T cells. The study provided preliminary evidence of appropriate cytotoxic T lymphocytes trafficking to tumor sites; however, the investigators were not able to confirm this hypothesis given noticeable false-positive signals in preinfusion scans.

EGFRvIII Trials

Two in-human EGFRvIII-directed CAR trials have been conducted to date that provide support for further clinical advancement of CAR-T therapeutics that target this oncogenic variant. A phase I trial at the University of Pennsylvania with a single, intravenous infusion of EGFRvIII-directed CAR-T cells included 10 patients with EGFRvIII+ recurrent GBM.[5] Based on a preclinical trial of an anti-EGFRvIII CAR that demonstrated antitumor activity and minimal reactivity to human skin grafts in immunodeficient mice,[57] the research group leveraged this construct for the first in-human trial of an EGFRvIII-directed CAR. Substantial tumor regression was not observed in any patients based on MRI imaging. However, one patient had residual stable disease for more than 18 months postinfusion and all seven patients reoperated on postinfusion demonstrated a decrease or complete loss of the target antigen. The poor prognostic characteristics associated with the patient sample in this trial are of interest, because 9 out of 10 patients had multifocal disease and all patients were MGMT promoter unmethylated, which has been implicated as a predictive marker of poor survival outcomes.[58] Most patients had a postinfusion resection, enabling a comparative analysis of CAR-T cell trafficking in the peripheral blood and the tumor site. For two patients, CAR-T DNA sequence copies in brain tumor specimens were 3 and 100 times greater than their pairwise peripheral blood specimens, suggesting CAR-T cell trafficking to the appropriate compartment.

In contrast, a phase I dose-escalation trial for patients with recurrent EGFRvIII+ GBM using a third-generation construct incorporated lymphodepletion and systemic IL-2 administration, similar to protocols that have resulted in clinical responses for patients with melanoma and synovial sarcoma.[25] Eighteen patients ultimately received the CAR-T infusion product that included 4-1BB and CD28 costimulatory domains. There were no objective responses by MRI imaging and most

Table 1
Summary of in-human CAR-T trials for GBM patients

Study, Year	No. of Patients	Target Antigen	CAR-T	Route of Administration	TME Response	Max Dose (Cells)	Safety and Tolerability	Outcomes
Goff et al,[25] 2019	18	EGFRvIII	EGFRvIII-CD28-41BBζ (third generation)	Intravenous	N/A	2.6×10^{10}	2 DLTs. 1 patient developed acute dyspnea and severe hypotension with subsequent treatment-related mortality (grade 5). 1 patient developed dyspnea that was successfully managed with CPAP.	Median OS: 6.9 mo. Median progression-free survival: 1.3 mo. 1 patient alive at 59 mo. 2 additional patients survived >1 y.
O'Rourke et al,[5] 2017	10	EGFRvIII	EGFRvIII-4-1BB CD3ζ Bulk T cells (second generation)	Intravenous	Increased expression of IDO1, FoxP3, IL-10, PD-L1, TGF-β 5 of 10 patients with 10-fold or greater increase in IL-6 postinfusion	5×10^{8}	No DLTs. Grade 3–4 Possibly related adverse events: left ventricular systolic dysfunction (n = 1), left-sided muscle weakness (n = 1), facial muscle weakness (n = 1), headache (n = 1), intracranial hemorrhage (n = 1), seizure (n = 2).	Median OS: 251 d. Post-treatment EGFRvIII loss in 5 out of 7 patients.

Reference	N	Target	Construct	Route	Immune response	Dose	Toxicity	Outcome
Ahmed et al.,[21] 2017	17	HER2	HER2-FRP5.CD28ζ VST (EBV-CMVpp65-AD) (second generation)	Intravenous	N/A	1×10^8	No DLTs. Grade 2–4 Possibly related adverse events: headache (n = 1), seizure (n = 2).	Median OS: 11.1 mo (24.5 mo from diagnosis), 1/16 patients partial response (>9 mo), 7/16 patients stable disease (8 wk–29 mo), 8/16 patients progressive disease. Patients with no salvage therapy before infusion had significantly longer median OS (27.2 mo) than those with previous salvage therapy (6.7 mo).
Keu et al.,[31] 2017	7		IL13 (E13Y)-CD3ζ [18F]FHBG-HSV1-TK-HPH- GR- deleted CD8+ CTLs (second generation)	Intracerebral	N/A	1×10^8	No DLTs. No major or life-threatening events related to [18F] FHBG and/or CTL infusions.	[18F]FHBG gene reporter used in novel PET-based imaging approach to in vivo CTL monitoring. Survival between 4 and 59 following first infusion of CTL product.
Brown et al,[32] 2016	1	IL13Rα2	IL13(E13Y)-41BBζ-CD19 t Memory T cells (second generation)	Intracavitary, intra-ventricular	Increased CD-3+ CD-14+ CD-15+, CD-19+ immune cells and 10-fold or greater increase in inflammatory cytokines (IFN-γ, TNF-α, IL-2, IL-5, IL-6, IL-8, IL-10) and chemokines (CXCL9, CXCL10, CCR2, IL-1Rα)	10×10^6	No DLTs. No grade 3–4 possibly related adverse events related to CAR-T administration.	Case report of 50-year-old patient demonstrating 7.5 clinical response, including complete elimination of spinal metastases following intraventricular delivery of the CAR construct. Disease progression at 228 d.

(continued on next page)

Table 1
(continued)

Study, Year	No. of Patients	Target Antigen	CAR-T	Route of Administration	TME Response	Max Dose (Cells)	Safety and Tolerability	Outcomes
Brown et al,[17] 2015	3	IL13Rα2	IL13(E13Y)-CD3ζ CD8⁺ CTLs (first generation)	Intracavitary, intratumoral	Transient inflammatory response and increase in necrotic volume at tumor site, confirmed by elevated lactate and lipid peaks and a low choline/creatinine ratio	1×10^8	No DLTs. Grade 3 adverse events: headache (n = 1), neurologic event shuffling gait and tongue deviation (n = 1).	Median postrelapse survival:10.3 mo. Significant decrease in IL13Rα2 expression vs pretreatment levels (1 patient). No tumor recurrence at border of resection cavity (2 out of 3 patients)

Abbreviations: CMV, cytomegalovirus; CPAP, continuous positive airway pressure; CTL, cytotoxic T lymphocytes; DLT, dose-limiting toxicity; EBV, Epstein-Barr virus; IFN, interferon; OS, overall survival; TGF, transforming growth factor; TME, tumor microenvironment; TNF, tumor necrosis factor; VST, virus-specific T cells.

patients had progressive disease at the first follow-up. With progression-free survival of 1.3 months, the investigators suggested that the anti-EGFRvIII CAR-T product provided minimal to no clinically meaningful benefit to patients, even with notable persistence of the CAR$^+$ cells at the 1-month postinfusion timepoint for 14 of the patients. Dose-limiting toxicities were associated with the highest dosage ($\geq 10^{10}$ cells), with one patient developing acute dyspnea and pulmonary edema and ultimately succumbing to severe hypotension and the other developing severe dyspnea that was managed successfully with continuous positive airway pressure. Refinement of EGFRvIII-directed CAR-T therapy, with respect to antitumor activity and its safety, may support ongoing clinical advancement of bispecific and trispecific CAR-T constructs that incorporate EGFRvIII targeting as a part of the therapeutic mechanism and anti-EGFRvIII antibody development.[59]

HER2 Trials

The first in-human anti-HER2 CAR-T product for GBM patients used a second-generation construct using a CD28 costimulatory domain.[21] Of note, the investigators expressed the CAR construct in virus-specific T cells (VSTs) to facilitate adoption of the infusion product. These VSTs not only provide antitumor activity, but also receive a sufficient costimulatory signal following native receptor engagement by latent virus antigens presented by endogenous professional antigen-presenting cells.[21,60] The Baylor team generated HER2-directed CAR-T cells that were specific for cytomegalovirus, Epstein-Barr virus, or adenovirus. Expansion, measured by interferon-γ Elispot assays, was not observed in vivo in GBM patients, in contrast to the significant expansion of VSTs in hematopoietic stem cell transplant recipients who are extremely lymphodepleted.[61,62] With respect to persistence, the CAR$^+$ cells were detectable in the peripheral blood for up to 12 months. This is a notable increase from persistence recorded in EGFRvIII- and IL13Rα2-directed CAR-T trials in GBM patients and provides additional support for the exploration of VST-based approaches to increasing CAR-T longevity in vivo.

EMERGENT CLINICAL TRIALS AND FUTURE DIRECTIONS

Currently, there are 16 trials that involve CAR-T therapy as a treatment modality for GBM on clinicaltrials.gov. Of these trials, seven are actively recruiting patients, one trial is active and not recruiting, and one trial has been terminated with results (**Table 2**).

Exploration of attractive antigen targets that can improve CAR-T engraftment, persistence, and efficacy is a prominent theme in emergent GBM CAR-T clinical trials. Targets of interest include more conventional IL-13Rα2 and HER2 and novel antigens of interest, such as B7-H3 (CD276), an antigen that is not normally expressed in CNS tissue, but has enriched expression in GBM patients (NCT04385173, NCT04077866). Erythropoietin-producing hepatocellular carcinoma A2 (EphA2), a receptor tyrosine kinase that is overexpressed in GBM and is associated with poor outcomes,[66-68] is also a promising target. A phase I/II trial explored the effectiveness and safety of an anti-EphA2 CAR-T therapy in GBM patients; however, the study was recently withdrawn (NCT02575261).

Combination therapy of CAR-T immunotherapy used in conjunction with immune checkpoint blockade and antiangiogenic therapy is an emergent area in GBM therapeutic development. Upregulation of immunosuppressive factors, including programmed death-ligand 1 (PD-L1), IDO1, FoxP3, and transforming growth factor-β, has been implicated in the GBM tumor microenvironment,[12] demonstrating a role for checkpoint blockade and other therapeutics that can potentiate the host response through reversal of T-cell exhaustion. An ongoing single-arm, open-label study at The University of Pennsylvania builds on a prior phase I study that established the safety and tumor localization profiles of an EGFRvIII-direct CAR (NCT02209376). The group is now combining 2.0 × 10^8 cell doses of the anti-EGFRvIII construct with 200-mg pembrolizumab, a humanized antibody directed against programmed cell death protein (PD-1) following adjuvant radiotherapy (NCT03726515). Strategies that target the abnormal vascularization of the GBM TME are also promising in the context of combination therapy.[69] CAR-T administration in combination with bevacizumab, an anti-VEGF monoclonal antibody, may counteract the immunosuppressive effects modulated by VEGF, such as the recruitment of regulatory T cells and myeloid-derived suppressor cells and disrupted dendritic cell activation[70] and has shown to strengthen the antitumor efficacy of an anti-GD2 CAR-T therapy in a preclinical study.[71]

In addition to a marked immunosuppressive signature, the GBM tumor microenvironment also presents challenges with respect to antigen escape. Loss of target antigen represents the paradox of effective CAR-T treatment; postinfusion antigen loss is indicative of effective antitumor

Table 2
Active trials of CAR-T cell therapies for glioblastoma

NCT#/Institution	Study Name	Phase	Target Antigen	ROA	Comments
NCT04385173, Second Affiliated Hospital of Zhejiang University School of Medicine, Hangzhou, China	Pilot Study of B7-H3 CAR-T in Treating Patients With Recurrent and Refractory Glioblastoma	I	B7-H3	Intratumoral/intracerebroventricular	No lymphodepleting chemotherapy. Locoregional administration. Inclusion criteria require B7-H3-positive tumor by IHC with H-score $\geq$ 50.
NCT04077866, Second Affiliated Hospital of Zhejiang University School of Medicine, Hangzhou, China	B7-H3 CAR-T for Recurrent or Refractory Glioblastoma	I/II	B7-H3	Intratumoral/intracerebroventricular	Randomized parallel-arm study to evaluate head-to-head safety and efficacy of B7-H3 CAR-T to temozolomide alone in relapsed/refractory GBM patients.
NCT04045847, Xijing Hospital, Xi'an, Shaanxi, China	CD147-CART Cells in Patients With Recurrent Malignant Glioma	I	CD147	Intracavitary	Estimated enrollment n = 31 patients.
NCT04214392, City of Hope Medical Center, Duarte, California	Chimeric Antigen Receptor (CAR) T Cells With a Chlorotoxin Tumor-Targeting Domain for the Treatment of MPP2+ Recurrent or Progressive Glioblastoma	I	MPP2	Dual delivery	Recognition domain of CAR derived from CTLX, a natural peptide from the nontoxic venom component of death stalker scorpion venom. Orthotopic xenograft mice models have demonstrated antitumor activity of CTLX-directed CAR therapy for MPP2+ tumors.[63]
NCT04003649, City of Hope Medical Center, Duarte, California	IL13Ralpha2-Targeted Chimeric Antigen Receptor (CAR) T Cells With or Without Nivolumab and Ipilimumab in Treating Patients With Recurrent or Refractory Glioblastoma	I	IL13Rα2	Intratumoral/intraventricular	CAR-T combination with immune checkpoint blockade therapy (nivolumab and ipilimumab).

Location	Title	Phase	Target	ROA	Notes
NCT02208362, City of Hope Medical Center, Duarte, California	Genetically Modified T-cells in Treating Patients With Recurrent or Refractory Malignant Glioma	I	IL13Rα2	Intracavitary/intratumoral, intraventricular	Published cohort of 3 patients suggests second-generation IL13Rα2 CAR has antitumor activity.[64]
NCT03389230, City of Hope Medical Center, Duarte, California	Memory-Enriched T Cells in Treating Patients With Recurrent or Refractory Grade III-IV Glioma	I	HER2	Intratumoral/intracavitary, intraventricular	Locoregional delivery of HER2-directed CAR to the brain for GBM patients.
NCT02664363, The Preston Robert Tisch Brain Tumor Center at Duke, Durham, North Carolina	EGFRvIII CAR T Cells for Newly-Diagnosed WHO Grade IV Malignant Glioma (ExCeL)	I	EGFRvIII	Intravenous	Dose-intensified lymphodepletion preconditioning to grade 3 lymphopenia with TMZ. Dose-escalation study with ^{111}In-labeled CARs.
NCT03726515, Abramson Cancer Center of the University of Pennsylvania, Philadelphia, Pennsylvania	CART-EGFRvIII + Pembrolizumab in GBM	I	EGFRvIII	Intravenous	Based on upregulation of anti-inflammatory molecules including PD-L1 in this group's previous study,[5] pembrolizumab (PD-1 inhibitor) treatment added in combination EGFRvIII-directed CAR.[65]

Abbreviations: CTLX, chlorotoxin; IHC, Immunohistochemistry; ROA, Route of administration; WHO, World Health Organization.
Data accessed from clinicaltrials.gov on November 6, 2020.

activity, but simultaneously impairs the honing mechanism of CAR-T cells and enables tumor escape, because the reengineered immune cells have lost their target on the GBM tumor cell surface that ensures appropriate localization, engagement, and activation of the T-cell construct. Bivalent and trivalent CARs that incorporate multiple well-characterized GBM antigen targets including IL13Rα2, EGFRvIII, HER2, and EphA2 are currently under investigation in preclinical animal models.[12] A preclinical trial at Baylor College of Medicine, using a trispecific CAR directed against IL13Rα2 and HER2 and EphA2 demonstrated significant antitumor activity and broader therapeutic activity[41] than a similar bivalent construct targeting IL13Rα2 and HER2 also designed by the group.[72] However, loss of target antigen was common in surviving GBM cells suggesting tumor escape.[12,41,72]

Ongoing and future trials that investigate the safety, tolerability, and activity of CAR-T cells that target novel antigens, invoke combination therapy, and address GBM tumor microenvironment considerations may provide new avenues for therapeutic development. VSTs, lymphodepletion regimens, and immune checkpoint blockade represent a few of the emergent strategies that are under investigation in active trials. Given the high unmet clinical need for relapsed/refractory GBM patients and increasingly well-characterized role of the immune system in GBM pathogenesis, clinical advancement CAR-T cell therapies from preclinical models to pivotal-stage trials is top-of-mind for clinicians and investigators because these immunotherapies may substantially improve clinical outcomes for this patient population.

CLINICS CARE POINTS

- Persistence and expansion of CAR-T cells post-infusion is limited in most patients, with lymphodepletion preconditioning and use of VSTs as potential strategies to overcome this limitation to durable therapeutic response.

- Dose-limiting toxicities with CAR-T administration, although rare, can result in potentially fatal complications including acute dyspnea and severe hypotension and patients should be closely monitored when titrating a patient to higher CAR-T cell doses.

- Preliminary evidence suggests intraventricular administration may be relevant for the treatment of leptomeningeal disease and spinal metastases and able to attenuate tumor growth at sites distant to the point of administration.

- A single study indicates that patients with no salvage therapy before CAR-T administration may have substantially longer median overall survival compared with their counterparts who did receive prior salvage therapy, suggesting that prior disease course and treatment history is relevant to a patient's course.

ACKNOWLEDGMENT

Funding for the work was provided by the GBM Translational Center of Excellence grant from the Abramson Cancer Center.

DISCLOSURE

D.M. O'Rourke and Z.A. Binder are inventors on patents related to CAR-T cells that have been filed by the University of Pennsylvania.

REFERENCES

1. Ostrom QT, Gittleman H, Xu J, et al. CBTRUS statistical report: primary brain and other central nervous system tumors diagnosed in the United States in 2009-2013. Neuro Oncol 2016;18(suppl_5):v1–75.

2. Gilbert MR, Wang M, Aldape KD, et al. Dose-dense temozolomide for newly diagnosed glioblastoma: a randomized phase III clinical trial. J Clin Oncol 2013;31(32):4085–91.

3. Stupp R, Mason WP, van den Bent MJ, et al. Radiotherapy plus concomitant and adjuvant temozolomide for glioblastoma. N Engl J Med 2005;352(10):987–96.

4. Patil CG, Yi A, Elramsisy A, et al. Prognosis of patients with multifocal glioblastoma: a case-control study: clinical article. J Neurosurg 2012;117(4):705–11.

5. O'Rourke DM, Nasrallah MP, Desai A, et al. A single dose of peripherally infused EGFRvIII-directed CAR T cells mediates antigen loss and induces adaptive resistance in patients with recurrent glioblastoma. Sci Transl Med 2017;9(399). https://doi.org/10.1126/scitranslmed.aaa0984.

6. Chuntova P, Downey KM, Hegde B, et al. Genetically engineered T-cells for malignant glioma: overcoming the barriers to effective immunotherapy. Front Immunol 2019;9. https://doi.org/10.3389/fimmu.2018.03062.

7. Hombach A, Wieczarkowiecz A, Marquardt T, et al. Tumor-specific T cell activation by recombinant immunoreceptors: CD3ζ signaling and CD28

costimulation are simultaneously required for efficient IL-2 secretion and can be integrated into one combined CD28/CD3ζ signaling receptor molecule. J Immunol 2001;167(11):6123–31.

8. Maude SL, Laetsch TW, Buechner J, et al. Tisagenlecleucel in children and young adults with B-cell lymphoblastic leukemia. N Engl J Med 2018; 378(5):439–48.

9. Neelapu SS, Locke FL, Bartlett NL, et al. Axicabtagene ciloleucel CAR T-cell therapy in refractory large B-cell lymphoma. N Engl J Med 2017;377(26): 2531–44.

10. Schmidts A, Maus MV. Making CAR T cells a solid option for solid tumors. Front Immunol 2018;9:2593.

11. Bagley SJ, Desai AS, Linette GP, et al. CAR T-cell therapy for glioblastoma: recent clinical advances and future challenges. Neuro Oncol 2018;20(11): 1429–38.

12. Akhavan D, Alizadeh D, Wang D, et al. CAR T cells for brain tumors: lessons learned and road ahead. Immunol Rev 2019;290(1):60–84.

13. Zhang C, Liu J, Zhong JF, et al. Engineering CAR-T cells. Biomark Res 2017;5. https://doi.org/10.1186/s40364-017-0102-y.

14. June CH, O'Connor RS, Kawalekar OU, et al. CAR T cell immunotherapy for human cancer. Science 2018;359(6382):1361–5.

15. Milone MC, Fish JD, Carpenito C, et al. Chimeric receptors containing CD137 signal transduction domains mediate enhanced survival of T cells and increased antileukemic efficacy in vivo. Mol Ther 2009;17(8):1453–64.

16. Vormittag P, Gunn R, Ghorashian S, et al. A guide to manufacturing CAR T cell therapies. Curr Opin Biotechnol 2018;53:164–81.

17. Brown CE, Badie B, Barish ME, et al. Bioactivity and safety of IL13Rα2-redirected chimeric antigen receptor CD8+ T cells in patients with recurrent glioblastoma. Clin Cancer Res 2015;21(18):4062–72.

18. Wang X, Rivière I. Clinical manufacturing of CAR T cells: foundation of a promising therapy. Mol Ther Oncolytics 2016;3:16015.

19. Sahin A, Sanchez C, Bullain S, et al. Development of third generation anti-EGFRvIII chimeric T cells and EGFRvIII-expressing artificial antigen presenting cells for adoptive cell therapy for glioma. PLoS One 2018;13(7). https://doi.org/10.1371/journal.pone.0199414.

20. Guerrero AD, Moyes JS, Cooper LJ. The human application of gene therapy to re-program T-cell specificity using chimeric antigen receptors. Chin J Cancer 2014;33(9):421–33.

21. Ahmed N, Brawley V, Hegde M, et al. HER2-specific chimeric antigen receptor-modified virus-specific T cells for progressive glioblastoma: a phase 1 dose-escalation trial. JAMA Oncol 2017;3(8): 1094–101.

22. Roddie C, O'Reilly M, Dias Alves Pinto J, et al. Manufacturing chimeric antigen receptor T cells: issues and challenges. Cytotherapy 2019;21(3): 327–40.

23. Kaneko S, Mastaglio S, Bondanza A, et al. IL-7 and IL-15 allow the generation of suicide gene–modified alloreactive self-renewing central memory human T lymphocytes. Blood 2009;113(5):1006–15.

24. Suryadevara CM, Desai R, Abel ML, et al. Temozolomide lymphodepletion enhances CAR abundance and correlates with antitumor efficacy against established glioblastoma. Oncoimmunology 2018;7(6). https://doi.org/10.1080/2162402X.2018.1434464.

25. Goff SL, Morgan RA, Yang JC, et al. Pilot trial of adoptive transfer of chimeric antigen receptor-transduced T cells targeting EGFRvIII in patients with glioblastoma. J Immunother 2019;42(4):126–35.

26. Engelhardt B, Ransohoff RM. Capture, crawl, cross: the T cell code to breach the blood–brain barriers. Trends Immunol 2012;33(12):579–89.

27. Zhu X, Fallert-Junecko BA, Fujita M, et al. Poly-ICLC promotes the infiltration of effector T cells into intracranial gliomas via induction of CXCL10 in IFN-α and IFN-γ dependent manners. Cancer Immunol Immunother 2010;59(9):1401–9.

28. Baron JL, Madri JA, Ruddle NH, et al. Surface expression of alpha 4 integrin by CD4 T cells is required for their entry into brain parenchyma. J Exp Med 1993;177(1):57–68.

29. Sarkaria JN, Hu LS, Parney IF, et al. Is the blood–brain barrier really disrupted in all glioblastomas? A critical assessment of existing clinical data. Neuro Oncol 2018;20(2):184–91.

30. Watkins S, Robel S, Kimbrough IF, et al. Disruption of astrocyte–vascular coupling and the blood–brain barrier by invading glioma cells. Nat Commun 2014;5(1):4196.

31. Keu KV, Witney TH, Yaghoubi S, et al. Reporter gene imaging of targeted T-cell immunotherapy in recurrent glioma. Sci Transl Med 2017;9(373). https://doi.org/10.1126/scitranslmed.aag2196.

32. Brown CE, Alizadeh D, Starr R, et al. Regression of glioblastoma after chimeric antigen receptor T-cell therapy. N Engl J Med 2016;375(26):2561–9.

33. Hao C, Parney IF, Roa WH, et al. Cytokine and cytokine receptor mRNA expression in human glioblastomas: evidence of Th1, Th2 and Th3 cytokine dysregulation. Acta Neuropathol (Berl) 2002; 103(2):171–8.

34. Mirzaei R, Sarkar S, Yong VW. T cell exhaustion in glioblastoma: intricacies of immune checkpoints. Trends Immunol 2017;38(2):104–15.

35. Hussain SF, Yang D, Suki D, et al. The role of human glioma-infiltrating microglia/macrophages in mediating antitumor immune responses. Neuro Oncol 2006;8(3):261–79.

36. Dubinski D, Wölfer J, Hasselblatt M, et al. CD4+ T effector memory cell dysfunction is associated with the accumulation of granulocytic myeloid-derived suppressor cells in glioblastoma patients. Neuro Oncol 2016;18(6):807–18.

37. Colwell N, Larion M, Giles AJ, et al. Hypoxia in the glioblastoma microenvironment: shaping the phenotype of cancer stem-like cells. Neuro Oncol. 2017; 19(7):887–96.

38. Agarwal P, Pajor MJ, Anson DM, et al. Elucidating immunometabolic targets in glioblastoma. Am J Cancer Res 2017;7(10):1990–5.

39. Eder K, Kalman B. Molecular heterogeneity of glioblastoma and its clinical relevance. Pathol Oncol Res 2014;20(4):777–87.

40. Eskilsson E, Røsland GV, Solecki G, et al. EGFR heterogeneity and implications for therapeutic intervention in glioblastoma. Neuro Oncol 2018;20(6): 743–52.

41. Bielamowicz K, Fousek K, Byrd TT, et al. Trivalent CAR T cells overcome interpatient antigenic variability in glioblastoma. Neuro Oncol 2018;20(4): 506–18.

42. Nickel GC, Barnholtz-Sloan J, Gould MP, et al. Characterizing mutational heterogeneity in a glioblastoma patient with double recurrence. PLoS One 2012;7(4). https://doi.org/10.1371/journal.pone. 0035262.

43. Debinski W, Gibo DM, Slagle B, et al. Receptor for interleukin 13 is abundantly and specifically overexpressed in patients with glioblastoma multiforme. Int J Oncol 1999;15(3):481–6.

44. Brown CE, Warden CD, Starr R, et al. Glioma IL13Rα2 is associated with mesenchymal signature gene expression and poor patient prognosis. PLoS One 2013;8(10):e77769.

45. Haynik DM, Roma AA, Prayson RA. HER-2/neu expression in glioblastoma multiforme. Appl Immunohistochem Mol Morphol 2007;15(1):56–8.

46. Mineo J-F, Bordron A, Quintin-Roué I, et al. Increasing of HER2 membrane density in human glioblastoma U251MG cell line established in a new nude mice model. J Neurooncol 2006;76(3): 249–55.

47. Koka V, Potti A, Forseen SE, et al. Role of Her-2/neu overexpression and clinical determinants of early mortality in glioblastoma multiforme. Am J Clin Oncol 2003;26(4):332–5.

48. Schneider JR, Kwan K, Boockvar JA. Use of HER2-specific chimeric antigen receptor-modified virus-specific T cells as a potential therapeutic for progressive HER2-positive glioblastoma. Neurosurgery 2017;81(5):N42–3.

49. Ahmed N, Salsman VS, Kew Y, et al. HER2-specific T cells target primary glioblastoma stem cells and induce regression of autologous experimental tumors. Clin Cancer Res 2010;16(2):474–85.

50. Brennan CW, Verhaak RGW, McKenna A, et al. The somatic genomic landscape of glioblastoma. Cell 2013;155(2):462–77.

51. Padfield E, Ellis HP, Kurian KM. Current therapeutic advances targeting EGFR and EGFRvIII in glioblastoma. Front Oncol 2015;5. https://doi.org/10.3389/ fonc.2015.00005.

52. Li G, Wong AJ. EGF receptor variant III as a target antigen for tumor immunotherapy. Expert Rev Vaccin 2008;7(7):977–85.

53. Feldkamp MM, Lala P, Lau N, et al. Expression of activated epidermal growth factor receptors, Ras-guanosine triphosphate, and mitogen-activated protein kinase in human glioblastoma multiforme specimens. Neurosurgery 1999;45(6):1442–53.

54. Shinojima N, Tada K, Shiraishi S, et al. Prognostic value of epidermal growth factor receptor in patients with glioblastoma multiforme. Cancer Res 2003; 63(20):6962–70.

55. Pelloski CE, Ballman KV, Furth AF, et al. Epidermal growth factor receptor variant III status defines clinically distinct subtypes of glioblastoma. J Clin Oncol 2007;25(16):2288–94.

56. Struve N, Binder ZA, Stead LF, et al. EGFRvIII upregulates DNA mismatch repair resulting in increased temozolomide sensitivity of MGMT promoter methylated glioblastoma. Oncogene 2020;39(15): 3041–55.

57. Johnson LA, Scholler J, Ohkuri T, et al. Rational development and characterization of humanized anti–EGFR variant III chimeric antigen receptor T cells for glioblastoma. Sci Transl Med 2015;7(275): 275ra22.

58. Hegi ME, Liu L, Herman JG, et al. Correlation of O6-methylguanine methyltransferase (MGMT) promoter methylation with clinical outcomes in glioblastoma and clinical strategies to modulate MGMT activity. J Clin Oncol 2008;26(25):4189–99.

59. Johns TG, Stockert E, Ritter G, et al. Novel monoclonal antibody specific for the de2-7 epidermal growth factor receptor (EGFR) that also recognizes the EGFR expressed in cells containing amplification of the EGFR gene. Int J Cancer 2002;98(3): 398–408.

60. Pule MA, Savoldo B, Myers GD, et al. Virus-specific T cells engineered to coexpress tumor-specific receptors: persistence and antitumor activity in individuals with neuroblastoma. Nat Med 2008;14(11): 1264–70.

61. Leen AM, Bollard CM, Mendizabal AM, et al. Multicenter study of banked third-party virus-specific T cells to treat severe viral infections after hematopoietic stem cell transplantation. Blood 2013;121(26): 5113–23.

62. Leen AM, Myers GD, Sili U, et al. Monoculture-derived T lymphocytes specific for multiple viruses expand and produce clinically relevant effects in

immunocompromised individuals. Nat Med 2006; 12(10):1160–6.

63. Wang D, Starr R, Chang W-C, et al. Chlorotoxin-directed CAR T cells for specific and effective targeting of glioblastoma. Sci Transl Med 2020; 12(533). https://doi.org/10.1126/scitranslmed. aaw2672.

64. Brown CE, Starr R, Weng L, et al. 247. Phase I study of second generation chimeric antigen receptor-engineered T cells targeting IL13Rα2 for the treatment of glioblastoma. Mol Ther 2016;24:S97.

65. Bagley S, Desai A, Binder Z, et al. RBTT-12. A phase I study of EGFRvIII-directed Car T cells combined with PD-1 inhibition in patients with newly, diagnosed, MGMT-unmethylated glioblastoma: trial in progress. Neuro Oncol. 2019;21(Suppl 6):vi221.

66. Wykosky J, Gibo DM, Stanton C, et al. EphA2 as a novel molecular marker and target in glioblastoma multiforme. Mol Cancer Res 2005;3(10):541–51.

67. Liu F, Park PJ, Lai W, et al. A genome-wide screen reveals functional gene clusters in the cancer genome and identifies EphA2 as a mitogen in glioblastoma. Cancer Res 2006;66(22):10815–23.

68. Wang L-F, Fokas E, Bieker M, et al. Increased expression of EphA2 correlates with adverse outcome in primary and recurrent glioblastoma multiforme patients. Oncol Rep 2008;19(1):151–6.

69. Amoozgar Z, Jain RK, Duda DG. Role of apelin in glioblastoma vascularization and invasion after anti-VEGF therapy: what is the impact on the immune system? Cancer Res 2019;79(9):2104–6.

70. Yang J, Yan J, Liu B. Targeting VEGF/VEGFR to modulate antitumor immunity. Front Immunol 2018; 9. https://doi.org/10.3389/fimmu.2018.00978.

71. Bocca P, Di Carlo E, Caruana I, et al. Bevacizumab-mediated tumor vasculature remodelling improves tumor infiltration and antitumor efficacy of GD2-CAR T cells in a human neuroblastoma preclinical model. Oncoimmunology 2017;7(1):e1378843.

72. Hegde M, Corder A, Chow KK, et al. Combinational targeting offsets antigen escape and enhances effector functions of adoptively transferred T cells in glioblastoma. Mol Ther 2013;21(11):2087–101.

Immunovirotherapy for the Treatment of Glioblastoma and Other Malignant Gliomas

Dagoberto Estevez-Ordonez, MD[a], Gustavo Chagoya, MD[a], Arsalaan Salehani, MD[a], Travis J. Atchley, MD[a], Nicholas M.B. Laskay, MD[a], Matthew S. Parr, MD[a], Galal A. Elsayed, MD[a], Anil K. Mahavadi, MD[a], Sage P. Rahm, MD[a], Gregory K. Friedman, MD[a,b], James M. Markert, MD, MPH[c,*]

KEYWORDS

- Glioblastoma • Immunovirotherapy • Oncolytic virus • Herpes simplex virus (HSV-1) • Brain tumors
- Oncolytic virotherapy

KEY POINTS

- Immunovirotherapy has emerged as a promising targeted approach for treatment of GBM and other malignant gliomas.
- There are multiple viral prototypes for targeted oncolytic virotherapy and targeted drug delivery in various stages of clinical development with promising results.
- Herpes Simplex Virus type 1 offers numerous advantages as an oncolytic virus with several genetic enhancements currently being tested in clinical trials in adults and children.

INTRODUCTION

Glioblastoma multiforme (GBM) represents nearly half of all primary malignant brain tumors in adults, and malignant gliomas are a leading cause of cancer-related morbidity and mortality in children.[1–3] Outcomes for patients with GBM are poor, and effective treatment options are limited with individuals having a median survival of approximately 15 months.[2,4] The current treatment protocol focuses on maximal safe resection, radiotherapy, and concurrent tumor-treating fields/chemotherapy with temozolomide (TMZ) with only a modest effect on outcomes.[4–8] There are multiple factors that contribute to treatment resistance and recurrence of GBM. It is highly invasive, with glioma cells spreading widely within normal brain tissue at early stages.[9–11] GBMs contain tumorigenic glioma stem cells that contribute to tumor initiation, therapeutic resistance, and recurrence.[12] GBM also exhibits both intertumoral and intratumoral heterogeneity, which contributes to diagnostic complexity and limits the application of personalized, targeted therapies.[12]

There is a substantial need for novel therapeutic approaches that address several of these challenges. Immunovirotherapy has emerged as a targeted approach for treatment of GBM and other malignant gliomas with promising results.[5,13,14] Multiple viral vectors have been genetically altered and developed as oncolytic viruses and for targeted drug delivery. There are currently several ongoing clinical trials for the treatment of GBM with immunovirotherapy.[12,15,16] In this review, we

a Department of Neurosurgery, The University of Alabama at Birmingham, 1060 Faculty Office Tower 510 20th Street South, Birmingham, AL, USA; b Department of Pediatrics, Division of Pediatric Hematology-Oncology, The University of Alabama at Birmingham; c Department of Neurosurgery, Neurosurgery, Pediatrics, and Cell, Developmental and Integrative Biology, The University of Alabama at Birmingham, 1060 Faculty Office Tower 510 20th Street South, Birmingham, AL, USA
* Corresponding author.
E-mail address: jmarkert@uabmc.edu

Neurosurg Clin N Am 32 (2021) 265–281
https://doi.org/10.1016/j.nec.2020.12.008
1042-3680/21/© 2021 Elsevier Inc. All rights reserved.

discuss the recent advances and current state of viral vectors developed for the targeted treatment of GBM and malignant gliomas including their mechanism of action and clinical applications.

HUMAN ONCOLYTIC VIRUS MODELS
Adenovirus

Adenovirus (Adv) is a double-stranded nonenveloped DNA virus causing mild upper respiratory symptoms in humans that typically self-resolve. Within the realm of immunovirotherapy, recombinants of Adv that show conditional replication are some of the most studied oncolytic viruses.[16,17] The key to the multiple immunovirotherapy applications of the oncolytic Adv comes from its E1A gene, which is essential in its replication and is the first gene expressed on viral infection.[18] The Ki67 promoter for E1A expression can be upregulated in conjunction with arming the oncolytic Adv with interleukin (IL)-15 gene expression against GBM cells with resultant enhanced anti-GBM efficacy via activation of microglial cells.[18] Adenovirus can also be used to deliver suicide gene therapy.[19] These suicide genes have successfully induced apoptosis via conversion of the prodrug 5-FC into 5-fluorouracil in the presence of Escherichia coli cytosine deaminase (CD) and have encoded proteins that terminate protein synthesis within tumor cells.[19] Adenovirus, therefore, represents a multifaceted vector in the immunovirotherapy arsenal against GBM.

In 2018, Lang and colleagues[20] published landmark results from a Phase I, dose-escalation, biologic-end-point study investigating Delta-24-RGD oncolytic virus. Participants were separated into 2 groups, with group A receiving a single intratumoral injection of the virus into biopsy-confirmed recurrent tumor and group B undergoing intratumoral injection through an implanted catheter followed by en bloc resection days postimplantation to evaluate posttreatment specimens. The study demonstrated quite promising clinical results, with 20% of group A patients surviving more than 3 years posttreatment and 12% of patients demonstrating greater than 95% enhancing tumor reduction with associated more than 3 years of progression-free survival. Analysis of group B specimens postresection demonstrated direct virus-induced oncolysis with tumor infiltration by CD8 cells. Subsequent analyses of cell lines derived from these patients showed induction of immunogenic cell death after virus insertion into tumor cells. Overall, this Phase I study provided promising results demonstrating increased long-term survival in patients with recurrent high-grade gliomas due to the direct oncolytic effects of DNX-2401 adenovirus.[20]

A promising study recently published in Neuro-Oncology Advances found potentiating effects of the Adv Delta24-RGD on the response of a murine GBM model to anti-PD1 therapy overcoming tumor-induced immune suppression via significant recruitment of dendritic cells resulting in a robust antitumor response and survival benefit, suggesting the potential benefit of combination therapy.[21,22] Other mechanisms of action affect the function of T cells, specifically decreasing tumor-infiltrating T regulatory (Treg) cells and increasing interferon-gamma producing CD8 T cells. In addition, the oncolytic AdCMVdelta24 virus can augment systemic tumor antigen specific T cells and reprogram Treg cells to a stimulatory rather than immunosuppressive state.[23]

Reduced expression in immortalized cells/ Dickkopf-3 (REIC/Dkk-3) is a tumor suppressor and therapeutic gene in many human cancers, including malignant glioma with promising results with adenovirus oncolytic therapy.[24] An adenovirus REIC vector was developed to increase REIC/Dkk-3 expression (Ad-SGE-REIC), which is currently undergoing a Phase I/IIa clinical trial for treatment of recurrent malignant glioma.[25]

Not only can the Adv vector be used to stimulate the antitumor immune response, but it also has possible applications to enhance intraoperative discernment of tumor tissue from normal brain. In 2015, Yano and colleagues[26] reported the successful use of a green fluorescent protein expressing adenovirus OBP-401 to label GBM cells to allow fluorescence guided surgery techniques to resect the murine GBM with nearly undetectable residual macroscopic tumor in the surgical bed.

Herpes Simplex Virus Type-1

Genetically engineered oncolytic Herpes Simplex Virus type 1 (oHSV), in particular, has been the focus of extensive preclinical and clinical research, offering several advantages as a therapeutic vector.[14] It is an enveloped icosahedral virus with double-stranded linear DNA that belongs to the Herpesviridae family. It is intrinsically neurotropic and does not integrate into the host cell DNA, making it an ideal vector for targeting primary brain tumors.[27,28] The deletion of essential genes required for replication in normal cells in combination with replacement of nonessential genes with foreign DNA can provide therapeutic advantages.[14,28] In addition, engineered oHSVs remain sensitive to antivirals, which contributes to its safety profile in the event of unanticipated adverse reactions.

The introduction of inactivating mutations in the $\gamma_1 34.5$ neurovirulence gene, an essential gene for viral replication in normal cells in the central nervous system, has been extensively used in oncolytic viral models.[29,30] In response to herpes simplex virus (HSV)-1 infection, normal cells activate the double-stranded RNA–dependent protein kinase R (PKR) system. This leads to phosphorylation of eukaryotic initiation factor (eIF) 2α inducing translational arrest and resulting in severe impairment of viral protein synthesis.[29] Infected cell protein 34.5 (ICP34.5), the product of $\gamma_1 34.5$, reverses this process and is thus essential for successful viral replication in the central nervous system. Deletion of $\gamma_1 34.5$ results in conditional viral replication within tumor cells that have low intrinsic PKR activity, such as human glioma.[5,29,30] This prevents productive infection in normal cells in the brain through PKR-mediated translational arrest while still maintaining oncolytic activity against glioma cells, which have defective signaling pathways and/or activating RAS mutations that suppress antiviral responses.[5,29,30] Clinical trials of $\gamma_1 34.5$-deleted oHSV G207 (**Table 1**) have demonstrated safety with evidence of efficacy in both adults and children (**Table 2**).[14,31–37] Markert and colleagues[32] conducted a phase I trial on 21 adult patients and demonstrated safety at doses up to 3×10^9 pfu with 9 patients showing evidence of neuropathologic or radiographic response. A follow-up phase 1b trial on 6 patients with recurrent GBM receiving 2 doses of G207 totaling 1.15×10^9 pfu, with 13% of this total dose injected before tumor resection via a catheter placed stereotactically into enhancing portion of the tumor, also demonstrated safety and confirmed viral replication.[34] A third study demonstrated safety of vG207 in combination a single 5 Gy radiation dose in 9 adults with recurrent high-grade gliomas to provide in vivo synergistic viral replication based on preclinical data.[33] A clinical trial in pediatric supratentorial HGG trial is now complete and demonstrated safety of a controlled-rate infusion of intratumoral G207 up to 1×10^8 pfu (maximum planned dose) alone and combined with 5 Gy of radiation. Radiographic, neuropathologic, and/or clinical responses were seen in 11 of 12 patients. Matched pretreatment and posttreatment tissue in several patients demonstrated marked increase in tumor-infiltrating lymphocyte months after treatment with G207 (data not yet published).[31] A first-in-human trial assessing the safety of G207 alone and combined with 5 Gy of radiation in malignant cerebellar tumors, including malignant gliomas, is currently ongoing.[37]

Placing ICP34.5 or its human ortholog GADD34 under nestin promoter control (rQNestin34.5 and NG34) resulted in enhanced selectivity and efficacy compared with control virus in preclinical models.[38,39] Nestin encodes for the intermediate filament, which is a protein expressed during neuronal embryogenesis but not in the adult brain and it has been shown to be upregulated in malignant glioma, resulting in selective production of ICP34.5.[38,40] An ongoing Phase I clinical trial is currently ongoing to test the safety of these viral constructs (see **Table 1**). Another approach uses oHSV G47Δ constructed by deleting the $\alpha 47$ gene, responsible for inhibiting the transporter associated with antigen presentation, from $\gamma 34.5$-deficient HSV-1 vectors; leading to increased MHC class I expression in infected human cells and enhanced viral replication. Ongoing phase I-IIa clinical trials in Japan are assessing the safety and efficacy of G47Δ for the treatment of GBM.[41,42] Interim analysis of these showed that the 1-year survival rate of 13 patients was 92.3%.[42]

Pathophysiological hypoxia is a hallmark of high-grade gliomas. It fosters the glioma stemlike cell (GSC) phenotype and has been linked to tumor development, invasiveness, and resistance to chemotherapy and radiation. Although GSCs demonstrated no inherent resistance to oHSV, hypoxia may limit the oncolytic effect of some oHSVs.[43–46] To improve replication in such hostile environments without increasing neurovirulence, chimeric HSV C134 was developed to express the human cytomegalovirus (HCMV) PKR-evasion gene.[43,47] C134 is able to evade PKR-mediated protein shutoff and maintain late viral protein synthesis to significantly enhance virus replication, including in hypoxic conditions.[43] There is an ongoing clinical trial assessing the safety and therapeutic benefit of C134.[48]

In addition to direct oncolytic effects, oHSV can elicit a robust antitumor immune response.[1] Viruses with insertion of proinflammatory cytokine genes have been described, such as IL-12, which results in intratumoral production of IL-12 during viral replication to enhance targeted immune destruction.[13] IL-12 has potent antitumor properties that enhance the cytolytic activity of natural killer cells and cytotoxic T cells.[49] It also promotes the development of T_H-1 immune response, potentially eliciting a more durable antitumor effect.[49] Treatment with oHSV models producing IL-12 in combination with immune checkpoints (CTLA-4 and PD-1) have also shown promising results.[50] There are several completed and ongoing trials assessing the safety and therapeutic benefit of second-generation oHSVs (eg, IL-12 producing oHSV M032) in adults.[13,14]

Measles Virus

Measles virus (MV) is a single-stranded, negative-sense, enveloped RNA virus within the *Morbillivirus* genera of the Paramyxoviridae family. MV

Table 1
Ongoing and completed clinical trials[a]

Virus	GBM Type	Study Title	Phase	Biological	n	Duration	NCT Number and Reference	Status
Adenovirus	Recurrent	DNX-2401 (Formerly Known as Delta-24-RGD-4C) for Recurrent Malignant Gliomas	Phase I	DNX-2401	37	February 2009–February 2015	NCT00805376 [20]	Completed
	Recurrent	Safety Study of Replication-competent Adenovirus (Delta-24-RGD) in Patients With Recurrent Glioblastoma	Phase I-II	DNX-2401	20	June 2010–December 2014	NCT01582516	Completed
	Recurrent	Virus DNX2401 and Temozolomide in Recurrent Glioblastoma	Phase I	DNX2401	31	September 2013–March 2017	NCT01956734	Completed
	Recurrent	DNX-2401 With Interferon Gamma (IFN-γ) for Recurrent Glioblastoma or Gliosarcoma Brain Tumors	Phase I	DNX-2401	37	September 11, 2014–March 15, 2018	NCT02197169	Completed
	Recurrent	Combination Adenovirus + Pembrolizumab to Trigger Immune Virus Effects	Phase II	DNX-2401	49	June 2016–June 2021	NCT02798406	Active, not recruiting
	Recurrent	DNX-2440 Oncolytic Adenovirus for Recurrent Glioblastoma	Phase I	DNX-2440	24	October 16, 2018–October 16, 2022	NCT03714334	Recruiting
	Recurrent	Oncolytic Adenovirus DNX-2401 in Treating Patients With Recurrent High-Grade Glioma	Phase I	DNX-2401	36	February 12, 2019–May 31, 2022	NCT03896568	Recruiting
Herpes	Recurrent	Conditionally replicating herpes simplex virus mutant, G207 for the treatment of malignant glioma	Phase I	G207	21	February 1998–May 1999	NCT00036699 [32]	Completed
	Recurrent	Phase Ib trial of mutant herpes simplex virus G207 inoculated pre-and post-tumor resection for recurrent GBM	Phase Ib	G207	6	January 2002–August 2003	NCT00028158 [34]	Completed
	Recurrent	G207 Followed by Radiation Therapy in Malignant Glioma	Phase I	G207	9	May 2005–December 2008	NCT00157703 [33]	Completed

Virus	Tumor	Title	Phase	Agent	Number	Dates	NCT	Status
	Recurrent	Oncolytic HSV-1716 in Treating Younger Patients With Refractory or Recurrent High-Grade Glioma That Can Be Removed By Surgery	Phase I	HSV-1716	2	December 2013–May 2016	NCT02031965	Terminated
	Recurrent	Genetically Engineered HSV-1 Phase 1 Study for the Treatment of Recurrent Malignant Glioma	Phase I	M032 (NSC 733972)	15 of 26	September 2014–September 2023	NCT02062827	Recruiting
	Recurrent	HSV G207 Alone or With a Single Radiation Dose in Children With Progressive or Recurrent Supratentorial Brain Tumors	Phase I	G207	12	May 2016–April 2021	NCT02457845	Active, not recruiting
	Recurrent	A Study of the Treatment of Recurrent Malignant Glioma With rQNestin34.5v.2	Phase I	rQNestin34.5v.2	108	July 18, 2017–July 2022	NCT03152318	Recruiting
	Recurrent	HSV G207 in Children With Recurrent or Refractory Cerebellar Brain Tumors	Phase I	G207	15	September 12, 2019–September 1, 2024	NCT03911388	Recruiting
	Recurrent	Trial of C134 in Patients With Recurrent GBM	Phase I	C134	24	September 23, 2019–September 2024	NCT03657576	Active, not recruiting
	Recurrent	HSV G207 With a Single Radiation Dose in Children With Recurrent High-Grade Glioma	Phase II	G207	30	October 1, 2020–October 1, 2024	NCT04482933	Not yet recruiting
Measles	Recurrent	Viral Therapy in Treating Patients With Recurrent Glioblastoma Multiforme	Phase I	MV-CEA	23	October 23, 2006–November 30, 2019	NCT00390299	Completed, results not published yet
NDV	Recurrent	New Castle Disease Virus (NDV) in Glioblastoma Multiforme (GBM), Sarcoma and Neuroblastoma	Phase I-II	HUJ	0	July 2011–July 2011	NCT01174537	Withdrawn
Polio	Recurrent	PVSRIPO for Recurrent Glioblastoma (GBM)	Phase I	PVSRIPO	61	April 25, 2012–June 2021	NCT01491893 [75]	Active, not recruiting
	Recurrent	PVSRIPO in Recurrent Malignant Glioma	Phase II	PVSRIPO	122	June 1, 2017–December 2023	NCT02986178	Active, not recruiting
	Recurrent	Phase 1b Study PVSRIPO for Recurrent Malignant Glioma in Children	Phase I	PVSRIPO	12	December 5, 2017–July 1, 2021	NCT03043391	Recruiting

(continued on next page)

Table 1
(continued)

Virus	GBM Type	Study Title	Phase	Biological	n	Duration	NCT Number and Reference	Status
Parvovirus	Recurrent	Parvovirus H-1 (ParvOryx) in Patients With Progressive Primary or Recurrent Glioblastoma Multiforme	Phase I-IIa	H-1PV	18	September 2011–May 2015	NCT01301430	Completed
Reovirus	Recurrent	A Phase I Trial of Intratumoral Administration of Reovirus in Patients With Histologically Confirmed Recurrent Malignant Gliomas	Phase I	Reolysin	12	June 2002–July 2005	N/A[89]	Completed
	Recurrent	Safety and Efficacy Study of REOLYSIN® in the Treatment of Recurrent Malignant Gliomas	Phase I	Reolysin	18	July 2006–June 2010	NCT00528684 [90]	Completed
	Recurrent	Wild-Type Reovirus in Combination With Sargramostim in Treating Younger Patients With High-Grade Relapsed or Refractory Brain Tumors	Phase I	Reolysin	6	June 21, 2015–January 1, 2025	NCT02444546	Active, not recruiting
Vaccinia	Recurrent	Safety and Efficacy of the Oncolytic Virus Armed for Local Chemotherapy, TG6002/5-FC, in Recurrent Glioblastoma Patients	Phase I-II	TG6002	78	October 12, 2017–September 2021	NCT03294486	Recruiting

Abbreviations: HSV, herpes simplex virus; MV-CEA, measles virus carcinoembryonic antigen.
[a] Citations are included only for clinical trials with published results.

Table 2
Summary viral constructs for the treatment of glioblastoma and other malignant gliomas

Viral Vector	Mechanism/Pathway Involved	Effect(s) on Tumor Cell
Adenovirus		
REIC/Dkk-3 + cRGD	Activation caspase-9; reduced expression B-catenin	Decreased proliferation rate
Antisense MMP-9	Downregulation of MMP-9 activity	Impaired tumor invasiveness
DNX-2401 + pembrolizumab	Increased epitope presentation to CD8+ T cells	Induced antiglioma immune response
AAV8 and AAV9 +IFN-B	Increase in tumor-associated microglia	Improved tumor sensitivity to chemoradiation; improved median survival
dsAAV2	Downregulation of TGF-B	Suppressed tumor growth; reduced tumor immunosuppressive effects
Herpes Virus		
G47Δ	Deletion of the γ134.5 and α47 genes and a disabling lacZ insertion within ICP6; Murine angiostatin insertion	Gain of function mutation leading to increased MHC class I expression in infected cells this resulting in enhanced viral replication
HSVtk + Flt3L	Release of HMGB1	Phagocytosis of tumor; activation of immune response
HSV-M032	Deletion in both copies of $\gamma_1$34.5 gene; Insertion of Human IL-12	Selective glioma cell replication and expression of IL-12 in infected glioma cells resulting in enhanced immune response and tumor cell lysis
HSV-G207	Deletion in both copies of $\gamma_1$34.5 gene and disabling lacZ insertion in UL39	Selective glioma cell replication
HSV-C134	Deletion in both copies of $\gamma_1$34.5 gene, expression of the HCMV TRS1 gene product	Selective and enhanced glioma cell replication
rQNestin34.5v.2	Deletion in $\gamma_1$34.5 gene and UL39; ICP-34.5 under control of synthetic nestin promoter	Selective and enhanced glioma cell replication
Lentivirus		
Sh-SirT1	Downregulation SirT1	Increased tumor sensitivity to radiotherapy
Sh-TLX	Downregulation TLX; expression of TET3	Impaired tumor growth and tumorigenicity of stem cells
GAS1 + PTEN	Decreased AKT and ERK 1/2 expression	Impaired tumor growth
Paramoxyvirus		
Measles (MV-CEA)	Attenuated strain modified to express the carcinoembryonic antigen gene	Designed to track viral gene expression in vivo via serum analysis to optimize dosing and administration schedule without resorting to histologic tissue analysis

(continued on next page)

Table 2
(continued)

Viral Vector	Mechanism/Pathway Involved	Effect(s) on Tumor Cell
Measles (MV-NIS)	Attenuated strain modified to express human thyroidal sodium iodide symporter (NIS) gene	NIS can act as a reporter gene that enables the non-invasive tracking of viral localization, spread, gene expression and replication over time. NIS may also be used as a therapeutic transgene by allowing intracellular uptake of isotopes, such as ^{131}[I] (radiovirotherapy)
Picornavirus		
Poliovirus (PVSRIPO)	Enhanced immune cell infiltration; reduction of TIM-3 expression	Promote immune response and tumor inflammation
Retrovirus		
Toca 511	Increased delivery of 5-FC to tumor	Increased tumor sensitivity to radiotherapy

expresses a glycoprotein hemagglutinin protein H that has a high affinity for CD46 receptors shown to be overexpressed in GBM cells.[51,52] The MV Edmonston strain (MV-Edm), a well-known attenuated strain used to vaccinate humans against MV, has been further modified to express the carcinoembryonic antigen gene (MV-CEA).[53]

Phuong and colleagues[54] were the first to show that intravenous MV-CEA resulted in significantly prolonged survival and regression of in vivo glioblastoma tumor in mice bearing subcutaneous and orthotopic U87 tumors MV-CEA treated mice had no neurologic or clinical toxicity, which sparked further investigation. In subsequent studies, MV specificity for GBM was increased by developing retargeted oncolytic measles strains that invade via different receptors: epidermal growth factor receptor (MV-EGFR), EGF receptor variant III (MV-EGFRvIII), and IL-13Rα2 receptor.[55–58] Additional studies demonstrated that MV immunovirotherapy against GBMs can be enhanced with either adjuvant radiation therapy or anti-PD-1 antibody therapy.[59,60] Recombinant oncolytic MV (MV-NIS) is another example that was designed to express human thyroidal sodium iodide symporter (NIS) gene. NIS can act as a reporter gene via radiotracers and can also be used as a therapeutic transgene via radiovirotherapy, by allowing intracellular uptake 131[I] potentially enhancing the therapeutic efficacy.[61]

A phase 1 clinical trial treated 23 measles immune patients who were candidates for gross total or subtotal tumor resection of recurrent GBM with intracranial injection of MV-CEA.[62] One group received a total dose of MV-CEA ranging from 10^5 to 2×10^7 TCID50 via injection into the resection cavity. The second group of patients received one intratumoral MV-CEA injection and subsequently underwent tumor resection 5 days following this first intratumoral injection–time for projected maximum viral replication to be achieved– with a second MV-CEA injection into the resection cavity before closure. Resected tumor specimens were analyzed with in situ hybridization and immunohistochemistry.[63]

Poliovirus

Poliovirus is a positive-sense, single-stranded RNA encapsulated virus belonging to the Picornaviridae family known for its neurotoxic effects.[64] The prototype oncolytic poliovirus developed by Gromeier and colleagues,[65] PVS-RIPO, is the live attenuated poliovirus type 1 (Sabin) with its internal ribosome entry site (IRES) replaced by that of human rhinovirus type 2 (HRV2). Although this polio-rhinovirus chimera was found to possess neuronal incompetence, in vitro studies demonstrated its ability to infect and reduce glioma cell viability and trigger cytolysis of GBM primary cultures.[66–71] In subsequent animal studies, PVSRIPO was able to arrest tumor growth in both murine GBM flank tumor models and improve survival after intracranial virus administration in mice.[66,72] In addition, its efficacy was found to be correlated with CD155 expression, known to be overexpressed in human GBM.[73,74]

Indeed, its moderate success in preclinical models paved the way for a phase II clinical trial involving inoculation of 61 patients with recurrent GBM with PVS-RIPO. The results were published in a landmark article in 2018, which not only corroborated safety of intratumoral viral administration in humans but demonstrated an increase in patient survival rate from 4% to 21% at 36 months when compared with historical control groups.[75,76] Three other clinical trials on PVS-RIPO are currently ongoing assessing safety in children and combination therapy with lomustine (CCNU) and pembrolizumab.[76–78] Because clinical and radiographic responses were observed after the first cycle of chemotherapy administered for tumor progression in patients receiving PVSRIPO infusion, a second follow-up randomized trial of PVSRIPO alone or in combination with single-cycle CCNU in patients with recurrent World Health Organization grade IV malignant glioma is ongoing to further assess the potential of combination therapy CCNU.[76]

Reovirus

Another human virus that has shown oncolytic ability is the Respiratory Enteric Orphan virus or Reovirus, a segmented nonenveloped double-stranded RNA virus composed of 3 size groups. This naturally occurring virus, which is commonly isolated in the respiratory and gastrointestinal tracts of humans but causes mild to no symptoms, preferentially targets the activated RAS pathway.[79] The numerous downstream effectors induced by the RAS/RalGEF/p38 pathway in particular, have been implicated in promoting the reovirus life cycle and leading to cell death.[80–84]

Animal studies in severe combined immunodeficient (SCID) mice containing subcutaneous MG cell lines U251 N and intracerebral cell lines U251 N and U87lacZ showed a reduction in tumor burden after infection with serotype 3 (strain Dearing) live virus.[85,86] Lethality was also demonstrated in vitro in 83% of 24 established malignant glioma cell lines. The susceptibility of cells to reovirus may in part be attributed to the various ways reovirus circumvents cell defense mechanisms. For example, when 3-dimensional cultures of stem cell-like cells (GSC) from grade IV gliomas (glioblastoma) expressing junction adhesion molecule-A (JAM-A) were infected by the wild-type (wt) variant and the JAM-A independent jin-1 reovirus variant, viral entry and protein synthesis were similar.[87] JAM-A is typically used by wt reovirus for cell entry and level of expression is correlated with infectivity. These results suggest that reovirus may use alternative entry pathways for infectivity that avoid the JAM-A adhesion route. Interestingly, reovirus has been found to also upregulate PD-L1 expression lending credence to its use as part of a multifaceted tumor killing strategy with the use of PD-1/PD-L1 inhibitors.[88]

The first clinical trial using reovirus in recurrent malignant glioma demonstrated that intratumoral injection was safe.[89] Although the trial's purpose was not to show efficacy, 6 patients lived more than 6 months, 3 patients lived more than 1 year, and 1 continued to survive at 54 months. A subsequent study using convection-enhanced delivery also confirmed safety and noticed improved survival >2 years in select patients.[90] Intravenous administration of reovirus has also been evaluated in preclinical studies with promising results.[91]

ZOONOTIC ONCOLYTIC VIRUS MODELS
Newcastle Disease Virus

Newcastle disease virus (NDV) is a chicken pathogen with selective oncolytic properties applicable to various types of human cancer.[92] Molecularly, NDV is an avian paramyxovirus with a negative-stranded RNA genome.[17] Although the tumor-suppressive abilities of NDV have been extensively demonstrated through in vivo models and clinical trials, the exact mechanism is not fully understood. It is theorized that NDV achieves oncolysis via activation of a Ras pathway in addition to inducing secretion of tumor necrosis factor alpha (TNF-alpha) by mononuclear cells resulting in an enhanced antitumor immune response.[17] More recent studies suggest that the Ras-related C3 botulism toxin substrate 1 (Rac1) pathway may be the target of NDV.[92] Rac1 is involved in proliferation signaling by regulating gene transcription and G1 cell cycle progression. In GBM, Rac1 is therefore a crucial contributor to cell survival. NDV interactions with Rac1 are believed to induce cell cycle arrest along with degradation of the actin cytoskeleton and ultimately cell death.[92] Murine models have shown increased long-term survival after NDV injection due to cytotoxic T-cell infiltration.[16] However, this long-term survival benefit was not seen in immunodeficient murine models with depleted CD8 cells, stressing the importance of an intact host immune system for maximal benefit.[16] Type I interferon (IFN) expression in GBM cells also greatly impacts the effectiveness of NDV given the role of IFN in promoting an antiviral state and decreasing viral replication.[93] Nonetheless, recombinant NDV expression of an IFN antagonistic protein can overcome this protective role of IFN in GBM cells.[93]

NDV delivery to GBM cells can be targeted via mesenchymal stem cells (MSCs). This technique takes advantage of the natural ability of MSCs to target sites of injury and inflammation, including tumors.[94] Higher rates of apoptosis were demonstrated in glioma cells when MSCs were used as the vector for NDV delivery as compared with direct NDV infection with similar virus titers. Moreover, TNF-related apoptosis-inducing ligand (TRAIL) has been identified as a key mediator in the antitumor effects of these hybrid MSCs due to synergy between TRAIL and NDV in the induction of apoptosis.[94] NDV can also potentiate the effects of TMZ. Bai and colleagues[95] found that when combined with TMZ, NDV inhibits AKT and activates AMPK, ultimately resulting in enhanced antitumor effects of TMZ and extended survival in a murine model. Clinical trials have demonstrated therapeutic efficacy and safety of autologous NDV-modified cellular vaccines or oncolytic effects in clinical trials but larger clinical trials are necessary to confirm efficacy.[96] In a phase I/II clinical trial, Freeman and colleagues[97] showed that the toxicity of NDV strain (HUJ, lentogenic) was minimal and a maximal tolerated dose was not achieved when administered intravenously to 14 patients with GBM using intrapatient dose escalation (1–11 billion infectious units) followed by 3 cycles of 55 billion infectious units with 1 patient achieving a complete response, and the others developed progressive disease.

Rodent Parvovirus

Certain members of the Parvoviridae family, a group of nonenveloped icosahedral single-stranded DNA viruses, can selectively kill malignant glioma cells while sparing normal cells in preclinical studies. These include rodent oncolytic viruses such as the Minute Virus of Mice and the more extensively studied rat parvovirus H-1PV.[98] Intratumoral and intravenous injection of H-1PV into 12 immunodeficient rats containing the U87 human glioma cell line resulted in prolonged survival and decreased tumor burden compared with controls.[99] The efficacy was in part due to a secondary viremia that resulted from progeny particles after initial tumor infection and boosted infection of remaining tumor cells. The lethality of H-1PV also extends to malignant gliomas resistant to death ligands such as TRAIL and DNA-damaging agents such as cisplatin.[100] The virus triggers accumulation of lysosomal cathepsins and downregulating cathepsin inhibitors. The orientation of certain variable regions of the capsid protein of H-1PV has also been tied to its infectivity.[101]

Studies in short-term and low-passage cultures of human grade IV and gliosarcoma cell lines also showed increased susceptibility to H-1PV at low multiplicities of infection (MOI; 1–5 infectious units per cell).[102] These cell cultures more closely parallel clinically diseased cells than do cells from long-term in vitro cell cultures. Intranasal application of H-1PV has also been shown to prolong survival in immunodeficient rats containing U87 human glioma cells versus controls. A Phase I/IIa trial of H-1PV in 18 patients demonstrated no dose-limited toxicity and widespread distribution after intratumoral and intravenous injection.[103,104]

Other Viral Vectors

Several other potential viral vectors have been described, but have not been assessed in clinical trials for GBM. Pseudorabies virus (PRV) and the Seneca Valley Virus (SVV), 2 viruses in which pigs are the natural host, have shown potential as oncolytic targets. However, intravenous infusion of PRV did not result in uptake within intracranial glioma cells.[105,106] SVV improved survival in mice bearing GBM as well as medulloblastoma and retinoblastoma models, which led to phase 1 clinical trials in adults and children with neuroendocrine tumors, which demonstrated safety, but no clear antitumor responses, and all patients rapidly developed anti-SVV antibodies and cleared the virus.[107,108] Vesicular Stomatitis Virus (VSV) and Sindbis Virus (SIN) are mosquito-borne viruses that have also shown oncolytic potential. Chimeric VSV-lymphocytic choriomeningitis virus, and VSV-Chikungunya virus mutants with replacement of the VSV glycoprotein have demonstrated tumor lysis with decreased toxicity to normal cells in glioma and intracranial melanoma mouse models.[109,110] SIN has tropism for neural cells and can cause encephalitis in mice.[17] Tropism for tumor cells is believed to be related to the high affinity laminin receptor, which is overexpressed in many tumors.[111] SIN can be a vector for introduction of hyperfusogenic membrane glycoproteins that lead to formation of syncytia and apoptosis.[112] Myxoma virus and Vaccinia virus (VV), within the Poxviridae family are the most promising candidates for malignant glioma virotherapy because they are highly immunogenic and capable of creating antitumor immunity.[113–116]

NONONCOLYTIC VIRAL VECTORS FOR GENE THERAPY OR TARGETED DRUG DELIVERY

Gene therapy has emerged as a potential treatment for malignant gliomas, whereby a vector introduces tumor suppressing or growth regulating genes into malignant cells. Multiple approaches are used for gene therapy including suicide gene, oncolytic gene, and tumor suppressor gene therapies.[117]

Viruses are a prime candidate for the introduction of gene therapies. They create a potent cytotoxic effect and are easily modified to facilitate genetic engineering.[19] Current approaches are attempting to target proteins commonly mutated or upregulated in GBM, including EGFR, PTEN, IDH-1, and p53.[118] The most common viral vectors include neurotropic retrovirus and adenoviruses. Retroviral vectors were among the first studied, and the first trial began in 1992 with a retroviral HSV-thymidine kinase (HSV-tk) with ganciclovir. HSV-tk acts as a suicide gene and converts the prodrug ganciclovir into its active form to inhibit cell division and DNA replication. The efficacy of this treatment was limited to small tumor sizes given its poor transfection efficiency.[119]

Adenoviral vectors have been used in clinical trials. An early study of an adenoviral vector with wt p53 gene (Ad-p53) showed efficacious transfection of tumor cells with minimal toxicity; however, similar to retroviral vectors, Ad-p53 demonstrated poor ability to penetrate tumor tissue widely.[120] Sandmair and colleagues[121] demonstrated increased survival time in patients receiving ganciclovir with adenovirus-delivered HSV-tk as compared with retrovirus delivery, again demonstrating poor retroviral transfection and tumor penetrance. In addition, adenovirus and HSV vectors have been used to introduce CD, which convert the prodrug 5-fluorocytosine into 5-flurouracil, inducing apoptosis.[122] A phase I study in patients with recurrent glioma with aglatimagene besadenovec (AdV-tk), which adenoviral vector engineered to express the HSV thymidine kinase (HSV-tk) gene in conjunction with a synthetic anti-herpetic prodrug acyclic guanosine analogue administration demonstrated a safe dose range with 3 of 13 patients surviving more than 24 months.[123] A subsequent phase I trial in children treated with AdV-tk as adjuvant to surgery and radiation for pediatric malignant glioma and recurrent ependymoma also showed safety and potential efficacy.[124]

Lentiviral vectors have been used to introduce small-hairpin RNA (shRNA) to silence sirtuin 1 expression in GBM, which results in increased radiosensitivity with resultant increased tumor death.[125] Similarly, lentiviral delivery of human orphan nuclear receptor tailless (TLX) shRNA resulted in tumor growth inhibition and decreased tumorigenicity.[126,127]

CHALLENGES, LIMITATIONS, AND FUTURE DIRECTIONS

Although clinical trials have been completed or are ongoing for several oncolytic viruses, only a few have moved beyond a Phase I clinical trial.[16] Finding the ideal balance to achieve safety but also virulence to maximize efficacy remains a significant challenge.

Moreover, viral delivery remains a significant challenge, as most clinical trials have focused on intratumoral delivery. Recent trials have used stereotactic techniques to place a localized catheter into the tumor to use for administration of virus.[31,33,35,37,128] This requires a neurosurgical procedure and may limit additional doses. Thus, innovative routes of administration need to be devised, such as systemic, intrathecal, intracavitary, and intraventricular delivery. However, the challenges of systemic delivery are considerable due to the blood-brain-barrier and virus neutralizing antibodies, and the safety of these routes needs to be confirmed.[16]

Although the clinical results of several oncolytic viruses have been promising including HSV, poliovirus, and adenovirus, these studies have all been in recurrent, often heavily pretreated patients. Thus, it will be important to test immunovirotherapy in upfront regimens. Furthermore, future studies are needed to combine oncolytic viruses with other potentially synergistic approaches to maximize oncolysis an antitumor immune response such as immune checkpoint inhibitors, CAR-T therapy enhanced with bispecific T-cell engagers (BiTE), vaccines, and other immunotherapies.[14,50,129–131] For example, Saha and colleagues[129] demonstrated durable responses in an orthotopic GBM model by combining anti-PD-1 and anti-CTLA-4 antibodies with oHSV expressing IL-12. An alternate approach to systemic delivery of checkpoint inhibitors is by using oncolytic viruses carrying genetic material to express the immune checkpoint inhibitors locally.[103,132,133] In addition, CAR-T-cell therapy with bicistronic constructs can convert gliomas who have difficult-to-target surface topology to more familiar, targetable topology or help trigger enhanced immune responses with targeted, localized CD3 expression to facilitate local immunomodulation.[130]

SUMMARY

Immunovirotherapy has shown significant promise as a targeted therapy for malignant gliomas, and attempts to address several of the challenges often encountered in treatment, such as ability to treat unresectable lesions or addressing challenges encountered hypoxia, anti-inflammatory effects, and consequences of intratumoral and intertumoral heterogeneity in treatment. However, barriers related to therapeutic delivery, viral entry and replication, and immunosuppressed patients must be overcome. Strategies such as arming viral vectors with enhancements (therapeutic trans-genes, checkpoint inhibition, host antiviral immune response, improved and selective replication) and combining viruses with synergistic agents must continue to be developed and tested in the clinics so that the great therapeutic potential of oncolytic immunovirotherapy can be realized.

CLINICS CARE POINTS

- To date, no oncolytic virus has been approved by the FDA for the treatment of malignant glioma and all remain investigational treatments.

- Multiple ongoing clinical trials are currently enrolling participants, most of them available for patients with recurrent malignant gliomas.

- Oncolytic viral models engineered to alter/modulate various cellular and inflammatory pathways leading to selective replication in tumor cells, enhanced immune response, impaired tumor angiogenesis, amongst others.

- Multiple non-oncolytic viral vectors have been studied as gene therapy vectors in glioma; these varied approaches include increasing radiosensitity via gene silencing and induction of tumor cell apoptosis in conjunction with various prodrug administrations.

- Talimogene laherparepvec (T-VEC) is the first US Food and Drug Administration (FDA)-approved oncolytic virus; and is currently indicated for advanced melanoma. T-VEC is an oHSV that and expresses human granulocyte macrophage colony-stimulating factor (GM-CSF) to active the immune system and has specific genetic deletions that result in improved capacity for MHC presentation.

ACKNOWLEDGMENT

The manuscript was supported in part by National Cancer Institute grants R01CA222903, R01CA217179 and a grant from Gateway for Cancer Research (all JMM -Last Author). And supported in part by the National Institutes of Health (Training Grant R25 TW009337) funded by the Fogarty International Center, National Institutes of Health Office of the Director, and National Institute of Mental Health. (DEO - First author).

DISCLOSURES

Dr J.M. Markert holds equity (<8%) in Aettis, Inc. (a company that holds stocks of oncolytic virus); Treovir, Inc (25%), a company holding intellectual property and funding clinical trials of oncolytic virus for pediatric brain tumors. A company that Dr J.M. Markert formerly held equity in (<8%) Catherex, Inc., was purchased in a structured buyout. Dr J.M. Markert has served as a consultant for Imugene. He also holds a fraction of the IP associated with oncolytic virus C134, which is licensed by Mustang Biotech.

REFERENCES

1. Louis David N, Hiroko O, Wiestler Otmar D, et al. The 2007 WHO classification of tumours of the central nervous system. Acta Neuropathol 2007; 114(2):97–109.
2. Ostrom Quinn T, Gino C, Gittleman H, et al. CBTRUS statistical report: primary brain and other central nervous system tumors diagnosed in the United States in 2012–2016. Neuro Oncol 2019; 21(Supplement_5):v1–100.
3. Mackay A, Anna B, Carvalho D, et al. Integrated molecular meta-analysis of 1,000 pediatric high-grade and diffuse intrinsic pontine glioma. Cancer Cell 2017;32(4):520–37.e5.
4. Wen Patrick Y, Santosh K. Malignant gliomas in adults. N Engl J Med 2008;359(5):492–507.
5. Andreansky SS, He B, Gillespie GY, et al. The application of genetically engineered herpes simplex viruses to the treatment of experimental brain tumors. Proc Natl Acad Sci U S A 1996;93(21): 11313–8.
6. Roger S, Mason Warren P, van den Bent Martin J, et al. Radiotherapy plus concomitant and adjuvant temozolomide for glioblastoma. N Engl J Med 2005;352(10):987–96.
7. Omuro A, DeAngelis Lisa M. Glioblastoma and other malignant gliomas: a clinical review. JAMA 2013;310(17):1842–50.
8. Cohen KJ, Pollack Ian F, Zhou T, et al. Temozolomide in the treatment of high-grade gliomas in children: a report from the Children's Oncology Group. Neuro Oncol 2011;13(3):317–23.
9. Cheng L, Wu Q, Guryanova Olga A, et al. Elevated invasive potential of glioblastoma stem cells. Biochem Biophys Res Commun 2011;406(4):643–8.
10. Hirokazu S, Yoshikawa K, Makoto I, et al. Pathological features of highly invasive glioma stem cells in a mouse xenograft model. Brain Tumor Pathol 2014;31(2):77–84.
11. Aboody Karen S, Brown A, Rainov Nikolai G, et al. Neural stem cells display extensive tropism for pathology in adult brain: evidence from intracranial gliomas. Proc Natl Acad Sci U S A 2000;97(23): 12846–51.
12. Bernstock Joshua D, Mooney James H, Ilyas A, et al. Molecular and cellular intratumoral

heterogeneity in primary glioblastoma: clinical and translational implications. J Neurosurg 2019;1–9. https://doi.org/10.3171/2019.5.JNS19364.

13. Patel Daxa M, Foreman Paul M, Burt NL, et al. Design of a phase I clinical trial to evaluate M032, a genetically engineered HSV-1 Expressing IL-12, in patients with recurrent/progressive glioblastoma multiforme, anaplastic astrocytoma, or gliosarcoma. Hum Gene Ther Clin Dev 2016; 27(2):69–78.

14. Totsch Stacie K, Charles S, Kang KD, et al. Oncolytic herpes simplex virus immunotherapy for brain tumors: current pitfalls and emerging strategies to overcome therapeutic resistance. Oncogene 2019;38(34):6159–71.

15. Foreman Paul M, Friedman Gregory K, Cassady Kevin A, et al. Oncolytic virotherapy for the treatment of malignant glioma. Neurotherapeutics 2017;14(2):333–44.

16. Martikainen M, Magnus E. Virus-based immunotherapy of glioblastoma. Cancers (Basel) 2019; 11(2). https://doi.org/10.3390/cancers11020186.

17. Guido W, Koray O, van den Pol Anthony N. Oncolytic virus therapy of glioblastoma multiforme – concepts and candidates. Cancer J 2012;18(1): 69–81.

18. Zhang Q, Zhang J, Tian Y, et al. Efficacy of a novel double-controlled oncolytic adenovirus driven by the Ki67 core promoter and armed with IL-15 against glioblastoma cells. Cell Biosci 2020;10. https://doi.org/10.1186/s13578-020-00485-1.

19. Manikandan C, Kaushik A, Sen D. Viral vector: potential therapeutic for glioblastoma multiforme. Cancer Gene Ther 2020;27(5):270–9.

20. Lang Frederick F, Conrad C, Gomez-Manzano C, et al. Phase I Study of DNX-2401 (Delta-24-RGD) oncolytic adenovirus: replication and immunotherapeutic effects in recurrent malignant glioma. J Clin Oncol 2018;36(14):1419–27.

21. Kim Julius W, Jason M, Young Jacob S, et al. A comparative study of replication-incompetent and -competent adenoviral therapy-mediated immune response in a murine glioma model. Mol Ther Oncolytics 2017;5:97–104.

22. Zineb B, Cor B, John C, et al. Low-dose oncolytic adenovirus therapy overcomes tumor-induced immune suppression and sensitizes intracranial gliomas to anti-PD-1 therapy. Neurooncol Adv 2020; 2(1). https://doi.org/10.1093/noajnl/vdaa011.

23. Qiao J, Dey M, Chang Alan L, et al. Intratumoral oncolytic adenoviral treatment modulates the glioma microenvironment and facilitates systemic tumor-antigen-specific T cell therapy. Oncoimmunology 2015;4(8). https://doi.org/10.1080/2162402X.2015.1022302.

24. Oka T, Kazuhiko K, Shimazu Y, et al. A super gene expression system enhances the anti-glioma effects of adenovirus-mediated REIC/Dkk-3 gene therapy. Sci Rep 2016;6:33319.

25. Kazuhiko K, Fujii K, Shimazu Y, et al. Study protocol of a Phase I/IIa clinical trial of Ad-SGE-REIC for treatment of recurrent malignant glioma. Future Oncol 2020;16(6):151–9.

26. Yano S, Miwa S, Kishimoto H, et al. Experimental curative fluorescence-guided surgery of highly invasive glioblastoma multiforme selectively labeled with a killer-reporter adenovirus. Mol Ther 2015;23(7):1182–8.

27. Friedman Gregory K, Pressey Joseph G, Reddy Alyssa T, et al. Herpes simplex virus oncolytic therapy for pediatric malignancies. Mol Ther 2009; 17(7):1125–35.

28. Shah Amish C, Dale B, Yancey GG, et al. Oncolytic viruses: clinical applications as vectors for the treatment of malignant gliomas. J Neurooncol 2003;65(3):203–26.

29. Wilcox Douglas R, Richard L. The herpes simplex virus neurovirulence factor γ34.5: revealing virus–host interactions. PLoS Pathog 2016;12(3). https://doi.org/10.1371/journal.ppat.1005449.

30. Toshihiro M, Rabkin Samuel D, Yazaki T, et al. Attenuated multi–mutated herpes simplex virus–1 for the treatment of malignant gliomas. Nat Med 1995;1(9):938–43.

31. Waters Alicia M, Johnston James M, Reddy Alyssa T, et al. Rationale and design of a Phase 1 clinical trial to evaluate HSV G207 alone or with a single radiation dose in children with progressive or recurrent malignant supratentorial brain tumors. Hum Gene Ther Clin Dev 2017;28(1):7–16.

32. Markert JM, Medlock MD, Rabkin SD, et al. Conditionally replicating herpes simplex virus mutant, G207 for the treatment of malignant glioma: results of a phase I trial. Gene Ther 2000;7(10):867–74.

33. Markert James M, Razdan Shantanu N, Hui-Chien K, et al. A phase I trial of oncolytic HSV-1, G207, given in combination with radiation for recurrent GBM demonstrates safety and radiographic responses. Mol Ther 2014;22(5):1048–55.

34. Markert James M, Liechty Peter G, Wang W, et al. Phase Ib trial of mutant herpes simplex virus G207 inoculated pre-and post-tumor resection for recurrent GBM. Mol Ther 2009;17(1):199–207.

35. Bernstock Joshua D, Wright Z, Bag Asim K, et al. Stereotactic placement of intratumoral catheters for continuous infusion delivery of herpes simplex virus -1 G207 in pediatric malignant supratentorial brain tumors. World Neurosurg 2019;122:e1592–8.

36. Bernstock Joshua D, Nunzio V, Rong Li, et al. A novel in situ multiplex immunofluorescence panel for the assessment of tumor immunopathology and response to virotherapy in pediatric glioblastoma reveals a role for checkpoint protein inhibition. Oncoimmunology 2019;8(12):e1678921.

37. Bernstock Joshua D, Bag Asim K, Fiveash J, et al. Design and rationale for first-in-human phase 1 immunovirotherapy clinical trial of oncolytic HSV G207 to treat malignant pediatric cerebellar brain tumors. Hum Gene Ther 2020;31(19–20):1132–9.

38. Kambara H, Okano H, Chiocca E, et al. An oncolytic HSV-1 mutant expressing ICP34.5 under control of a nestin promoter increases survival of animals even when symptomatic from a brain tumor. Cancer Res 2005;65(7):2832–9.

39. Nakashima H, Nguyen T, Kasai K, et al. Toxicity and efficacy of a Novel GADD34-expressing Oncolytic HSV-1 for the treatment of experimental glioblastoma. Clin Cancer Res 2018;24(11):2574–84.

40. Dahlstrand J, Collins VP, Lendahl U. Expression of the class VI intermediate filament nestin in human central nervous system tumors. Cancer Res 1992;52(19):5334–41.

41. Taguchi S, Fukuhara H, Todo T. Oncolytic virus therapy in Japan: progress in clinical trials and future perspectives. Jpn J Clin Oncol 2019;49(3):201–9.

42. Tomoki T. ATIM-14. results of phase II clinical trial of oncolytic herpes virus G47Δ in patients with glioblastoma. Neuro Oncol 2019;21(Suppl 6):vi4.

43. Friedman GK, Nan L, Haas MC, et al. γ₁34.5-deleted HSV-1-expressing human cytomegalovirus IRS1 gene kills human glioblastoma cells as efficiently as wild-type HSV-1 in normoxia or hypoxia. Gene Ther 2015;22(4):348–55.

44. Jensen Randy L. Brain tumor hypoxia: tumorigenesis, angiogenesis, imaging, pseudoprogression, and as a therapeutic target. J Neurooncol 2009;92(3):317–35.

45. Friedman Gregory K, Langford Catherine P, Coleman Jennifer M, et al. Engineered herpes simplex viruses efficiently infect and kill CD133+ human glioma xenograft cells that express CD111. J Neurooncol 2009;95(2):199–209.

46. Friedman Gregory K, Haas Marilyn C, Kelly VM, et al. Hypoxia moderates γ134.5-deleted herpes simplex virus oncolytic activity in human glioma xenoline primary cultures. Transl Oncol 2012;5(3):200–7.

47. Cassady Kevin A. Human cytomegalovirus TRS1 and IRS1 gene products block the double-stranded-RNA-activated host protein shutoff response induced by herpes simplex virus type 1 infection. J Virol 2005;79(14):8707–15.

48. Markert James M. Trial of C134 in patients with recurrent GBM - Full Text View - ClinicalTrials.gov. Available at: https://clinicaltrials.gov/ct2/show/NCT03657576. Accessed September 17, 2020.

49. Parker JN, Gillespie GY, Love CE, et al. Engineered herpes simplex virus expressing IL-12 in the treatment of experimental murine brain tumors. Proc Natl Acad Sci U S A 2000;97(5):2208–13.

50. Saha D, Martuza Robert L, Rabkin Samuel D. Macrophage polarization contributes to glioblastoma eradication by combination immunovirotherapy and immune checkpoint blockade. Cancer Cell 2017;32(2):253–67.e5.

51. Dörig Ruth E, Anne M, Chopra A, et al. The human CD46 molecule is a receptor for measles virus (Edmonston strain). Cell 1993;75(2):295–305.

52. MaenpAa A, Sami J, Hakulinen J, et al. Expression of complement membrane regulators membrane cofactor protein (CD46), decay accelerating factor (CD55), and protectin (CD59) in human malignant gliomas. Am J Pathol 1996;148(4):14.

53. Peng Kah-Whye, Facteau S, Wegman T, et al. Noninvasive in vivo monitoring of trackable viruses expressing soluble marker peptides. Nat Med 2002;8(5):527–31.

54. Phuong LK, Allen C, Peng KW, et al. Use of a vaccine strain of measles virus genetically engineered to produce carcinoembryonic antigen as a novel therapeutic agent against glioblastoma multiforme. Cancer research 2003;63(10):2462–9.

55. Allen C, Vongpunsawad S, Nakamura T, et al. Retargeted oncolytic measles strains entering via the EGFRvIII receptor maintain significant antitumor activity against gliomas with increased tumor specificity. Cancer Res 2006;66(24):11840–50.

56. Allen C, Paraskevakou G, Iankov I, et al. Interleukin-13 displaying retargeted oncolytic measles virus strains have significant activity against gliomas with improved specificity. Mol Ther 2008;16(9):1556–64.

57. Allen C, Opyrchal M, Aderca I, et al. Oncolytic measles virus strains have significant antitumor activity against glioma stem cells. Gene Ther 2013;20(4):444–9.

58. Georgia P, Allen C, Nakamura T, et al. Epidermal growth factor receptor (EGFR)–retargeted measles virus strains effectively target EGFR- or EGFRvIII expressing gliomas. Mol Ther 2007;15(4):677–86.

59. Liu C, Sarkaria JN, Petell CA, et al. Combination of measles virus virotherapy and radiation therapy has synergistic activity in the treatment of glioblastoma multiforme. Clin Cancer Res 2007;13(23):7155–65.

60. Hardcastle J, Mills L, Malo Courtney S, et al. Immunovirotherapy with measles virus strains in combination with anti–PD-1 antibody blockade enhances antitumor activity in glioblastoma treatment. Neuro Oncol 2017;19(4):493–502.

61. Pavlos M, Dispenzieri A, Evanthia G. Clinical testing of engineered oncolytic measles virus strains in the treatment of cancer: An overview. Curr Opin Mol Ther 2009;11(1):43–53.

62. Evanthia G. Viral therapy in treating patients with recurrent glioblastoma multiforme - full text view -

ClinicalTrials.gov. Available at: https://clinicaltrials.gov/ct2/show/NCT00390299. Accessed November 29, 2020.

63. Pavlos M, Mateusz O, Dispenzieri A, et al. Clinical trials with oncolytic measles virus: current status and future prospects. Curr Cancer Drug Targets 2018;18(2). https://doi.org/10.2174/1568009617666170222125035.

64. Man Mohan M, Mehndiratta P, Pande R. Poliomyelitis: historical facts, epidemiology, and current challenges in eradication. Neurohospitalist 2014; 4(4):223–9.

65. Gromeier M, Alexander L, Wimmer E. Internal ribosomal entry site substitution eliminates neurovirulence in intergeneric poliovirus recombinants. Proc Natl Acad Sci U S A 1996;93(6):2370–5.

66. Gromeier M, Lachmann S, Rosenfeld MR, et al. Intergeneric poliovirus recombinants for the treatment of malignant glioma. Proc Natl Acad Sci U S A 2000;97(12):6803–8.

67. Merrill Melinda K, Dobrikova Elena Y, Matthias G. Cell-type-specific repression of internal ribosome entry site activity by double-stranded RNA-binding protein 76. J Virol 2006;80(7):3147–56.

68. Merrill Melinda K, Matthias G. The double-stranded RNA binding protein 76:NF45 heterodimer inhibits translation initiation at the rhinovirus type 2 internal ribosome entry site. J Virol 2006; 80(14):6936–42.

69. Dobrikova Elena Y, Goetz C, Walters Robert W, et al. Attenuation of neurovirulence, biodistribution, and shedding of a poliovirus:rhinovirus chimera after intrathalamic inoculation in Macaca fascicularis. J Virol 2012;86(5):2750–9.

70. Yang X, Chen E, Jiang H, et al. Evaluation of IRES-mediated, cell-type-specific cytotoxicity of poliovirus using a colorimetric cell proliferation assay. J Virol Methods 2009;155(1):44–54.

71. Merrill Melinda K, Bernhardt G, Sampson John H, et al. Poliovirus receptor CD155-targeted oncolysis of glioma. Neuro Oncol 2004;6(3):208–17.

72. Dobrikova Elena Y, Trevor B, Poiley-Nelson J, et al. Recombinant oncolytic poliovirus eliminates glioma in vivo without genetic adaptation to a pathogenic phenotype. Mol Ther 2008;16(11): 1865–72.

73. Vidyalakshmi C, Bryant Jeffrey D, Piao H, et al. Validation of an immunohistochemistry assay for detection of CD155, the poliovirus receptor, in malignant gliomas. Arch Pathol Lab Med 2017; 141(12):1697–704.

74. Goetz C, Dobrikova E, Mayya S, et al. Oncolytic poliovirus against malignant glioma. Future Virol 2011;6(9):1045–58.

75. Annick D, Matthias G, Herndon James E, et al. Recurrent glioblastoma treated with recombinant poliovirus. N Engl J Med 2018;379(2):150–61.

76. Istari Oncology, Inc. PVSRIPO for recurrent glioblastoma (GBM) - full text view–ClinicalTrials.gov. Available at: https://clinicaltrials.gov/ct2/show/NCT01491893. Accessed November 23, 2020.

77. Istari Oncology, Inc. A phase 2, open-label, single arm study evaluating the efficacy, safety and tolerability of PVSRIPO and the immune checkpoint inhibitor pembrolizumab in the treatment of patients with recurrent glioblastoma.- full text view–ClinicalTrials.gov. Available at: https://clinicaltrials.gov/ct2/show/NCT04479241. Accessed November 23, 2020.

78. Istari Oncology, Inc. Phase 1b Study PVSRIPO for recurrent malignant glioma in children–full text view–ClinicalTrials.gov. Available at: https://clinicaltrials.gov/ct2/show/NCT03043391. Accessed November 23, 2020.

79. Prior Ian A, Hood Fiona E, Hartley James L. The frequency of ras mutations in cancer. Cancer Res 2020;80(14):2969–74.

80. Gong J, Mita Monica M. Activated ras signaling pathways and reovirus oncolysis: an update on the mechanism of preferential reovirus replication in cancer cells. Front Oncol 2014;4:167.

81. Norman Kara L, Lee Patrick WK. Reovirus as a novel oncolytic agent. J Clin Invest 2000;105(8): 1035–8.

82. Norman Kara L, Lee Patrick WK. Not all viruses are bad guys: the case for reovirus in cancer therapy. Drug Discov Today 2005;10(12):847–55.

83. Smakman N, van der Bilt JDW, van den Wollenberg DJM, et al. Immunosuppression promotes reovirus therapy of colorectal liver metastases. Cancer Gene Ther 2006;13(8):815–8.

84. Strong JE, Coffey MC, Tang D, et al. The molecular basis of viral oncolysis: usurpation of the Ras signaling pathway by reovirus. EMBO J 1998; 17(12):3351–62.

85. Wilcox ME, Yang W, Senger D, et al. Reovirus as an oncolytic agent against experimental human malignant gliomas. J Natl Cancer Inst 2001;93(12): 903–12.

86. Radhashree M, Ghalib Mohammad H, Goel S. Reovirus: a targeted therapeutic – progress and potential. Mol Cancer Res 2012;10(12). https://doi.org/10.1158/1541-7786.MCR-12-0157.

87. van den Hengel SK, Balvers RK, Dautzenberg IJC, et al. Heterogeneous reovirus susceptibility in human glioblastoma stem-like cell cultures. Cancer Gene Ther 2013;20(9):507–13.

88. Samson A, Scott Karen J, Taggart D, et al. Intravenous delivery of oncolytic reovirus to brain tumor patients immunologically primes for subsequent checkpoint blockade. Sci Transl Med 2018;10(422). https://doi.org/10.1126/scitranslmed.aam7577.

89. Forsyth P, Gloria R, George D, et al. A Phase I trial of intratumoral administration of reovirus in patients

with histologically confirmed recurrent malignant gliomas. Mol Ther 2008;16(3):627–32.

90. Kicielinski Kimberly P, Chiocca EA, Yu John S, et al. Phase 1 clinical trial of intratumoral reovirus infusion for the treatment of recurrent malignant gliomas in adults. Mol Ther 2014;22(5):1056–62.

91. Romit C, Tran H, Giovanni S, et al. The oncolytic virus, pelareorep, as a novel anticancer agent: a review. Invest New Drugs 2015;33(3):761–74.

92. Jafri Malin A, Mustafa Z, Aini I. Newcastle disease virus interaction in targeted therapy against proliferation and invasion pathways of glioblastoma multiforme. Biomed Res Int 2014;2014. https://doi.org/10.1155/2014/386470.

93. García-Romero N, Palacín-Aliana I, Esteban-Rubio S, et al. Newcastle disease virus (NDV) oncolytic activity in human glioma tumors is dependent on CDKN2A-Type I IFN gene cluster codeletion. Cells 2020;9(6). https://doi.org/10.3390/cells9061405.

94. Gila K, Jiang W, Shimon S, et al. Mesenchymal stem cells enhance the oncolytic effect of Newcastle disease virus in glioma cells and glioma stem cells via the secretion of TRAIL. Stem Cell Res Ther 2016;7. https://doi.org/10.1186/s13287-016-0414-0.

95. Bai Y, Chen Y, Hong X, et al. Newcastle disease virus enhances the growth-inhibiting and proapoptotic effects of temozolomide on glioblastoma cells in vitro and in vivo. Sci Rep 2018;8. https://doi.org/10.1038/s41598-018-29929-y.

96. Shi J, Sun P, Zhang Y, et al. The antitumor effects of Newcastle disease virus on glioma. Biocell 2019; 43(3):119–28.

97. Freeman Arnold I, Zichria ZR, Gomori John M, et al. Phase I/II Trial of Intravenous NDV-HUJ oncolytic virus in recurrent glioblastoma multiforme. Mol Ther 2006;13(1):221–8.

98. Paglino Justin C, Koray O, van den Pol Anthony N. LuIII parvovirus selectively and efficiently targets, replicates in, and kills human glioma cells. J Virol 2012;86(13):7280–91.

99. Geletneky K, Kiprianova I, Ayache A, et al. Regression of advanced rat and human gliomas by local or systemic treatment with oncolytic parvovirus H-1 in rat models. Neuro Oncol 2010;12(8):804–14.

100. Piazza MD, Carmen M, Geletneky K, et al. Cytosolic activation of cathepsins mediates parvovirus H-1-induced killing of cisplatin and TRAIL-resistant glioma cells. J Virol 2007;81(8):4186–98.

101. Cho I-R, Kaowinn S, Song J, et al. VP2 capsid domain of the H-1 parvovirus determines susceptibility of human cancer cells to H-1 viral infection. Cancer Gene Ther 2015;22(5):271–7.

102. Calle Marta Herrero y, Cornelis Jan J, Herold-Mende C, et al. Parvovirus H-1 infection of human glioma cells leads to complete viral replication

and efficient cell killing. Int J Cancer 2004;109(1):76–84.

103. Geletneky Karsten, Johannes H, Rommelaere J, et al. Phase I/IIa study of intratumoral/intracerebral or intravenous/intracerebral administration of Parvovirus H-1 (ParvOryx) in patients with progressive primary or recurrent glioblastoma multiforme: ParvOryx01 protocol. BMC Cancer 2012;12:99.

104. Geletneky K, Hajda J, Angelova Assia L, et al. Oncolytic H-1 parvovirus shows safety and signs of immunogenic activity in a first phase I/IIa Glioblastoma Trial. Mol Ther 2017;25(12):2620–34.

105. Guido W, Tattersall P, Pol Anthony N. Targeting human glioblastoma cells: comparison of nine viruses with oncolytic potential. J Virol 2005;79(10):6005–22.

106. Koray O, Guido W, Piepmeier Joseph M, et al. Systemic vesicular stomatitis virus selectively destroys multifocal glioma and metastatic carcinoma in brain. J Neurosci 2008;28(8):1882–93.

107. Rudin Charles M, Poirier John T, Senzer Neil N, et al. Phase I clinical study of seneca valley virus (SVV-001), a replication-competent picornavirus, in advanced solid tumors with neuroendocrine features. Clin Cancer Res 2011;17(4):888–95.

108. Burke MJ, Charlotte A, Weigel Brenda J, et al. Phase I trial of seneca valley virus (NTX-010) in children with relapsed/refractory solid tumors: a report of the Children's Oncology Group. Pediatr Blood Cancer 2015;62(5):743–50.

109. Alexander Muik, Kneiske Inna, Marina Werbizki, et al. Pseudotyping vesicular stomatitis virus with lymphocytic choriomeningitis virus glycoproteins enhances infectivity for glioma cells and minimizes neurotropism. J Virol 2011;85(11):5679–84.

110. Zhang X, Mao G, van den Pol Anthony N. Chikungunya-vesicular stomatitis chimeric virus targets and eliminates brain tumors. Virology 2018;522:244–59.

111. Wang KS, Kuhn RJ, Strauss EG, et al. High-affinity laminin receptor is a receptor for Sindbis virus in mammalian cells. J Virol 1992;66(8):4992–5001.

112. Zhang J, Frolov I, Russell Stephen J. Gene therapy for malignant glioma using Sindbis vectors expressing a fusogenic membrane glycoprotein. J Gene Med 2004;6(10):1082–91.

113. Villa Nancy Y, Wasserfall Clive H, Meacham Amy M, et al. Myxoma virus suppresses proliferation of activated T lymphocytes yet permits oncolytic virus transfer to cancer cells. Blood 2015; 125(24):3778–88.

114. Torres-Domínguez Lino E, Grant McF. Poxvirus oncolytic virotherapy. Expert Opin Biol Ther 2019; 19(6):561–73.

115. Lun XQ, Jang J-H, Tang N, et al. Efficacy of systemically administered oncolytic vaccinia virotherapy for malignant gliomas is enhanced by

combination therapy with rapamycin or cyclophosphamide. Clin Cancer Res 2009;15(8):2777–88.

116. Lun X, Yang W, Tommy A, et al. Myxoma virus is a novel oncolytic virus with significant antitumor activity against experimental human gliomas. Cancer Res 2005;65(21):9982–90.

117. Hidehiro O, Smith Christian A, Rutka James T. Gene therapy for malignant glioma. Mol Cell Ther 2014;2:21.

118. Breanne C, Lee JS, Alexander-Bryant Angela A. Vectors for glioblastoma gene therapy: viral & non-viral delivery strategies. Nanomaterials (Basel) 2019;9(1). https://doi.org/10.3390/nano9010105.

119. Rainov NG. A phase III clinical evaluation of herpes simplex virus type 1 thymidine kinase and ganciclovir gene therapy as an adjuvant to surgical resection and radiation in adults with previously untreated glioblastoma multiforme. Hum Gene Ther 2000;11(17):2389–401.

120. Lang Frederick F, Bruner Janet M, Fuller Gregory N, et al. Phase I trial of adenovirus-mediated p53 gene therapy for recurrent glioma: biological and clinical results. J Clin Oncol 2003; 21(13):2508–18.

121. Sandmair AM, Loimas S, Puranen P, et al. Thymidine kinase gene therapy for human malignant glioma, using replication-deficient retroviruses or adenoviruses. Hum Gene Ther 2000;11(16): 2197–205.

122. Kazuhiko K, Tamiya T, Ono Y, et al. Apoptosis induction with 5-fluorocytosine/cytosine deaminase gene therapy for human malignant glioma cells mediated by adenovirus. J Neurooncol 2004; 66(1–2):117–27.

123. Trask TW, Trask RP, Aguilar-Cordova E, et al. Phase I study of adenoviral delivery of the HSV-tk gene and ganciclovir administration in patients with current malignant brain tumors. Mol Ther 2000;1(2): 195–203.

124. Kieran Mark W, Goumnerova L, Peter M, et al. Phase I study of gene-mediated cytotoxic immunotherapy with AdV-tk as adjuvant to surgery and radiation for pediatric malignant glioma and recurrent ependymoma. Neuro Oncol 2019;21(4):537–46.

125. Chang C-J, Hsu C-C, Ming-Chi Y, et al. Enhanced radiosensitivity and radiation-induced apoptosis in glioma CD133-positive cells by knockdown of SirT1 expression. Biochem Biophys Res Commun 2009;380(2):236–42.

126. Cui Q, Yang S, Ye P, et al. Downregulation of TLX induces TET3 expression and inhibits glioblastoma stem cell self-renewal and tumorigenesis. Nat Commun 2016;7:10637.

127. Guffey MB, Parker JN, Luckett WS, et al. Engineered herpes simplex virus expressing bacterial cytosine deaminase for experimental therapy of brain tumors. Cancer Gene Ther 2007;14(1):45–56.

128. Markert James M. A Phase 1 Study of M032 (NSC 733972), a Genetically Engineered HSV-1 Expressing IL-12, in Patients with recurrent/progressive glioblastoma multiforme, Anaplastic Astrocytoma, or Gliosarcoma. - full text view–ClinicalTrials.gov. Available at: https://clinicaltrials.gov/ct2/show/NCT02062827. Accessed November 23, 2020.

129. Saha D, Martuza Robert L, Rabkin Samuel D. Oncolytic herpes simplex virus immunovirotherapy in combination with immune checkpoint blockade to treat glioblastoma. Immunotherapy 2018;10(9): 779–86.

130. Choi Bryan D, Yu X, Castano Ana P, et al. CAR-T cells secreting BiTEs circumvent antigen escape without detectable toxicity. Nat Biotechnol 2019; 37(9):1049–58.

131. Eleonora P, Maria Ruggero De, Haas TL. Identification of targets to redirect CAR T cells in glioblastoma and colorectal cancer: an arduous venture. Front Immunol 2020;11:565631.

132. Senior M. Checkpoint inhibitors go viral. Nat Biotechnol 2019;37(1):12–7.

133. Yin Y, Boesteanu Alina C, Binder Zev A, et al. Checkpoint blockade reverses anergy in IL-13Rα2 humanized scFv-based CAR T cells to treat murine and canine gliomas. Mol Ther Oncolytics 2018;11:20–38.

Targeting Glioma Stem Cells

Yagmur Muftuoglu, MD, PhD[a], Frank Pajonk, MD, PhD[b,c,*]

KEYWORDS

- Glioblastoma • Glioblastoma-initiating cells • Intratumoral heterogeneity • Plasticity

KEY POINTS

- The concept of tumor-initiating cells is an old concept in oncology that was recently revived with the discovery of markers, able to enrich for tumor-initiating cells.
- Intratumoral heterogeneity and plasticity during undisturbed growth and in response to anticancer effect the efficacy of the standard-of-care in glioblastoma.
- Targeting cellular plasticity in glioblastoma emerges as a means to improve treatment outcome in glioblastoma.

INTRODUCTION

Glioblastoma (GBM) remains the deadliest brain cancer in adults, with almost all patients succumbing to the disease. The current standard of care, surgery followed by radiotherapy and temozolomide, prolongs the median survival from 2 to 3 months to 12 to 14 months.[1] Reasons for treatment failure in GBM are multiple and include the dispersion of cancer cells into the normal brain parenchyma far beyond the bulk tumor detected by clinical imaging modalities, the almost always incomplete surgical resection of the tumor, the lack of blood-brain barrier penetration for many systemic therapies, and the normal tissue radiation tolerance of the brain. Mounting evidence suggests that GBMs contain a small number of glioma-initiating cells (GICs)[2–4] (often called glioma stem cells). The relative resistance of these GICs to chemotherapy and radiotherapy further contributes to the treatment resistance of GBM, making GICs an attractive target for novel treatment approaches against this disease.[5,6]

THE HISTORY OF THE CANCER STEM CELL HYPOTHESIS

Tumor cell heterogeneity in cancer has been recognized since 1875 when Julius Conheim published a case report on a sarcoma of the kidney[7] and laid the groundwork for the cancer stem cell (CSC) hypothesis. It argues that tumors are organized hierarchically with a small number of CSCs at the apex of this hierarchy, able to self-renew, repopulate a tumor after sublethal treatment, and give rise to the differentiated progeny, which lack these defining features of CSCs.[8] Given the resistance of CSCs to radiation[5,9] and chemotherapy[6,10] and their low frequency in many solid tumors including GBM,[11] bulk tumor responses in these cancers do not necessarily reflect responses of CSCs to treatment. Although this is and always has been a well-understood phenomenon in radiation therapy, the efficacy of chemotherapeutic agents is often evaluated based on bulk tumor responses, and current classical radiosensitizers offer only marginal improvements in local control while adding significant toxicity.[12]

[a] Department of Neurosurgery, David Geffen School of Medicine, University of California Los Angeles, 300 Stein Plaza Driveway, Suite 420, Los Angeles, CA 90095-1714, USA; [b] Department of Radiation Oncology, David Geffen School of Medicine, University of California Los Angeles, 10833 Le Conte Avenue, Los Angeles, CA 90095-1714, USA; [c] Jonsson Comprehensive Cancer Center, University of California Los Angeles, Los Angeles, CA, USA
* Corresponding author. Department of Radiation Oncology, David Geffen School of Medicine at UCLA, 10833 Le Conte Avenue, Los Angeles, CA 90095-1714.
E-mail address: pajonk@ucla.edu

Neurosurg Clin N Am 32 (2021) 283–289
https://doi.org/10.1016/j.nec.2021.01.002
1042-3680/21/© 2021 Elsevier Inc. All rights reserved.

With the lack of marker systems to identify CSCs, the CSC hypothesis was mainly a theoretic concept until in 2003 Michael Clarke, Peter Dirks, and Harley Kornblum independently reported surface marker combinations that could prospectively identify tumor cell populations, highly enriched for tumor-initiating cells in breast[13] and brain cancers.[2,4]

In 1976, Nowell[14] introduced the clonal evolution model of tumor organization. Similar to the CSC hypothesis, the model assumes a clonal origin of cancers, without proposing a hierarchical organization. The clonal evolution model postulates that the genetic instability of cancer cells leads to different clones of cells that contribute to the cellular heterogeneity of cancers; in turn, subsequent acquisition of additional mutations that favor cellular proliferation generate cells that outcompete other cell populations and become the driving cell population in a tumor. Considering the stochastic nature of acquiring additional genetic mutations, this model predicts that every cell in the tumor can acquire CSC traits through genetic changes, rather than epigenetic modifications. There is indisputable evidence supporting the genetically unstable nature of solid cancers and its role on the genetic heterogeneity of solid tumors, even if they originate from specific cell clones. What is less clear is whether or not CSC traits are shifting from one clone to another in a stochastic manner. There is evidence that the clonal evolution model may hold true for some cancers[15]; however, most solid tumors seem to follow a hierarchical model.[11]

Finally, a lesser known interconversion model assumes multiple cellular states with differing tumorigenicities and growth rates depending on the context in which the process of differentiation is bidirectional. Evidence supporting interconversion of differentiated cells into leukemogenic cells has been reported for acute myeloid leukemia.[16] More recently, it has been increasingly recognized that these three models are not necessarily exclusive and that stemness is less of a binary state but rather a continuous variable contributing to the heterogeneity of tumors.[17]

DEFINITIONS/BACKGROUND

Normal neural stem/progenitor cells in the central nervous system have been rigorously defined, and stem cell state and differentiation steps into neurons can be followed by well-defined marker combinations that have been carefully validated in functional assays.[18] The definition of GICs is less uniform in the literature and ranges from correlating rigorous functional testing of patient-derived cells with marker profiles[4] to less stringent studies that establish gliomaspheres from cell lines that have been cultures as monolayers for decades and labeling them glioma stem cell lines. The functional identification of tumor-initiating cells, including GICs, is traditionally performed using in vivo limiting dilution assays in which the frequency of GICs can be calculated retrospectively.[19] Time-intensive and resource-consuming, this assay is now often replaced or complemented with in vitro limiting dilution assays, where cells form clonal gliomaspheres from single cells under conditions that favor cells able to grow serum-free and where cells prone to die from anoikis are eliminated.[20] Gliomaspheres in this assay do not necessarily derive exclusively from GICs but can give an approximation on the self-renewal capacity of GBM cell subpopulations.

In many studies, the prospective identification of GIC relies on the surface protein CD133 (AC133 or prominin-1), a pentaspan transmembrane glycoprotein that was first described on cellular protrusions of hematopoietic stem cells.[21] Its validity to identify GICs in GBM is discussed controversially[22,23] with some studies viewing it as a measure of a bioenergetic stress, unrelated to stemness.[24] Despite the controversy surrounding CD133, it is widely applied to enrich for tumorigenic GBM cells. Additional surface markers for GIC enrichment include stage-specific embryonic antigen-1 (SSEA-1)[23]; a surface antigen expressed by glia and neural progenitors called A2B5[25]; stem cell markers, such as nestin[26] and CD15[27]; and integrin-α6, often coexpressed with other markers and thought to contribute to tumorsphere generation in vitro and tumor growth in vivo.[28] Functional markers include high ALDH1 activity and lack of proteasome activity.[29] An excellent review of surface and functional markers of GICs is found in the article by Ludwig and Kornblum.[30]

DISCUSSION
Clinical Relevance of Glioma-Initiating Cells

GICs constitute a small fraction of the tumor bulk[31] but quietly play multiple critical roles in promoting relentless tumor progression. They resemble noncancerous progenitor cells normally found in brain tissue and can produce neurons and other cell types, in vitro and in vivo. By definition, they promote development of the initial lesion by producing differentiated cancer cells that possess the ability to rapidly divide. Additionally, when injected into immunologically deficient mice via secondary transplantation, GICs cause development of tumors phenotypically similar to the donor tissue.[31] Recent studies have demonstrated the role of GICs in promoting invasiveness, especially subpopulations expressing A2B5 with or without CD133 expression.[25,32]

In addition to their direct actions, GICs also manipulate and benefit from their microenvironment for optimal tumorigenesis. Residing in the perivascular space allows GICs to retain their stem cell properties via a steady supply of nutrients and vascular-derived signaling factors that promote self-renewal,[33] and GICs further secrete extracellular matrix proteins to develop a specific microenvironment conducive to their proliferation and differentiation.[34] Cross-signaling between GICs and other cell types also propagates tumor development.[35] As another example, GICs effectively evade the immune system by inhibiting the proliferation of T cells; by expressing defective antigen-processing machinery; and by only weakly expressing MHC-I, MHC-II, and NKG2D ligand, important players in antigen recognition by T cells and natural killer cells.[36]

Finally, GICs remain infamous for their ability to survive chemotherapy and radiation. Traditional chemotherapies target rapidly dividing cells by taking advantage of unstable DNA repair mechanisms, but GICs remain rather quiescent relative to these typical tumor cells. GICs also overexpress important players in the DNA repair pathway, such as O-6 methylguanine-DNA-methyltransferase (MGMT).[37] This allows them to more efficiently correct DNA damage caused by temozolomide, which functions by methylating guanine moieties at the O-6 position, normally resulting in serious DNA damage. In fact, protein expression of MGMT in GIC cell lines predicts resistance to chemotherapy, although MGMT methylation status curiously does not strongly correlate with resistance.[38] GICs may also express drug transporters, such as multidrug resistance 1 of the ABC transporter family, at higher levels to pump out therapeutic molecules.[39] Radiation seems to actively enrich the percentage of CD133[+] GICs remaining after conventional fractionation,[5] and the GIC population that remains serves to heighten DNA repair efforts, via more efficient homologous recombination and aberrancies in the checkpoints that govern cell growth.[40] As such, slowly dividing GICs allow for the universal recurrence that ultimately dampens patient survival.

Given their role in promoting recurrence, studies have shown prognostic value in the characterization of tumor GIC populations.[41,42] A recent massive meta-analysis proved that higher levels of CD133 expression correlate with worse progression-free survival and worse overall survival, particularly among patients with grade IV, but not grade II or III, glioma, whereas higher levels of nestin expression correlate with worse overall survival among patients with only grade II or III glioma.[43] In addition, GICs can serve as a model for high-throughput experiments to identify molecules that target this quiescent population. One such study successfully cultured GICs as neurospheres with heterogeneity matching that of the original tumor and developed a high-throughput proliferation assay to identify multiple compounds with anti-GIC activity from a pilot experiment. Not all results of in vitro assays translate well in vivo, however, partly because multiple GIC lines have been identified and developed over time.[44]

In reality, the phenotype of these powerful stem cells varies among patients, and a single tumor can harbor a handful of different phenotypes. For example, GIC subpopulations even without CD133 expression also demonstrate similar properties. The A2B5[+]/CD133[-] subpopulation retains motility, invasiveness, and tumorigenic properties,[22,25,32] as alluded to previously. The SSEA-1/CD15[+] subpopulation of GICs reportedly can also form tumor spheres, albeit typically smaller than CD133[+] tumor spheres and yet positive for Ki-67, rendering these smaller formations likely more proliferative than those positive for CD133.[45] Such a diversity offers a mere glimpse into the complexity of various GIC subpopulations and harkens back to the heterogeneous nature of GBM, further encouraging the development of personalized combinatorial therapies for combating inevitable recurrence. The challenge of targeting GICs may present the most impactful existing opportunity to improve the standard-of-care for GBM, elucidated in greater depth next.

Glioma-Initiating Cells and the Standard-of-Care

The standard-of-care, surgery followed by radiotherapy and temozolomide, fails to provide cure for patients with GBM and only prolongs median survival by about 12 months.[46]

The benefit of surgery in patients with GBM is well-established and gross-total resection undeniably prolongs survival.[47] Like all surgeries, every brain tumor resection creates a wound and sets a repair program into motion that is triggered by cytokines and hypoxia. However, hypoxia in particular is a key feature of GBM, associated with the niche requirements of GICs[48,49] and known for supporting phenotypic plasticity of GBM cells.[50] It remains to be seen if pathways engaged in GBM cells in those hypoxic resection margins can be used against GICs.

One of the many reasons for treatment failure in GBM is that the standard-of-care differentially affects GICs and their progeny. First reported by Jeremy Rich's laboratory, GICs exhibit relative radioresistance as a result of a more efficient repair of DNA double-strand breaks.[5] It is important to point out that this resistance is relative to that of more differentiated GBM cells, that GICs still respond to radiation, and that radiotherapy prolongs median survival in a dose-dependent manner[51] by about 6 to 9 months, thus making it the most effective agent against GBM so far. The dose-dependency of the response of GBM to radiation would imply that further dose escalation or alternative fractionation schemes could improve treatment outcome. However, standard fractionation schemes applying 2-Gy fractions, five times per week were empirically established and do not necessarily present an optimum. In fact, experimental evidence suggests that taking the heterogeneity of GBM into consideration, more unconventional fractionation schemes could improve the efficacy of radiotherapy against GBM.[52] Yet, clinical attempts at improving the impact of radiotherapy have so far largely failed[53] and dose escalation up to a total dose of 90 Gy did not improve survival.[54,55]

A large number of groups have demonstrated resistance of GICs to many commonly used chemotherapeutic agents,[6,56] including temozolomide.[38,57] Several different mechanisms contribute to this resistance including the overexpression of ABC transporter proteins, which can be exploited to enrich GICs in side-population assays[58] and are responsible for an active efflux of chemotherapeutic agents; the preference to reside not only in a perivascular niche but also inside the hypoxic microenvironment of the tumor core,[59,60] in which the efficacy of chemotherapy is drastically reduced[61,62]; and overexpression of free radical scavenging systems[63] able to detoxify drugs. Furthermore, a large number of targeted therapies against bulk tumor cell populations in GBM have largely failed to improve outcome.[64]

Taken together, the standard-of-care against GBM and many of its iterations have hit a critical barrier and their inefficacy to eliminate GICs suggests that specific targeting of GICs could further improve treatment outcome for patients with GBM.

Targeting Glioma-Initiating Cells

From the identification of tumor-initiating cells came considerable enthusiasm for novel therapies aimed at this rare population. With this in mind, the discussion of how gliomas are organized becomes of less academic and more of practical importance because it dictates possible intervention points to target GICs. A hierarchical model of GBM implies a finite number of GICs, responsible for the repopulation of the tumor, and suggests that their successful elimination will improve treatment outcome. The understanding that those tumor-initiating cells potentially derive from normal stem cells implied to target developmental signaling pathways including the Wnt, BMP, and c-Met pathways in GICs,[65] known to govern stem cell traits in normal neural/progenitor stem cells. However, if GICs are driven by the same pathways that maintain neural stem cells or progenitor cells, every attempt to target these pathways for therapeutic gain will then rely on the existence of a therapeutic window[66] that limits current established antitumor therapies. For example, whereas CD133[+] GBM cells can be targeted by inhibition of the Notch pathway by γ-secretase inhibitors in patients,[67] normal stem cell compartments like that of the gastrointestinal tract rely on the same pathway and exhibit significant toxicity. In fact, clinical results fall short of the encouraging experimental findings that motivated the clinical trials.[68]

If in fact the clonal evolution model more accurately describes the organizational structure of GBM, targeting GICs becomes more complicated. Different driver mutations in individual clones will emerge over time,[69] leading to dysregulation of multiple pathways that potentially can maintain stemness. Although the number of these mutations is most likely finite, surgical specimens will only provide snapshots of the evolutionary landscape of these mutations and will not be informative enough to select treatments against individual clones over time unless an overarching feature of GICs can be identified and targeted.

The problem of targeting GICs is further complicated when one factors the effects of cancer therapies[70] and the response of surviving tumor cells into the equation. Microenvironmental stress,[71] chemotherapy, and radiation[72] induce interconversion of non-GICs into induced GICs, thus replenishing the pool of treatment-resistant GICs and fueling recurrences. In the case of ionizing radiation, this process involves re-expression of developmental transcription factors and global epigenetic changes.[73] In a recent unbiased high-throughput screen, we were able to identify compounds that can interfere with the process of radiation-induced phenotype conversion.[74] One group of compounds identified in this screen was that of dopamine receptor antagonists that easily cross the blood-brain barrier and not only prevent the induction of GICs but also target intrinsic GICs and non-GICs,[73] thereby significantly prolonging survival in a mouse model of GBM. With novel dopamine receptor antagonists harboring more favorable side effect profiles in clinical development,[75] this strategy could offer a novel approach to improve the efficacy of the standard-of-care in GBM.

SUMMARY

GICs accomplish several tasks critical to tumor growth and recurrence by promoting invasiveness, immune system evasion, and resistance to existing therapeutic options via conversion of non-GICs into new GICs following radiation. Although GICs are identified by a handful of different markers (CD133, SSEA-1, A2B5, nestin, and integrin-α6), the scientific community still lacks a complete understanding of different such subtypes. Furthermore, translating the excitement surrounding experimental therapies into successful clinical outcomes has proved difficult. Hampering the effect of GICs may be possible, however, by inhibiting the treatment-induced phenotype conversion that replenishes residual tumor of its GIC population and helps promote recurrence.

CLINICS CARE POINTS

- GICs drive recurrences and are a potential target against GBM.
- Prospective identification of GICs is hampered by the fact that marker systems only enrich for GICs.
- Intratumoral heterogeneity and plasticity of GBM allow tumors to escape therapies aimed at GICs.

DISCLOSURE

Dr. Pajonk was supported by grants from the National Cancer Institute (R01CA200234, P50CA211015). Dr. Muftuoglu has nothing to disclose.

REFERENCES

1. Stupp R, Mason WP, van den Bent MJ, et al. Radiotherapy plus concomitant and adjuvant temozolomide for glioblastoma. N Engl J Med 2005;352(10): 987–96.
2. Singh SK, Clarke ID, Terasaki M, et al. Identification of a cancer stem cell in human brain tumors. Cancer Res 2003;63(18):5821–8.
3. Singh SK, Hawkins C, Clarke ID, et al. Identification of human brain tumour initiating cells. Nature 2004; 432(7015):396–401.
4. Hemmati HD, Nakano I, Lazareff JA, et al. Cancerous stem cells can arise from pediatric brain tumors. Proc Natl Acad Sci U S A 2003;100(25): 15178–83.
5. Bao S, Wu Q, McLendon RE, et al. Glioma stem cells promote radioresistance by preferential activation of the DNA damage response. Nature 2006;444(7120): 756–60.
6. Eramo A, Ricci-Vitiani L, Zeuner A, et al. Chemotherapy resistance of glioblastoma stem cells. Cell Death Differ 2006;13(7):1238–41.
7. Cohneim J. Congenitales, quergestreiftes Muskelsarkom der Nieren. Virchows Archiv 1875;65(1):64–9.
8. Reya T, Morrison SJ, Clarke MF, et al. Stem cells, cancer, and cancer stem cells. Nature 2001; 414(6859):105–11.
9. Phillips TM, McBride WH, Pajonk F. The response of CD24(-/low)/CD44+ breast cancer-initiating cells to radiation. J Natl Cancer Inst 2006;98(24):1777–85.
10. Li X, Lewis MT, Huang J, et al. Intrinsic resistance of tumorigenic breast cancer cells to chemotherapy. J Natl Cancer Inst 2008;100(9):672–9.
11. Ishizawa K, Rasheed ZA, Karisch R, et al. Tumor-initiating cells are rare in many human tumors. Cell Stem Cell 2010;7(3):279–82.
12. Overgaard J. Chemoradiotherapy of head and neck cancer: can the bumble bee fly? Radiother Oncol 2009;92(1):1–3.
13. Al-Hajj M, Wicha MS, Benito-Hernandez A, et al. Prospective identification of tumorigenic breast cancer cells. Proc Natl Acad Sci U S A 2003;100:3983–8.
14. Nowell PC. The clonal evolution of tumor cell populations. Science 1976;194(4260):23–8.
15. Quintana E, Shackleton M, Sabel MS, et al. Efficient tumour formation by single human melanoma cells. Nature 2008;456(7222):593–8.
16. McKenzie MD, Ghisi M, Oxley EP, et al. Interconversion between tumorigenic and differentiated states in acute myeloid leukemia. Cell Stem Cell 2019; 25(2):258–72.e9.
17. MacArthur BD, Lemischka IR. Statistical mechanics of pluripotency. Cell 2013;154(3):484–9.
18. Bazan E, Alonso FJ, Redondo C, et al. In vitro and in vivo characterization of neural stem cells. Histol Histopathol 2004;19(4):1261–75.
19. Hu Y, Smyth GK. ELDA: extreme limiting dilution analysis for comparing depleted and enriched populations in stem cell and other assays. J Immunol Methods 2009;347(1–2):70–8.
20. Frisch SM, Francis H. Disruption of epithelial cell-matrix interactions induces apoptosis. J Cell Biol 1994;124(4):619–26.
21. Yin AH, Miraglia S, Zanjani ED, et al. AC133, a novel marker for human hematopoietic stem and progenitor cells. Blood 1997;90(12):5002–12.
22. Ogden AT, Waziri AE, Lochhead RA, et al. Identification of A2B5+CD133- tumor-initiating cells in adult

human gliomas. Neurosurgery 2008;62(2):505–14 [discussion: 514–5].

23. Son MJ, Woolard K, Nam DH, et al. SSEA-1 is an enrichment marker for tumor-initiating cells in human glioblastoma. Cell stem cell 2009;4(5):440–52.

24. Griguer CE, Oliva CR, Gobin E, et al. CD133 is a marker of bioenergetic stress in human glioma. PLoS One 2008;3(11):e3655.

25. Tchoghandjian A, Baeza N, Colin C, et al. A2B5 cells from human glioblastoma have cancer stem cell properties. Brain Pathol 2010;20(1):211–21.

26. Jin X, Jin X, Jung JE, et al. Cell surface Nestin is a biomarker for glioma stem cells. Biochem Biophys Res Commun 2013;433(4):496–501.

27. Mao XG, Zhang X, Xue XY, et al. Brain tumor stem-like cells identified by neural stem cell marker CD15. Transl Oncol 2009;2(4):247–57.

28. Lathia JD, Gallagher J, Heddleston JM, et al. Integrin alpha 6 regulates glioblastoma stem cells. Cell stem cell 2010;6(5):421–32.

29. Vlashi E, Kim K, Lagadec C, et al. In vivo imaging, tracking, and targeting of cancer stem cells. J Natl Cancer Inst 2009;101(5):350–9.

30. Ludwig K, Kornblum HI. Molecular markers in glioma. J Neurooncol 2017;134(3):505–12.

31. Lathia JD, Gallagher J, Myers JT, et al. Direct in vivo evidence for tumor propagation by glioblastoma cancer stem cells. PLoS One 2011;6(9):e24807.

32. Sun T, Chen G, Li Y, et al. Aggressive invasion is observed in CD133(-)/A2B5(+) glioma-initiating cells. Oncol Lett 2015;10(6):3399–406.

33. Calabrese C, Poppleton H, Kocak M, et al. A perivascular niche for brain tumor stem cells. Cancer cell 2007;11(1):69–82.

34. Niibori-Nambu A, Midorikawa U, Mizuguchi S, et al. Glioma initiating cells form a differentiation niche via the induction of extracellular matrices and integrin αV. PLoS One 2013;8(5):e59558.

35. Jeon HM, Kim SH, Jin X, et al. Crosstalk between glioma-initiating cells and endothelial cells drives tumor progression. Cancer Res 2014;74(16):4482–92.

36. Di Tomaso T, Mazzoleni S, Wang E, et al. Immuno-biological characterization of cancer stem cells isolated from glioblastoma patients. Clin Cancer Res 2010;16(3):800–13.

37. Kitange GJ, Carlson BL, Schroeder MA, et al. Induction of MGMT expression is associated with temozolomide resistance in glioblastoma xenografts. Neuro Oncol 2009;11(3):281–91.

38. Blough MD, Westgate MR, Beauchamp D, et al. Sensitivity to temozolomide in brain tumor initiating cells. Neuro Oncol 2010;12(7):756–60.

39. Nakai E, Park K, Yawata T, et al. Enhanced MDR1 expression and chemoresistance of cancer stem cells derived from glioblastoma. Cancer Invest 2009;27(9):901–8.

40. Lim YC, Roberts TL, Day BW, et al. A role for homologous recombination and abnormal cell-cycle progression in radioresistance of glioma-initiating cells. Mol Cancer Ther 2012;11(9):1863–72.

41. Zeppernick F, Ahmadi R, Campos B, et al. Stem cell marker CD133 affects clinical outcome in glioma patients. Clin Cancer Res 2008;14(1):123–9.

42. Zhang M, Song T, Yang L, et al. Nestin and CD133: valuable stem cell-specific markers for determining clinical outcome of glioma patients. J Exp Clin Cancer Res 2008;27(1):85.

43. Wu B, Sun C, Feng F, et al. Do relevant markers of cancer stem cells CD133 and Nestin indicate a poor prognosis in glioma patients? A systematic review and meta-analysis. J Exp Clin Cancer Res 2015;34(1):44.

44. Mock A, Chiblak S, Herold-Mende C. Lessons we learned from high-throughput and top-down systems biology analyses about glioma stem cells. Curr Pharm Des 2014;20(1):66–72.

45. Ahmed AU, Auffinger B, Lesniak MS. Understanding glioma stem cells: rationale, clinical relevance and therapeutic strategies. Expert Rev Neurother 2013; 13(5):545–55.

46. Stupp R, Hegi ME, Mason WP, et al. Effects of radiotherapy with concomitant and adjuvant temozolomide versus radiotherapy alone on survival in glioblastoma in a randomised phase III study: 5-year analysis of the EORTC-NCIC trial. Lancet Oncol 2009;10(5):459–66.

47. Sanai N, Polley MY, McDermott MW, et al. An extent of resection threshold for newly diagnosed glioblastomas. J Neurosurg 2011;115(1):3–8.

48. Li Z, Bao S, Wu Q, et al. Hypoxia-inducible factors regulate tumorigenic capacity of glioma stem cells. Cancer Cell 2009;15(6):501–13.

49. Li Z, Rich JN. Hypoxia and hypoxia inducible factors in cancer stem cell maintenance. Curr Top Microbiol Immunol 2010;345:21–30.

50. Heddleston JM, Li Z, McLendon RE, et al. The hypoxic microenvironment maintains glioblastoma stem cells and promotes reprogramming towards a cancer stem cell phenotype. Cell Cycle 2009;8(20):3274–84.

51. Walker MD, Strike TA, Sheline GE. An analysis of dose-effect relationship in the radiotherapy of malignant gliomas. Int J Radiat Oncol Biol Phys 1979;5(10):1725–31.

52. Leder K, Pitter K, LaPlant Q, et al. Mathematical modeling of PDGF-driven glioblastoma reveals optimized radiation dosing schedules. Cell 2014;156(3):603–16.

53. Laperriere N, Zuraw L, Cairncross G. Cancer Care Ontario Practice Guidelines Initiative Neuro-Oncology Disease Site G. Radiotherapy for newly diagnosed malignant glioma in adults: a systematic review. Radiother Oncol 2002;64(3):259–73.

54. Badiyan SN, Markovina S, Simpson JR, et al. Radiation therapy dose escalation for glioblastoma

multiforme in the era of temozolomide. Int J Radiat Oncol Biol Phys 2014;90(4):877–85.

55. Wegner RE, Abel S, Horne ZD, et al. National trends in radiation dose escalation for glioblastoma. Radiat Oncol J 2019;37(1):13–21.

56. Kenig S, Faoro V, Bourkoula E, et al. Topoisomerase IIβ mediates the resistance of glioblastoma stem cells to replication stress-inducing drugs. Cancer Cell Int 2016;16:58.

57. Liu G, Yuan X, Zeng Z, et al. Analysis of gene expression and chemoresistance of CD133+ cancer stem cells in glioblastoma. Mol Cancer 2006;5: 67.

58. Hirschmann-Jax C, Foster AE, Wulf GG, et al. A distinct "side population" of cells with high drug efflux capacity in human tumor cells. Proc Natl Acad Sci U S A 2004;101(39):14228–33.

59. Smith SJ, Diksin M, Chhaya S, et al. The invasive region of glioblastoma defined by 5ALA guided surgery has an altered cancer stem cell marker profile compared to central tumour. Int J Mol Sci 2017; 18(11):2452.

60. Sattiraju A, Sai KKS, Mintz A. Glioblastoma stem cells and their microenvironment. Adv Exp Med Biol 2017;1041:119–40.

61. Teicher BA. Hypoxia and drug resistance. Cancer Metastasis Rev 1994;13(2):139–68.

62. Musah-Eroje A, Watson S. A novel 3D in vitro model of glioblastoma reveals resistance to temozolomide which was potentiated by hypoxia. J Neurooncol 2019;142(2):231–40.

63. Dokic I, Hartmann C, Herold-Mende C, et al. Gluta-thione peroxidase 1 activity dictates the sensitivity of glioblastoma cells to oxidative stress. Glia 2012; 60(11):1785–800.

64. Bai RY, Staedtke V, Riggins GJ. Molecular targeting of glioblastoma: drug discovery and therapies. Trends Mol Med 2011;17(6):301–12.

65. Mehta S, Lo Cascio C. Developmentally regulated signaling pathways in glioma invasion. Cell Mol Life Sci 2018;75(3):385–402.

66. Holthusen H. Erfahrungen über die Verträglichkeits-grenze für Röntgenstrahlen und deren Nutzanwendung zur Verhütung von Schäden. Strahlentherapie 1936;(57):254–69.

67. Xu R, Shimizu F, Hovinga K, et al. Molecular and clinical effects of notch inhibition in glioma patients: a phase 0/i trial. Clin Cancer Res 2016;22(19): 4786–96.

68. McCaw TR, Inga E, Chen H, et al. Gamma secretase inhibitors in cancer: a current perspective on clinical performance. Oncologist 2020. https://doi.org/10. 1002/onco.13627.

69. Abou-El-Ardat K, Seifert M, Becker K, et al. Comprehensive molecular characterization of multifocal glioblastoma proves its monoclonal origin and reveals novel insights into clonal evolution and heterogeneity of glioblastomas. Neuro Oncol 2017;19(4): 546–57.

70. Wang J, Cazzato E, Ladewig E, et al. Clonal evolution of glioblastoma under therapy. Nat Genet 2016;48(7):768–76.

71. Lee G, Auffinger B, Guo D, et al. Dedifferentiation of glioma cells to glioma stem-like cells by therapeutic stress-induced hif signaling in the recurrent GBM model. Mol Cancer Ther 2016;15(12):3064–76.

72. Safa AR, Saadatzadeh MR, Cohen-Gadol AA, et al. Glioblastoma stem cells (GSCs) epigenetic plasticity and interconversion between differentiated non-GSCs and GSCs. Genes Dis 2015;2(2):152–63.

73. Bhat K, Saki M, Vlashi E, et al. The dopamine receptor antagonist trifluoperazine prevents phenotype conversion and improves survival in mouse models of glioblastoma. Proc Natl Acad Sci U S A 2020; 117(20):11085–96.

74. Zhang L, Bochkur Dratver M, Yazal T, et al. Mebendazole potentiates radiation therapy in triple-negative breast cancer. Int J Radiat Oncol Biol Phys 2019;103(1):195–207.

75. Prabhu VV, Morrow S, Rahman Kawakibi A, et al. ONC201 and imipridones: anti-cancer compounds with clinical efficacy. Neoplasia 2020;22(12):725–44.

Therapeutic Delivery to Central Nervous System

Katherine E. Kunigelis, MD, Michael A. Vogelbaum, MD PhD*

KEYWORDS

- Glioblastoma • Clinical trials • Blood-brain barrier • Blood-brain-tumor barrier
- Convection-enhanced delivery

KEY POINTS

- The blood-brain barrier (BBB) and blood-tumor-barrier (BTB) present substantial barriers to delivery of therapeutic agents to the CNS.
- Intrinsic BBB mechanisms to passively or actively transport molecules severely restrict delivery of therapeutic agents.
- This hurdle is addressed by disrupting or bypassing the BBB to allow agents to enter central nervous system (CNS) tissue.
- Direct administration of agents to bypass the BBB include implantable controlled-release polymer systems, intracavitary drug delivery, direct injection of viral vectors, and convection-enhanced delivery (CED).
- CED uses direct pump-mediated continuous infusion into the tumor bed or tumor adjacent brain, circumventing the BBB. This approach has shown promising results with infusion of immunotoxins, chemotherapy, and viral vectors.

INTRODUCTION

In the United States, glioblastoma (GBM) has an incidence of 3.2 per 100,000 population.[1] Median overall survival (OS) for patients with newly diagnosed GBM is 12 months to 18 months,[2] with median progression-free survival (PFS) of only 6.9 months. Following recurrence, salvage treatment provides only 6 months to 8 months of additional survival.[3] The 3 major treatment modalities have not changed for over 3 decades.[2] Maximum safe resection with postoperative adjuvant radiation and chemotherapy via the Stupp protocol remains the standard of care.[4] The only new technology to have significantly changed outcomes is tumor treating fields. The addition of tumor treating fields to maintenance temozolomide in newly diagnosed GBM significantly increased PFS by 2.7 months and OS by 4.9 months.[5] There is no established standard for recurrent GBM.[6] Multiple therapeutic strategies have demonstrated minimal survival benefit but remission has yet to be achieved.[7]

CHALLENGES IN TREATING GLIOBLASTOMA

The effectiveness of therapeutics for GBM is limited due to the presence of blood-brain barrier (BBB) and blood-brain-tumor barrier (BTB) and cellular/genetic heterogeneity as well as an immunosuppressive tumor microenvironment.[8] Cellular pleomorphism associated with GBM provides a therapeutic challenge, even when drug delivery is achieved in target tissue. Four transcriptional profiles—classical (epidermal growth factor receptor [EGFR] drive), proneural (platelet-derived growth factor–driven), mesenchymal (neurofibromatosis type 1 driven), and neural—have been identified.

Department of Neuro-Oncology, Neuro-Oncology Program, Moffitt Cancer Center, 12902 USF Magnolia Drive, Tampa, FL 33612, USA
* Corresponding author. Moffitt Cancer Center, 12902 USF Magnolia Drive, Tampa, FL 33612.
E-mail address: Michael.Vogelbaum@moffitt.org

Neurosurg Clin N Am 32 (2021) 291–303
https://doi.org/10.1016/j.nec.2020.12.004
1042-3680/21/© 2020 Elsevier Inc. All rights reserved.

Once administered, therapeutic agents can select for proliferation of resistant cell types.[8] This phenomenon has been shown with temozolomide treatment of GBM.[9]

Although complete resection of the enhancing component of GBM is associated with increased survival, microinvasive infiltrating tumor cells throughout the normal parenchyma prevent surgical treatment from being curative.[6,7,10] Deeply infiltrative cells around the tumor periphery already may represent a more resilient cell population that initiates and drive tumor recurrence.[9,11] GBMs also contain discrete populations of cancer stem cells that are highly resistant to therapy and can redevelop into a large mass after the primary tumor is resected.[8,9] Furthermore, the cellular, genetic, and epigenetic biology of GBM is complex, and a single genetic or epigenetic target has not yet been discovered that would make targeted therapeutics more likely to be effective.[7] This heterogeneity likely increases over time and is revealed in biopsies of recurrent disease.[9]

Treatment of the residual, nonenhancing disease also is made difficult due to the presence of the BBB, which limits the ability of systemically delivered to achieve therapeutic concentrations within the tumor infiltrated brain. This issue extends to treatment of unresectable enhancing tumor, because the BTB may be partially open (to administered contrast agents) but not necessarily to therapeutic drugs. The full physiology and significance of the BBB and BTB on the growth and treatment resistance of GBM are not completely understood but present a substantial barrier to be overcome in the development of CNS directed therapeutics.[9]

THE BLOOD-BRAIN BARRIER

The restrictive function of the BBB remains one of the most significant challenges in treatment of GBM.[12] The BBB is formed by endothelial tight junctions, the basement membrane, and astrocyte foot processes, otherwise referred to as the neurovascular unit. Because the BBB relegates relatively unrestricted entry into the parenchyma to small (<400 Da) and lipophilic molecules, approximately 98% potential neurotherapeutics are unable to access the CNS.[8,10,13,14] To cross the BBB, lipid-mediated diffusion allows small molecules (with molecular weight <400 Da and <8 hydrogen bonds) to pass. Other endogenous transport systemics include carrier-mediated transport and receptor-mediated transport.[14] Membrane proteins act as transporters for small molecules, including ions, nutrients, and molecules for metabolism.[13] The BBB is not homogenous and there is variable permeability throughout the vasculature; there is more permeability in large vessels and less permeability due to tighter junctions in smaller ones. Permeability also changes over time, increasing with angiogenesis and with insults, such as ischemic injury.[15]

THE BLOOD-BRAIN-TUMOR BARRIER

The BTB forms after seeding of the parenchyma with tumor cells. The rapid expansion of colonizing cells quickly outgrows the existing blood supply, leading to tissue hypoxia. Up-regulated hypoxia-inducible factor 1 stimulates vascular endothelial growth factor (VEGF). VEGF causes breakdown of existing BBB cytoarchitecture as well as angiogenesis of structurally abnormal capillaries with increased permeability.[16–18] The combination of abnormal vasculature and tumor cells becomes the BTB.[18] Alteration in vascularization caused by growth of high-grade gliomas results in leakiness of the BTB, represented clinically by areas of contrast enhancement as well as surrounding vasogenic edema on magnetic resonance imaging (MRI).[16,17] These areas also lack typical structures of the BBB, including tight junctions.[18] Despite the disruption of the typical BBB architecture, the BTB continues to limit ingress of therapeutic molecules.[18] The BTB is heterogeneous, however, even within the same tumor, further complicating the therapeutic possibilities.[17]

STRATEGIES TO OVERCOME THE BLOOD-BRAIN BARRIER/BLOOD-BRAIN-TUMOR BARRIER

Strategies used to obtain adequate intratumoral drug concentrations may either take advantage of intrinsic BBB characteristics or disrupt or bypass the BBB to allow agents to pass through (**Table 1**). Passive targeting at sites of BBB disruption, active targeting via receptor-mediated transport, and immunotherapy take advantage of intrinsic properties of the BBB to deliver therapeutics. BBB disruption strategies include chemical—via osmotic agents or cytokines—and mechanical—via focused ultrasound (FUS) or laser interstitial thermal therapy (LITT). BBB bypass strategies include surgically implanted wafers, injections, and convection-enhanced delivery (CED).

Passive Targeting via Disrupted Blood-Brain Barrier at Glioblastoma Sites

GBM is associated with pathologic microvascular proliferation resulting in abnormal leaky tumor vessels, which disrupt the BBB at the tumor core and allow penetration of molecules up to 20 nm to

Table 1
Major categories of therapeutic strategies to overcome the blood-brain barrier and blood-brain-tumor barrier, along with specific examples

Passive BBB penetrating therapies	Traditional Chemotherapeutics (e.g. temozolomide)		19–23
Actively targeted BBB penetrating therapies	Receptor mediated transport	Transferrin	24–27
		Lipoprotein receptor related protein (LRP)	29
		Integrins	30
		D-glucose transporter (GLUT)	31
		Glial Fibrillary Acidic Protein (GFAP)	32
		Connexin 43	32
		Epidermal Growth Factor Receptor (EGFR)	33–35
		Interleukin 13 (IL-13)	36
		Fibroblast Growth Factor Inducible 14 (Fn14)	37
	Liposomes	Transferrin	39–43,85
		GFAP	32,39
		GLUT	39,44
Immunotherapy	Vaccines	DCVax-L	2,46
		EGFRvIII	47–50
	Chimeric Antigen Receptor (CAR) T-Cells	EGFR v III	46
		IL-23R alpha 2	51,52
Blood Brain Barrier Disruption	Osmotic - Mannitol		9,12,52,54
	Intra-Arterial		54,55
	Chemical, Bradykinin		12
	Ultrasound		12,52,56,57
	LITT		58–60
Directly Administered Therapeutics (implant or single injection)	Implantable Polymer Systems	Carmustine wafers (Gliadel)	6,9,10,12,52,61
	Direct Injection - Vectors	Toca511	2,64
		Parvovirus – ParvOnyx	6,64
		Adenovirus-HSVtk	65
		Adenovirus – DNX – 2401	66
		HSV – Mo32	67
		HSV – G207	68
Directly Administered Therapeutics (Convection Enhanced Delivery)	Immunotoxins	Transferrin – Diptheria	6,12,69
		Cintredekin Besudotox	12,45,70–72
		IL-4 conjugated to Pseudomonas exotoxin (PE38KDEL)	12,69
		TGF-alpha conjugated to Pseudomonas exotoxin (TP-38)	12,69
	Oligonucleotides	AP 12009	12
	Viral Vectors	Poliovirus (PVSRIPO)	2,46,62–64,73–75
	Chemotherapy	Paclitaxel	12,69
		Topotecan	3,12,77
		Temozolomide	69,78
	Nanoparticles	Magnetic Beads	6
		Liposomes	79

100 nm.[8] Passive targeting of molecules takes advantage of the at least partially disrupted BBB within the solid and enhancing portion of GBM; however, the infiltrating tumor cells in the periphery remain sequestered behind an intact BBB, largely impenetrable to systemic delivery of therapeutic agents.[7] This remains a challenge to traditional systemic chemotherapy regimens.[19–22]

A review of phase 0/window of opportunity clinical trials performing tissue-based assessments after systemic delivery of a drug showed that levels of drug accumulating in enhancing versus nonenhancing tumor tissue varied substantially with slower drug distribution in nonenhancing areas. Other studies, however, have shown similar drug levels within the tumor and the normal brain. Even when drug levels were found to accumulate in tissue, clinical activity of the drug often was lacking.[23]

Active Targeting via Receptor-Mediated Transport

Active nanotherapeutic targeting involves taking advantage of cell surface receptors preferentially expressed on GBM tumor cells. A specific targeting molecule and delivery system then must be designed. Several targets have been attempted in preclinical studies, including transferrin receptors,[24–28] lipoprotein receptor–related protein,[29] integrins,[30] D-glucose transporter (GLUT),[31] glial fibrillary acidic protein (GFAP),[32] connexin 43, EGFR,[33–35] interleukin (IL)-13,[36] and fibroblast growth factor–inducible 14 (Fn14),[37] with promising results.[8] Transferrin-conjugated nanobased drug delivery systems have been in human clinical trials without definitive results to this point.[8]

Macromolecule drug delivery systems, such as liposomes and polymers, increase efficacy, stability, and half-life of anticancer drugs while reducing toxicity to healthy tissues.[38] Liposomes can deliver small molecules with specificity to the nervous system by coupling to aptamers or monoclonal antibodies against transferrin receptors,[39–43] GFAP,[32,39] or GLUT4.[39,44] Liposomes have shown increased transport of both daunorubicin and doxorubicin to the brain.[39]

Biological Targeting of the Brain via Immunotherapy

One of the functions of the BBB is to help maintain the restricted immune environment of the CNS, and it has been well recognized that gliomas produce an immunosuppressive tumor microenvironment.[28] The immunosuppressive nature of the CNS and lack of a foundational mutations to target limit the efficacy of vaccines in GBM. Other considerations include the need for frequent steroid administration in this population, which can inactivate induced immune responses.[45] Nonetheless, a variety of types of systemic immunotherapeutics have been developed for GBM and rely on the ability of cellular and humoral elements of the immune system to effectively bypass or overcome restrictions imposed by the BBB.

Vaccines

Cancer vaccines aim to elicit T-cell responses with tumor cell killing properties. Vaccines investigated in GBM have either been peptide or dendritic cell vaccines. Peptide-targeted vaccines include the IMA950 peptide cocktail, a personalized peptide vaccination for recurrent GBM, and a peptide covering the IDH1R132H mutation in newly diagnosed grade III/IV tumors.[45] Dendritic cell therapy targets include the DCVax-L trial[2,46] and several ongoing clinical trials (NCT00323115 and NCT01280552).[46] Of particular note are the studies involving a dendritic vaccine targeting EGFRvIII, which progressed through phase I[47] and phase 2 in both newly diagnosed GBM[48] and recurrent[49] GBM with promising results but ultimately failed to increase survival in a phase 3 trial.[50]

Chimeric antigen receptor T cells

Chimeric antigen receptor (CAR) T cells are engineered to recognize tumor-associated antigens and bind to both antigens and activate T cells in a manner not dependent on MHC complexes.[10] CAR T-cell–based therapies have shown efficacy in murine glioma models. The patient's tumor sample is examined for tumor-specific antigens and a CAR is selected that is specific for that individual tumor. The lack of well-described and consistent tumor antigens in GBM has limited this technology. Three antigens have been targeted with clinical results—EGFRvIII, IL13Rα2, and HER2. EGFRvIII CARs showed improved survival in a preclinical mouse model. These are undergoing further investigation in a phase 2 trial (NCT01454596).[46] IL13Rα2 CAR can kill GBM and stem cells. It has shown promising clinical activity in clinical studies.[46] HER2 is a tyrosine kinase whose up-regulation portends a poor prognosis in GBM. Early clinical data show some clinical activity of CAR in recurrent HER2-positive GBM. Other targets are under investigation.[46] A case report of CAR–T cells targeting IL13Rα2 in recurrent GBM showed complete regression of all intracranial and spinal tumors lasting 7.5 months.[51] A phase I clinical trial is currently under way (NCT02208362).[51]

Blood-Brain Barrier Disruption Strategies

Several substances and states open tight junctions, including neurotransmitters, hormones, and inflammatory mediators; physiologic states, such as hypertension, hypoxia, or ischemia; or hypertonic substances, including mannitol, bradykinin, and angiotensin peptides.[12] This disruption increases spaces in between the tight junctions, thereby increasing drug permeability.[52] In GBM, the mostly commonly used of these are mannitol and FUS.

Osmotic

Mannitol Disrupting the BBB first was attempted more than 30 years ago via using hyperosmotic therapy to improve delivery of chemotherapy to brain tumors.[53] Osmotic BBB disruption can be achieved by intra-arterial (IA) infusion of a hyperosmotic agent, usually mannitol. Rapid diffusion of water out of cells causes shrinking of endothelial cells with opening of tight junctions for several hours. Subsequent administration of IA chemotherapy can increase concentrations of chemotherapeutic agents in the parenchyma up to 90-fold in animal models. Methotrexate delivery is increased 4-7-fold by addition of IA osmotic BBB disruption.[12] Retrospective studies demonstrated survival benefits with intraarterial mannitol infusion.[52] IA delivery of bevacizumab after BBB disruption with IA mannitol for recurrent GBM showed encouraging results in PFS (10 months), and all patients had radiographic response within 1 month with 8 showing decrease in tumor and 6 showing stable tumor.[54] This method remains limited, however, by toxicity and complexity of IA administration[52] and has not shown definitive efficacy in clinical trials.[9,55]

Bradykinin Mediators of the inflammatory response also disrupt tight junctions in vasculature. A bradykinin agonist RMP-7 selectively disrupts the BBB in regions of the BTB compared with nontumor BBB. Unfortunately, this agent has been associated with high levels of toxicity and further clinical development has been abandoned.[12]

Ultrasound

MRI-guided FUS (MRgFUS) disrupts BBB through targeted ultrasound beams that use thermal and mechanical stress to disrupt endothelial cells. The addition of microbubbles that expand and contract with ultrasound beams can transiently open the BBB.[52] MRgFUS causes focal openings that reverse within 23 hours.[12]

FUS has the potential to generate cytotoxicity within tumor tissue, enhance delivery of therapeutic agents, and improve extracellular distribution as well as stimulate an immune response in the tumor microenvironment, minimizing toxicity to normal tissue.[56] Multiple phase I clinical trials for GBM are under way.[9] In rat models, a combination of microbubbles and FUS-enhanced brain penetration of carmustine (BCNU).[52]

Currently, this technology requires a bone window in the skull, but recent advances in MRgFUS systems allow precise, temporally and spatially controllable, and safe externally delivered transcranial ultrasound energy, which is effective at disrupting the BBB as demonstrated by enhancement in white matter after gadolinium administration.[57] Technological advances like phased-array transducers and real-time temperature monitoring thus have made FUS more practical in treatment of glioma.[56] The actual impact of MRgFUS-induced BBB disruption on the ability of therapeutics to achieve adequate concentrations in brain or brain tumor tissue remains an area of active investigation.

Laser interstitial thermal therapy

Data from mouse models and patients who underwent laser ablation for GBM indicate that thermal therapy transiently increases BBB/BTB permeability from with a peak estimated at 1 week to 2 weeks post-treatment and lasting 4 weeks to 6 weeks.[58–60] In mouse modules, molecules up to 150 kDa are able to enter the CNS after LITT and infiltrate into a surround penumbra around the treated area and LITT in combination with doxorubicin was associated with increased survival.[58,60] A clinical trial investigating the combination of LITT and doxorubicin in adult populations recently has been completed (NCT01851733).[58]

Directly Administered Therapeutics

Another solution for this therapeutic delivery problem posed by the BBB is direct delivery of therapeutics into the tumor or post–resection cavity via bypassing the normal barrier. Multiple attempts at administration have been focused on implantable controlled-release polymer systems, various catheter devices for intracavitary drug delivery, direct injection of viral vectors, and CED.[6,12]

Implantable polymer systems

Implanted polymers aim to provide continuous drug delivery using a wafer with a controlled, sustained release rate.[12] Biodegradable polyanhydride wafers loaded with carmustine (Gliadel, Arbor Pharmaceuticals, Atlanta, Georgia) increase survival by 8 weeks when placed at recurrence and 2.3 months during primary resection.[10,61] The FDA approved carmustine wafers for use in recurrent high-grade glioma in 1996 and primary high-grade glioma in 2004.[8]

Phase 3 clinical trials have shown significant survival benefits with carmustine wafer placement intraoperatively but widespread use continues to be limited by toxicity concerns, wafer dislodgement, obstructive hydrocephalus, cyst formation, high infection rates, wound healing concerns, costs, and practical implications that carmustine wafer placement restricts patients from recruitment into clinical trials.[6,9,12,52]

Intraventricular/intracavitary catheters

Intraventricular or intracavitary approaches have been used to deliver bolus or infusion of chemotherapy directly into the ventricles or a tumor cyst or cavity. Agents, such as nitrosourea and methotrexate, have been tried. Concerns remain about infection, catheter obstruction, and inadequate drug distribution.[12] Intraventricular injection has limited use for parenchymal brain tumors because there is limited flow between the cerebrospinal fluid space and the intracellular space of the brain.[2] This strategy remains useful in some situations for treatment of leptomeningeal disease.

Direct injection

Viral therapy can be divided into 2 groups—replication-competent oncolytic viruses and replication-deficient viral vectors used as a delivery mechanism for therapeutic genes.[62] Oncolytic viruses transduce neoplastic cells and selectively replicates and induces systemic antitumor immunity.[63]

Toca 511 Toca 511 is a retroviral replication competent vector encoding the cytosine deaminase that converts the antifungal drug 5-fluorocytosine into the antineoplastic drug 5-fluorouracil. Phase I and preclinical studies indicated that this agent produced both antineoplastic activity and immune activation.[2] In a phase I trial (NCT01470794) of Toca 511 injected into the resection cavity of patients with recurrent high-grade gliomas followed by cycles of oral 5-fluorocytosine, median OS was 14.4 months. Five patients demonstrated complete response and were alive 33.9 months to 52.2 months after Toca 511 administration.[64] A randomized phase 2/3 trial versus standard of care (NCT02414165) used direct injection of retrovirus into the surgical resection cavity after bulk tumor removal to transduce the gene cytosine deaminase into infiltrating tumor cells.[2] This trial failed to meet its efficacy endpoint and further development was halted by the sponsor.

Oncolytic H-1 parvovirus (ParvOryx) In a phase I/IIa trial for recurrent GBM, an oncolytic parvovirus was administered via intratumoral or intravenous injection prior to resection and then again around the resection cavity after resection. Median OS was 15.5 months after oncolytic H-1 parvovirus whether it was administered IV or intratumoral.[64]

This technique also remains limited because intracerebral injection localizes delivery to cells at the site of the injection but does not penetrate tumor cells deep in parenchyma. The host immune response also limits viral transfection therapy beyond a few local cells.[6]

Adenovirus Adenovirus with herpes simplex virus (HSV) tyrosine kinase (sitimagene ceradenovec) followed by intravenous ganciclovir in patients with newly diagnosed resectable GBM underwent a phase 3 trial (EudraCT number 2004–000464–28) increased median time to death or reintervention but did not change OS.[65]

A phase I study of DNX-2401 (NCT00805376), a tumor-selective, replication-competent oncolytic adenovirus, was performed in patients with recurrent malignant glioma. This was administered via intratumoral injection or implanted catheter. Some patients (20%) had survival greater than 3 years from treatment and 12% showed a 95% or greater reduction in enhancing tumor.[66]

Herpes simplex virus M032 is an oncolytic HSV that selectively replicates in tumor cells. It also can act as a viral vector for molecules, such as IL-12.[67] This is now in a phase I clinical trial (NCT02062827).

Another HSV derivative (G207) was used with intratumoral inoculation into recurrent malignant glioma and was found to have no significant safety concerns.[68]

Convection-enhanced delivery

Overview First proposed in 1994,[3] CED uses direct pump-mediated continuous infusion into the tumor bed or tumor adjacent brain, circumventing the BBB. This strategy uses pressure-driven bulk flow via a small pressure gradient from a pump that pushes solute through a catheter targeted within the CNS. Stereotactically placed catheters are implanted through a burr hole near the therapeutic target—that is, enhancing tumor tissue—and attached to an infusion pump that directs the therapeutic agent at a predetermined concentration, rate, and duration.[12]

By creating a pressure gradient, CED can produce superior drug distribution compared with diffusion-based methods and allows adjustments to pressure and flow parameters to optimize distribution to the tumor area.[2,15] CED limits the potential for neurotoxicity because drug concentrations at the location of the delivery device do not need to be as high as if delivered via diffusion, which produces a steep concentration gradient.[3] CED can infuse agents regardless of their molecular size over clinically relevant distances, bypass the BBB, provide targeted delivery via catheter placement, and limit toxicity because distribution of drug drops off sharply in normal tissue.[15] This strategy avoids large boluses producing cerebral edema or intracranial pressure elevations.[12]

Multiple therapeutic agents have been investigated as potential CED infusates for glioma therapy, including immunotoxins, oligonucleotides, chemotherapy, and viral vectors.[3]

Immunotoxins Immunotoxins frequently have been investigated in conjunction with CED. Targeted immunotoxins are protein toxins produced by bacteria that are cytotoxic, which, coupled to carrier ligands used for cellular targeting, can become tumor selective complexes. They are more potent than traditional chemotherapeutic agents.

Transferrin–diphtheria   conjugates Conjugated toxins include transferrin–diphtheria conjugates (TF-CRM107). Phase I and phase 2 studies show promising tumor response in patients with malignant brain tumors and no significant neurotoxicity.[12] A phase I trial showed 50% decrease in tumor volume on MRI in 9/15 patients. Phase 2 trials, however, showed only a 39% response.[6] A phase 3 clinical trial of CED delivery into unresectable tumors compared with best medical therapy for GBM was halted due to an intermediate futility analysis.[12,69]

Cintredekin besudotox IL-13, which targets IL-13R α2 receptors overexpressed on malignant glioma cells, has been conjugated to truncated Pseudomonas exotoxin (PE38QQR)—a cytotoxin, to create cintredekin besudotox (CB). Phase I and phase 2 studies in the recurrent GBM setting showed that optimal CED infusion was via multiple catheters placed peritumorally status post–gross total resection.[12] A subsequent phase I study in the newly diagnosed setting was performed in which following gross total resection, CB was infused via 2 to 4 intraparenchymal catheters for 96 hours, with subsequent radiation with or without temozolomide in 22 patients. This was well tolerated without significant toxicity.[12,70]

The first completed phase 3 trial that used CED as the delivery approach was the NeoPharm PRECISE trial. It randomized 296 patients with recurrent GBM treated with gross total resection of recurrent enhancement to treatment with CB via CED or carmustine chemotherapy wafers implanted at the time of surgery.[71] There was no significant difference between the 2 groups in median survival—36.4 weeks for CED and 35.3 weeks for wafers.[72] PFS, however, favored the CED group at 17.7 weeks versus 11.4 weeks. A high rate of catheter misplacement was noted in this study.[36]

Interleukin 4 conjugated to Pseudomonas exotoxin IL-4 conjugated to Pseudomonas exotoxin (PE38KDEL) has been infused intratumorally into recurrent high-grade gliomas over 4 days to 8 days via 1 to 3 catheters and resulted in tumor necrosis in 6 of 9 patients. Phase I/2 trails of this agent have suggested an increase in overall median survival compared with historical controls.[12] Another study with 25 GBM patients showed tumor necrosis in a majority of patients. A case study of recurrent GBM treated with NBI-3001 showed survival of 36 months.[69]

TP-38 Malignant brain tumors overexpress EGFR via amplification of EGFR gene on chromosome 7p. Two ligands of EGFR are epidermal growth factor and Transforming growth factor (TGF)-α and can be used to target cytotoxic agents to EGFR expressing glioma cells. TP-38 is a recombinant toxin of TGF-α and an engineered Pseudomonas exotoxin—PE-38. This combination demonstrated therapeutic efficacy in murine models of intracranial epidermoid carcinoma, increasing survival. A phase I/2 trial using CED of TP-38 showed an acceptable safety profile.[12] In a case study of recurring GBM, PFS lasted 43 months. In 20 patients with recurrent or progressive malignant brain tumors, however, a high rate of failed intraparenchymal distribution with leaks into the subarachnoid space or ventricles was seen.[69]

Oligonucleotides
AP 12009 Overexpression of TGF-β2 in malignant tumors facilitates tumor development and metastasis. It has been targeted with AP 12009—an antisense oligonucleotide that targets the mRNA encoding TGF-β2. An open-label dose-escalation study showed median survival data greater than historical standards.[12] No further development has ensued, to date.

Viral vectors
Poliovirus An oncolytic polio-rhinovirus chimera (PVSRIPO) was developed for intratumoral injection into recurrent GBM.[2] PVSRIPO was derived from the live attenuated Sabin poliovirus vaccine.[62] It is a replication-competent attenuated poliovirus with its internal ribosome entry site substituted for that of rhinovirus type 2, preventing propagation in neurons.[64] The insertion of regulatory sequences derived from human rhinovirus allows the virus to selectively replicate within and destroy cancer cells.[73]

Poliovirus targets the poliovirus receptor CD155.[2] Analysis of high-grade malignant tissue found CD155 expressed in all cells and is upregulated, making this tissue very susceptible to the treatment.[73] In preclinical studies, PVSRIPO was shown to have cytotoxic effects on GBM cells in vitro.[46] Administration of PVSRIPO in mouse glioma models causes a rapid immune cell infiltrate at the site.[74]

A phase I clinical trial of intratumoral delivery of PVSRIPO in recurrent GBM via a surgically implanted catheter reported better survival rates at 24 months and 36 months compared with a historical control.[46,75] A phase I (NCT01491893) dose escalation trial used CED to infuse PVSRIPO into 61 recurrent supratentorial grade IV gliomas with median OS of 12.5 months.[64] Three patients had a sustained disease-free state 5 months to 12 months post-treatment.[63] Several limitations in the size and location of recurrent tumor were noted as well as development of significant cerebral edema.[2]

Combination therapy with PVSRIPO and lomustine showed a benefit in a subset of patients, leading to an ongoing randomized phase 2 trial of PVSRIPO alone or in combination with single-cycle lomustine in patients with recurrent GBM (NCT02986178).[2,64,76]

Chemotherapy A variety of conventional chemotherapies have been evaluated preclinically and in early-stage clinical trials; to date, none has gone on to full therapeutic development. Paclitaxel has been delivered by intratumoral CED in recurrent GBM with effective convection and a high antitumor radiographic response rate of 73% across 15 patients, although there were significant treatment-associated complications.[12,69] Topotecan in both free and liposomal-coated forms has been infused into rat models of GBM with improvement in survival and without significant neurotoxicity.[12] A phase Ib study of CED delivery of topotecan in patients with recurrent malignant gliomas found significant antitumor activity demonstrated by radiographic changes and prolonged OS with minimal associated toxicity.[77] Topotecan had favorable PFS and OS rates of 23 weeks and 60 weeks, respectively.[3] CED administration of temozolomide combined with whole-cell tumor immunizations in a mouse model of glioma significantly reduced tumor volume and increased T-cell intratumoral influx.[78] Translation to the clinical setting has been limited by the poor solubility of temozolomide in aqueous solution. A single 2015 study showed the bevacizumab administered via CED showed favorable survival compared intravenous bevacizumab in a highly selected patient population.[69]

Nanoparticles/liposomes Nanoparticles, such as magnetic beads measuring 15 nm to 80 nm, can be delivered with CED and loaded with bioactive molecules with high tissue clearance or reactivity rates.[3] Iron oxide nanoparticles delivered directly to the tumor bed in GBM patients have been stimulated by an alternating magnetic field, which causes production of heat. This was combined with fractionated stereotactic radiosurgery for synergistic cytotoxicity. This strategy demonstrated good outcomes but limited future care of the patient by making MRI unreliable due to artifact.[6]

Liposomes have been used to deliver nonreplicating adenoviruses containing the HSV–thymidine kinase (tk) gene into GBM with tumor reduction greater than 50% in 2/8 patients.[69] CED of HSV–tk failed to demonstrate survival benefits. A liposome encapsulated CED injection also did not show good benefit, because liposomes were retained at the site of injection, likely because they were large and positively charged.[79]

Practical considerations of convection-enhanced delivery The concept of CED was first introduced in 1994, but as of yet the limited number of agents to make it to phase 3 trials have not shown significant benefit. Areas for optimization of this strategy include technical considerations of catheter placement, catheter design, adequate distribution of agents, imaging of distribution, and timing of treatment.[9,52]

Catheter placement In the phase 3 PRECISE trial, position of nondedicated CED catheters (these were catheters that were designed to drain cerebrospinal fluid) was optimal in only 51% of patients, and drug distribution likely was adequate in less than 20% of patients. Optimal placement, defined somewhat arbitrarily based on limited clinical data, without imaging confirmation of distribution, was catheters placed 2.5 cm into the brain, at least 0.5 cm from the ependymal surface, and without pial or ventricular penetration.[61] Stereotactic implantation of catheters theoretically allows for precise targeting, but this also is affected by multiple clinical factors, including targeting accuracy, suitability of targets, locations of sulci, and other fluid spaces and (at the time of that study) inability to actively track catheter placement with image guidance. Clinically determined variables for catheter placement included intratumoral versus peritumoral locations, which can have an impact on the volume of drug distribution.[71,80]

Catheter design Catheter design considerations include materials, impact of design on placement procedure, and device dimensions. One issue with CED catheters is reflux—or the infusate moving back along the shaft of the cannula. Risk of reflux depends on fluid viscosity, flow rate, hydraulic resistance of tissue, the outer radius of the catheter, and the tissue deformation by catheter and infusion.[71] For nondedicated CED catheters, studies have shown that rates greater than 0.5 μL/min to 1 μL/min resulted in reflux.[3,61] There was a need for specialized catheters that could provide higher rates of infusion (up to 50 μL/min) with low risk of reflux in order to cover targets tissues that are on the order of tens to hundreds of cubic centimeters. Catheter materials must achieve a balance between rigidity for targeting and flexibility for prolonged administration outside the operating room (OR). Cannula size is one of the most easily modifiable factors determining effectiveness of CED. In general, smaller-bore cannulas perform better than larger ones and provide reflux-resistant fluid flow at a greater rate.[71] Past work suggests that a 27-gauge catheter provides an outer diameter needed to prevent reflux of infusate along the cannula, but cannulas this small are hard to position and manipulate. One solution for achieving this goal was with the development of rigid step-down catheters.[15] A step design cannula, in which the outer diameter of the cannula is progressively reduced, in steps, prevents reflux in vivo and maximizes distribution of agents delivered in the brain.[81] This design feature, which has been used by 2 commercialized devices (SmartFlow [MRI Interventions, Irvine, CA] and Alcyone MEMS Cannula [Alcyone Lifesciences, Lowell, MA]), demonstrates reflux-resistant flow but is limited to use in the OR only (and for the SmartFlow device, in an intraoperative MRI only) due to the rigid design of the cannulas, which are not amenable to use outside of the OR environment. A third commercialized device (SmartFlow [Brainlab]) makes use of the step-down tip design coupled to a flexible proximal catheter and a bone anchor. Another catheter design approach, which has yet to be commercialized, demonstrated a greater volume of distribution with use of a porous membrane along the distal part of the catheter as opposed to a step-down approach.[82] The fourth device to be commercialized, the Cleveland Multiport Catheter (Infuseon Therapeutics, Cleveland, OH), is a flexible device that can be secured for use outside of the OR and deploys 4 independent delivery microcatheters to provide a reliable, high-volume delivery of therapeutic agents to the brain. A pilot trial, published in 2019, in 3 patients demonstrated adequate delivery from all catheters and no significant complications.[80]

Volume of distribution The efficacy of a drug delivered by CED depends on ability to achieve sufficient concentrations within the targeted region.[6] Successful infusion relies on the cannula being inserted in a location where the infused agents achieve a predetermined volume and shape within a given amount of time.[71] Key factors

have been identified that affect the distribution of solutes delivered using CED, including infusion rate and volume, cannula size, the interstitial fluid pressure and tumor cytoarchitecture, and integrity of the BBB—a partially or fully opened BBB allows the infusate to diffuse out into the microcirculation, which acts as an infinite concentration sink.[12]

In CED, the bulk flow of interstitial fluid mediates drug distribution. Infusion rate and volume have an impact on this distribution. Because CED distributes infusate within interstitial space, the volume of distribution necessary varies depending on local conditions within the CNS, including edema, location, and white versus gray matter.[15] Because interstitial fluid pressure is higher in brain tumors (up to 50 mm Hg) compared with normal brain (1–2 mm Hg), this creates a pressure gradient, which moves infusate out of the tumor toward lower pressure in surrounding normal brain.[15] Affected tissue also tends to be heterogenous, limiting the homogenous distribution of infusate to all tumor tissue.[12] Additionally, in white matter regions, diffusion may follow existing white matter tracts, especially those already affected by edema.[3]

The concentration of a drug directly infused into brain parenchyma decreases logarithmically with each millimeter of distance from the CED catheter.[6] Also, because the drug undergoes positive pressure delivery to the area, drug residence time is short, decreasing the opportunity for water-soluble drugs to penetrate cell membranes or to interact with receptors.[15]

Monitoring Monitoring the distribution of an infusate delivered via CED remains an important consideration for determining whether an agent is likely to have reached its therapeutic target in the brain. Initial clinical work focused on indirect measures of distribution. Diffusion-weighted imaging on MRI showed early visualization of changes from CED infusions than traditional sequences.[79] Real-time visualization of the CED process in patients has been achieved with use of tracers that can be visualized with CT or MRI (eg, iodinated contrast agents or chelated gadolinium agents). This approach allows for real-time modification of the plan for reflux or otherwise suboptimal delivery.[12] These remain indirect methods, however, because they do not image the therapeutic agent itself. Direct imaging of the therapeutic agent has been achieved in limited situations, for example, in the development of a theragnostic drug for treating diffuse intrinsic pontine glioma.[83]

Long-term treatment A limitation of CED is that the currently commercialized catheters can be implanted only temporarily. Versions with accessible ports for long-term infusion are being explored in animal models and to some extent with customized systems in clinical patients.[3,84] CED infusions have been studied for up to 32 days in pig models using a single proximal ventricular catheter and topotecan. Although inflammation adjacent to the catheter tract at the time of placement is limited to a 50-μm radius,[3] long-term infusion via catheter is limited by gliosis around the catheter tip.[6] Drug stability and pump design also remain challenges for long-term infusion.[84]

SUMMARY

Therapeutic strategies for GBM face several hurdles, and development of novel therapeutics and delivery strategies must occur simultaneously to overcome physiologic barriers, such as the BBB and BTB. Use of strategies to disrupt or bypass the native BBB are necessary to deliver adequate concentrations of therapeutic agents. The ideal methods and agents to accomplish this goal, however, are yet to be determined. Therapeutic delivery via drug-embedded biodegradable wafers should be viewed as a proof of principle that establishes that direct delivery to the brain can provide clinical benefit. Further development of methods to break down or bypass the BBB and BTB is necessary in order to have reliable platforms on which to determine whether new therapeutic agents are likely to have meaningful activity in patients with GBM.

CLINICS CARE POINTS

- The BBB presents a substantial barrier to be overcome in the development of therapeutic delivery to the CNS.

- Strategies to obtain adequate intratumor drug concentrations may either take advantage of intrinsic BBB mechanisms to allow molecules to pass through or be transported or disrupt or bypass the BBB to allow agents to enter CNS tissue.

- Multiple attempts at direct administration of agents to bypass the BBB include implantable controlled-release polymer systems, various approaches for intracavitary drug delivery, direct injection of viral vectors, and CED.

- CED uses direct pump-mediated continuous infusion into the tumor bed or tumor adjacent brain, circumventing the BBB. This approach has shown promising results with infusion of immunotoxins, chemotherapy, and viral vectors.

DISCLOSURE

Dr M.A. Vogelbaum: indirect equity and royalty interests in Infuseon Therapeutics, Inc. Honoraria from Celgene, Blue Earth Diagnostics, and Tocagen.

REFERENCES

1. Ostrom Quinn T, Gittleman Haley, Liao Peter, et al. CBTRUS statistical report: primary brain and other central nervous system tumors diagnosed in the United States in 2010-2014. Neuro Oncol 2017; 19(5):v1–88.
2. Oberheim BNA, Hervey-Jumper SL, Berger Mitchel S. Management of glioblastoma, present and future. World Neurosurg 2019;131:328–38.
3. Vogelbaum Michael A, Aghi Manish K. Convection-enhanced delivery for the treatment of glioblastoma. Neuro Oncol 2015;17(December 2014):ii3–8.
4. Roger Stupp, Mason Warren P, van den Bent Martin J, et al. Radiotherapy plus concomitant and adjuvant temozolomide for glioblastoma. N Engl J Med 2005;352(10):987–96.
5. Roger Stupp, Taillibert Sophie, Kanner Andrew, et al. Effect of tumor-treating fields plus maintenance temozolomide vs maintenance temozolomide alone on survival in patients with glioblastoma. JAMA 2017;318(23):2306.
6. Mehta Ankit I, Linninger A, Lesniak MS, et al. Current status of intratumoral therapy for glioblastoma. J Neurooncol 2015;125(1):1–7.
7. Vogelbaum Michael A. Targeted therapies for brain tumors: will they ever deliver? Clin Cancer Res 2018;24(16):3790–1.
8. Wadajkar Aniket S, Dancy Jimena G, Hersh David S, et al. Tumor-targeted nanotherapeutics: overcoming treatment barriers for glioblastoma. Wiley Interdiscip Rev Nanomed Nanobiotechnol 2017;9(4):e1439.
9. Noch Evan K, Ramakrishna R, Rajiv M. Challenges in the treatment of glioblastoma: multisystem mechanisms of therapeutic resistance. World Neurosurg 2018;116:505–17.
10. Ferraris C, Roberta C, Pier Paolo P, et al. Overcoming the blood–brain barrier: successes and challenges in developing nanoparticle-mediated drug delivery systems for the treatment of brain tumours. Int J Nanomedicine 2020;15:2999–3022.
11. Satoru Osuka, Van Meir Erwin G. Overcoming therapeutic resistance in glioblastoma: the way forward. J Clin Invest 2017;127(2):415–26.
12. Bidros Dani S, Vogelbaum Michael A. Novel drug delivery strategies in neuro-oncology. Neurotherapeutics 2009;6(3):539–46.
13. Joan Abbott N. Blood-brain barrier structure and function and the challenges for CNS drug delivery. J Inherit Metab Dis 2013;36(3):437–49.

14. Pardridge William M. Drug transport across the blood-brain barrier. J Cereb Blood Flow Metab 2012;32(11):1959–72.

15. Vogelbaum Michael A. Convection enhanced delivery for the treatment of malignant gliomas: Symposium review. J Neurooncol 2005;73(1):57–69.

16. Van Tellingen O, Yetkin-Arik B, De Gooijer MC, et al. Overcoming the blood-brain tumor barrier for effective glioblastoma treatment. Drug Resist Updat 2015;19:1–12.

17. Evgenii B, Shaffer Kurt V, Lin C, et al. Blood-brain barrier, blood-brain tumor barrier, and fluorescence-guided neurosurgical oncology: delivering optical labels to brain tumors. Front Oncol 2020;10(June):1–27.

18. Sprowls SA, Arsiwala TA, Bumgarner JR, et al. Improving CNS Delivery to Brain Metastases by Blood-Tumor Barrier Disruption. Trends Cancer. 2019;5(8):495-505.

19. Jacus Megan O, Daryani Vinay M, Harstead KE, et al. Pharmacokinetic properties of anticancer agents for the treatment of central nervous system tumors: update of the literature. Clin Pharmacokinet 2016;55(3):297–311.

20. Rosso L, Brock CS, Gallo JM, et al. A new model for prediction of drug distribution in tumor and normal tissues: pharmacokinetics of temozolomide in glioma patients. Cancer Res 2009;69(1):120–7.

21. Portnow J, Badie B, Chen M, et al. The neuropharmacokinetics of temozolomide in patients with resectable brain tumors: potential implications for the current approach to chemoradiation. Clin Cancer Res 2009;15(22):7092–8.

22. Dréan A, Lauriane G, Maïté V, et al. Blood-brain barrier, cytotoxic chemotherapies and glioblastoma. Expert Rev Neurother 2016;16(11):1285–300.

23. Vogelbaum Michael A, Krivosheya D, Borghei-Razavi H, et al. Phase 0 and window of opportunity clinical trial design in neuro-oncology: a RANO review. Neuro Oncol 2020;(June):1–12. https://doi.org/10.1093/neuonc/noaa149.

24. Pang Z, Gao H, Yu Y, et al. Enhanced intracellular delivery and chemotherapy for glioma rats by transferrin-conjugated biodegradable polymersomes loaded with doxorubicin. Bioconjug Chem 2011;22(6):1171–80.

25. Li Y, He H, Jia X, et al. A dual-targeting nanocarrier based on poly(amidoamine) dendrimers conjugated with transferrin and tamoxifen for treating brain gliomas. Biomaterials 2012;33(15):3899–908.

26. Manuela P, Zappavigna S, Salzano G, et al. Medical treatment of orthotopic glioblastoma with transferrin-conjugated nanoparticles encapsulating zoledronic acid. Oncotarget 2014;5(21):10446–59.

27. Sang-Soo K, Antonina R, Kim E, et al. Encapsulation of temozolomide in a tumor-targeting nanocomplex enhances anti-cancer efficacy and reduces toxicity in a mouse model of glioblastoma. Cancer Lett 2015;369(1):250–8.

28. Nduom Edjah K, Weller M, Heimberger Amy B. Immunosuppressive mechanisms in glioblastoma: Neuro Oncol 2015;17(suppl 7):vii9–14.

29. Pang Z, Liang F, Hua R, et al. Lactoferrin-conjugated biodegradable polymersome holding doxorubicin and tetrandrine for chemotherapy of glioma rats. Mol Pharm 2010;7(6):1995–2005.

30. Jiang X, Xianyi S, Xin H, et al. Integrin-facilitated transcytosis for enhanced penetration of advanced gliomas by poly(trimethylene carbonate)-based nanoparticles encapsulating paclitaxel. Biomaterials 2013;34(12):2969–79.

31. Jiang X, Xin H, Ren Q, et al. Nanoparticles of 2-deoxy-d-glucose functionalized poly(ethylene glycol)-co-poly(trimethylene carbonate) for dual-targeted drug delivery in glioma treatment. Biomaterials 2014;35(1):518–29.

32. Chekhonin Vladimir P, Baklaushev Vladimir P, Yusubalieva Gaukhar M, et al. Targeted delivery of liposomal nanocontainers to the peritumoral zone of glioma by means of monoclonal antibodies against GFAP and the extracellular loop of Cx43. Nanomedicine 2012;8(1):63–70.

33. Milota K, Alexandros B, Machaidze R, et al. Targeted therapy of glioblastoma stem-like cells and tumor non-stem cells using cetuximab-conjugated iron-oxide nanoparticles. Oncotarget 2015;6(11):8788–806.

34. Hadjipanayis CG, Machaidze R, Kaluzova M, et al. EGFRvIII antibody-conjugated iron oxide nanoparticles for magnetic resonance imaging-guided convection-enhanced delivery and targeted therapy of glioblastoma. Cancer Res 2010;70(15):6303–12.

35. Alexandros B, Milota K, Hadjipanayis Costas G. Radiosensitivity enhancement of radioresistant glioblastoma by epidermal growth factor receptor antibody-conjugated iron-oxide nanoparticles. J Neurooncol 2015;124(1):13–22.

36. Madhankumar AB, Slagle-Webb B, Wang X, et al. Efficacy of interleukin-13 receptor-targeted liposomal doxorubicin in the intracranial brain tumor model. Mol Cancer Ther 2009;8(3):648–54.

37. Schneider Craig S, Perez Jimena G, Cheng E, et al. Minimizing the non-specific binding of nanoparticles to the brain enables active targeting of Fn14-positive glioblastoma cells. Biomaterials 2015;42:42–51.

38. Gupta Shiv K, Kizilbash Sani H, Daniels David J, et al. Editorial: targeted therapies for glioblastoma: a critical appraisal. Front Oncol 2019;9(November):1–4.

39. Glaser T, Han I, Wu L, et al. Targeted nanotechnology in glioblastoma multiforme. Front Pharmacol 2017;8(MAR):1–14.

40. Xue Ying, Wen He, Lu Wan-Liang, et al. Dual-targeting daunorubicin liposomes improve the therapeutic

efficacy of brain glioma in animals. J Control Release 2010;141(2):183–92.

41. QIN LI, WANG Cheng-Zheng, FAN Hui-Jie, et al. A dual-targeting liposome conjugated with transferrin and arginine-glycine-aspartic acid peptide for glioma-targeting therapy. Oncol Lett 2014;8(5): 2000–6.

42. Lam Fred C, Morton Stephen W, Wyckoff J, et al. Enhanced efficacy of combined temozolomide and bromodomain inhibitor therapy for gliomas using targeted nanoparticles. Nat Commun 2018;9(1):1991.

43. Eavarone David A, Yu X, Bellamkonda Ravi V. Targeted drug delivery to C6 glioma by transferrin-coupled liposomes. J Biomed Mater Res 2000; 51(1):10–4.

44. Fu Qiuyi, Zhao Yi, Yang Z, et al. Liposomes actively recognizing the glucose transporter GLUT 1 and integrin α v β 3 for dual-targeting of glioma. Arch Pharm (Weinheim) 2019;352(2):1800219.

45. Valérie D, Denis M, Dietrich PY. Current strategies for vaccination in glioblastoma. Curr Opin Oncol 2019;31(6):514–21.

46. Mooney J, Bernstock Joshua D, Ilyas A, et al. Current approaches and challenges in the molecular therapeutic targeting of glioblastoma. World Neurosurg 2019;129:90–100.

47. Sampson JH, Archer GE, Mitchell DA, et al. An epidermal growth factor receptor variant III-targeted vaccine is safe and immunogenic in patients with glioblastoma multiforme. Mol Cancer Ther 2009;8(10):2773–9.

48. Schuster J, Lai RK, Recht LD, et al. A phase II, multicenter trial of rindopepimut (CDX-110) in newly diagnosed glioblastoma: the ACT III study. Neuro Oncol 2015;17(6):854–61.

49. Reardon David A, Annick D, Vredenburgh James J, et al. Rindopepimut with Bevacizumab for Patients with Relapsed EGFRvIII-Expressing Glioblastoma (ReACT): results of a double-blind randomized phase II trial. Clin Cancer Res 2020;26(7):1586–94.

50. Weller M, Nicholas B, Tran David D, et al. Rindopepimut with temozolomide for patients with newly diagnosed, EGFRvIII-expressing glioblastoma (ACT IV): a randomised, double-blind, international phase 3 trial. Lancet Oncol 2017;18(10):1373–85.

51. Brown Christine E, Alizadeh D, Starr R, et al. Regression of glioblastoma after chimeric antigen receptor T-Cell therapy. N Engl J Med 2016;375(26):2561–9.

52. Rose JT, McDonald Kerrie L. The challenges associated with molecular targeted therapies for glioblastoma. J Neurooncol 2016;127(3):427–34.

53. Hersh David S, Wadjkar Aniket S, Roberts N, et al. Evolving drug delivery strategies to overcome the blood brain barrier. Curr Pharm Des 2016;22(9): 1177–93.

54. Jan-Karl B, Howard R, Shin Benjamin J, et al. Intra-arterial delivery of bevacizumab after blood-brain barrier disruption for the treatment of recurrent glioblastoma: progression-free survival and overall survival. World Neurosurg 2012;77(1):130–4.

55. Ellis Jason A, Banu M, Hossain Shaolie S, et al. Reassessing the role of intra-arterial drug delivery for glioblastoma multiforme treatment. J Drug Deliv 2015;2015:1–15.

56. Hersh David S, Kim Anthony J, Winkles Jeffrey A, et al. Emerging applications of therapeutic ultrasound in neuro-oncology. Neurosurgery 2016; 79(5):643–54.

57. Adomas B, McDannold Nathan J, Golby Alexandra J. Focused ultrasound strategies for brain tumor therapy. Oper Neurosurg (Hagerstown) 2020; 19(1):9–18.

58. Patel B, Yang Peter H, Kim Albert H. The effect of thermal therapy on the blood-brain barrier and blood-tumor barrier. Int J Hyperthermia 2020;37(2): 35–43.

59. Lee Ian, Kalkanis S, Hadjipanayis Constantinos G. Stereotactic laser interstitial thermal therapy for recurrent high-grade gliomas. Neurosurgery 2016; 79(suppl_1):S24–34.

60. Salehi A, Paturu Mounica R, Patel B, et al. Therapeutic enhancement of blood–brain and blood–tumor barriers permeability by laser interstitial thermal therapy. Neurooncol Adv 2020;2(1). https://doi.org/10. 1093/noajnl/vdaa071.

61. Healy A, Vogelbaum M. Convection-enhanced drug delivery for gliomas. Surg Neurol Int 2015;6(2): S59–67.

62. Foreman Paul M, Friedman Gregory K, Cassady Kevin A, et al. Oncolytic virotherapy for the treatment of malignant glioma. Neurotherapeutics 2017;14(2): 333–44.

63. Mehta AM, Sonabend AM, Bruce JN. Convection-enhanced delivery. Neurotherapeutics 2017;14(2): 358–71.

64. Stepanenko Aleksei A, Chekhonin Vladimir P. Recent advances in oncolytic virotherapy and immunotherapy for glioblastoma: a glimmer of hope in the search for an effective therapy? Cancers (Basel) 2018;10(12):1–24.

65. Westphal M, Ylä-Herttuala S, Martin J, et al. Adenovirus-mediated gene therapy with sitimagene ceradenovec followed by intravenous ganciclovir for patients with operable high-grade glioma (ASPECT): a randomised, open-label, phase 3 trial. Lancet Oncol 2013;14(9):823–33.

66. Lang Frederick F, Conrad C, Gomez-Manzano C, et al. Phase I Study of DNX-2401 (Delta-24-RGD) Oncolytic Adenovirus: Replication and Immunotherapeutic Effects in Recurrent Malignant Glioma. J Clin Oncol 2018;36(14):1419–27.

67. Patel Daxa M, Foreman Paul M, Burt NL, et al. Design of a phase I clinical trial to evaluate M032, a genetically engineered HSV-1 Expressing IL-12,

in patients with recurrent/progressive glioblastoma multiforme, anaplastic astrocytoma, or gliosarcoma. Hum Gene Ther Clin Dev 2016;27(2):69–78.

68. Markert JM, Medlock MD, Rabkin SD, et al. Conditionally replicating herpes simplex virus mutant, G207 for the treatment of malignant glioma: results of a phase I trial. Gene Ther 2000;7(10): 867–74.

69. Arman Jahangiri, Chin A, Patrick F, et al. Convection-enhanced delivery in glioblastoma: a review of preclinical and clinical studies. J Neurosurg 2017; 126(1):1–18.

70. Vogelbaum Michael A, Sampson John H, Kunwar S, et al. Convection-enhanced delivery of cintredekin besudotox (Interleukin-13-PE38QQR) followed by radiation therapy with and without temozolomide in newly diagnosed malignant gliomas: phase 1 study of final safety results. Neurosurgery 2007;61(5):1031–8.

71. Vogelbaum Michael A. Convection enhanced delivery for treating brain tumors and selected neurological disorders: Symposium review. J Neurooncol 2007;83(1):97–109.

72. Kunwar S, Chang S, Westphal M, et al. Phase III randomized trial of CED of IL13-PE38QQR vs Gliadel wafers for recurrent glioblastoma. Neuro Oncol 2010;12(8):871–81.

73. Merrill MK, Bernhardt G, Sampson JH, et al. Poliovirus receptor CD155-targeted oncolysis of glioma. Neuro Oncol 2004;6(3):208–17.

74. Matthias G, Nair Smita K. Recombinant poliovirus for cancer immunotherapy. Annu Rev Med 2018;69(1): 289–99.

75. Annick D, Matthias G, Herndon James E, et al. Recurrent glioblastoma treated with recombinant poliovirus. N Engl J Med 2018;379(2):150–61.

76. Abi-Aad Karl R, Turcotte Evelyn L, Welz Matthew E, et al. The use of recombinant poliovirus for the treatment of recurrent glioblastoma multiforme. World Neurosurg 2019;124:129 30.

77. Bruce Jeffrey N, Fine Robert L, Peter C, et al. Regression of recurrent malignant gliomas with convection-enhanced delivery of topotecan. Neurosurgery 2011;69(6):1272–80.

78. Julio EP, Kopecky J, Visse E, et al. Convection-enhanced delivery of temozolomide and whole cell tumor immunizations in GL261 and KR158 experimental mouse gliomas. BMC Cancer 2020;20(1):7.

79. Shi M, Léon S. Convection-enhanced delivery in malignant gliomas: a review of toxicity and efficacy. J Oncol 2019;2019. https://doi.org/10.1155/2019/9342796.

80. Vogelbaum Michael A, Brewer C, Barnett Gene H, et al. First-in-human evaluation of the cleveland multiport catheter for convection-enhanced delivery of topotecan in recurrent high-grade glioma: results of pilot trial 1. J Neurosurg 2019;130(2):476–85.

81. Krauze Michal T, Saito R, Charles N, et al. Reflux-free cannula for convection-enhanced high-speed delivery of therapeutic agents. J Neurosurg 2013; 103(5):1–12.

82. Brady Martin L, Raghavan R, Mata J, et al. Large-volume infusions into the brain: a comparative study of catheter designs. Stereotact Funct Neurosurg 2018;96(3):135–41.

83. Souweidane Mark M, Kramer K, Pandit-Taskar N, et al. Convection-enhanced delivery for diffuse intrinsic pontine glioma: a single-centre, dose-escalation, phase 1 trial. Lancet Oncol 2018;19(8): 1040–50.

84. Butowski Nicholas A, Bringas John R, Bankiewicz Krystof S, et al. Editorial. Chronic convection-enhanced delivery: the next frontier in regional drug infusion for glioblastoma. J Neurosurg 2019; 1–3. https://doi.org/10.3171/2019.4.JNS19614.

85. Sushant L, Singh J. Co-delivery of doxorubicin and erlotinib through liposomal nanoparticles for glioblastoma tumor regression using an in vitro brain tumor model. Colloids Surf B Biointerfaces 2019;173: 27–35.

Moving?

Make sure your subscription moves with you!

To notify us of your new address, find your **Clinics Account Number** (located on your mailing label above your name), and contact customer service at:

Email: journalscustomerservice-usa@elsevier.com

800-654-2452 (subscribers in the U.S. & Canada)
314-447-8871 (subscribers outside of the U.S. & Canada)

Fax number: 314-447-8029

Elsevier Health Sciences Division
Subscription Customer Service
3251 Riverport Lane
Maryland Heights, MO 63043

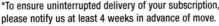
*To ensure uninterrupted delivery of your subscription, please notify us at least 4 weeks in advance of move.

ELSEVIER

Printed and bound by CPI Group (UK) Ltd, Croydon, CR0 4YY

08/05/2025

01864700-0016